EAT TO
LIVE

EAT TO LIVE

EAT TO LIVE

The Revolutionary Formula for Fast and Sustained Weight Loss

JOEL FUHRMAN, M.D.

With a Foreword by
Mehmet Oz, M.D.

Little, Brown and Company
Boston New York London

ISBN 0-316-82945-5

LCCN 2002114685

10   9   8

Q-MART

Text design Meryl Sussman Levavi/Digitext
Printed in the United States of America

To my mother, Isabel,

for all her love and sacrifice

and

in memory of my father, Seymour,

for instilling in me an interest in superior nutrition

Contents

Foreword

Although the United States is the most powerful nation on earth, the one area in which this country does not excel is health. And the future is not bright. Almost a third of our young children are obese, and many do not exercise. No matter how much information becomes available about the dangers of a sedentary lifestyle and a diet heavily dependent on processed foods, we don't change our ways. Ideally, Americans should be able to translate financial well-being into habits that lead to longer and better lives, untroubled by expensive and chronic medical illnesses. Yet, in the United States, as well as Western Europe, Russia, and many other affluent countries, the majority of adults are overweight and undernourished. While high-quality nutrition is readily available throughout the United States, the American public, rich and poor, is drawn to eating unhealthy food. Indeed, the list of top calorie sources for Americans includes many items I do not consider "real" foods, including milk, cola, margarine, white bread, sugar, and pasteurized processed American cheese.

Though smoking has received a lot of attention for the dangers it poses to public health, and cigarettes have been heavily lobbied against, obesity is a more important predictor of chronic ailments and quality of life than any other public scourge. In a recent survey of 9,500 Americans, 36 percent were overweight and 23 percent were obese, yet only 19 percent were daily smokers and 6 percent heavy drinkers. Several reasons for this epidemic of obesity in modern life have been offered. There is the pervasive role of advertising in Western society, the loss of family and social cohesiveness, the adoption of a sedentary lifestyle, and the lack of time to prepare fresh foods. In 1978, 18 percent of calories were eaten away from home; the figure is now 36 percent. In 1970, Americans ate 6 billion fast-food meals. By 2000, the figure was 110 billion.

Poor nutrition can also result in less productivity at work and school, hyperactivity among children and adolescents, and mood swings, all of which heighten feelings of stress, isolation, and insecurity. Even basic quality-of-life concerns such as constipation are affected, resulting in Americans spending $600 million annually on laxatives.

With time, the ravages of obesity predispose the typical American adult to depression, diabetes, and hypertension and increase the risks of death in all ages and in almost every ethnic and gender group. The U.S. Surgeon General has reported that 300,000 deaths annually are caused by or related to obesity. The incidence of diabetes alone has risen by a third since 1990, and treatment costs $100 billion a year. The illnesses caused by obesity also lead to more lost workdays than any other single ailment and increase pharmaceutical and hospital expenditures to palliate untreatable degenerative conditions.

Government policy has had limited power to stem the tide of obesity, yet our nation's leaders have supported formal reports calling for a national effort to raise awareness of the dangers of being overweight. As a part of the Healthy People 2010 initiative, the federal government has proposed several steps to reduce chronic diseases associated with diet and weight through the promotion of better health and nutritional habits. It has set dietary guidelines and has encouraged physical exercise, but these efforts have not managed to change the minds, or strengthen the hearts, of most Americans. It is clear to the public that a minor change in one's eating habits will hardly transform one's life so readily. So the public turns to magic cures, pills, supplements, drinks, and diet plans that simply don't work or are unsafe. After a few failures, they give up hope.

Unlike for many diseases, the cure for obesity is known. Studies with thousands of participants have demonstrated that the combination of a dramatic change in eating habits and daily exercise results in weight loss, including a 60 percent reduction in the chance of developing chronic ailments, such as diabetes. Disseminating detailed information on these barriers is relatively easy, yet the plethora of diet books and remedies have created a complex and contradictory array of choices for those who are desperate to lose weight. With the publication of Dr. Joel Fuhrman's book, outlining a perfectly rational, straightforward, and sustainable diet, I believe we are witnessing a medical breakthrough. If you give this diet your complete commitment, there is no question in my mind that it will work for you.

In creating this plan, Dr. Fuhrman, a world expert in nutrition and obesity research, has gone beyond the dietary guidelines set up by the National Institutes of Health and the American Heart Association. Importantly, *Eat to Live* takes these nationally endorsed standards a quantum step further. Whereas conventional standards are designed for mass consumption and offer modest adjustments to our present eating habits, Dr. Fuhrman's recommendations are designed for those seeking breakthrough results. I have referred my patients to Dr. Fuhrman and have seen firsthand how his powerful methods excite and motivate people, and have witnessed wonderful results for both weight reduction and health restoration.

I am a cardiovascular surgeon infatuated with the challenge and promise of "high-tech" medicine and surgery. Nonetheless, I have become convinced that the most overlooked tool in our medical arsenal is harnessing the body's own ability to heal through nutritional excellence.

Dr. Fuhrman is doctor as teacher; he makes applying nutritional science to our own lives easy to learn, compelling, practical, and fun. His own common sense and his scientifically supported solutions to many diet-induced ailments will enable many readers to achieve unexpected degrees of wellness quickly and easily. He reminds us that not all fats or carbohydrates are good or bad and that animal proteins catalyze many detrimental side effects to our health. He pushes us to avoid processed foods and to seek the rich nutrients and phytochemicals available in fresh foods. Finally, he offers a meal plan that is tasty and easy to follow. However, make no mistake, the information you will find in this book will challenge you; the scientific evidence he cites will make it harder for you to ignore the long-term impact of the typical American diet. Indeed, it is a wake-up call for all of us to make significant changes in our lives. Now is the time to put this information into action to bring optimal health to all Americans. Go for it!

Mehmet C. Oz, M.D.
Director, Cardiovascular Institute
Columbia-Presbyterian Medical Center

EAT TO
LIVE

Introduction

I couldn't play with my children; my fatigue was unbearable. I was becoming sicker and sicker and then I heard Dr. Fuhrman speak. I've lost sixty pounds, going from a size 22-plus to a size 8 and have remained at 125 pounds for three years. Dr. Fuhrman saved my life. My three teenage sons and my daughter witnessed the results I've attained and they all have adopted his plan, receiving dramatic health improvements as well. No more allergies and digestive problems.

— Lynne Bush

I thank my daughter Geri for insisting I go see Dr. Fuhrman. She said if anyone can help you, it's him. Well, she was right. After twenty-five years of taking insulin, I was off it completely in a few days. I was a great patient and did exactly as Dr. Fuhrman said, and it was well worth it. After losing sixty-five pounds, I have been medication-free for two years. I owe it all to him.

— Gerardo Petito

Let me tell you about a typical day in my private practice. I'll see anywhere from two to five new patients like Rosalee. When Rosalee first walked through my door, she weighed 215 pounds and was on two medications (Glucophage and Glucotrol) to control her diabetes, as well as two more (Accupril and Maxide) to control her high blood pressure. She'd tried every diet on the market and exercised but still couldn't manage to lose the weight she wanted to. She came to me desperate to regain a healthy weight and skeptical that my program could do anything more than what she achieved in the past — failure.

I asked her what in her wildest dreams she thought her ideal weight would be and how long it would take her to attain that goal. She thought that her ideal weight would be 125 and that she would like to be there within a year. I smiled and told her that I could design a diet for her to lose about five pounds the first month or twenty pounds the first month *and* reduce her medications. Not surprisingly, she picked the latter.

After hearing my explanation of the program I designed for her, Rosalee was psyched. With everything she had learned from reading about dieting, she had never realized how all the mixed messages had led her down the wrong path. The plan I outlined for Rosalee made sense to her. She said, "If I can eat all that good-tasting food and still lose that much weight, I will definitely follow your instructions precisely." When Rosalee returned to my office the following month, she had lost twenty-two pounds and had been off the Glucotrol for four weeks and the Maxide for two weeks. Her blood pressure was normal and her glucose was under better control on less medication. It was now time to reduce her medication even further and move to the next phase of the diet.

Rosalee is typical of the thousands of patients I have seen in my practice, men and women who are no longer overweight and chronically ill. I get such a thrill from helping these patients regain optimal health and weight that I decided to write this book to place all the most important information for weight loss and health recovery in one clear document. I needed to do this. If you implement the information in the pages that follow, you too will see potentially life-saving results.

I also see many young women who want to drop twenty to fifty pounds quickly in anticipation of an upcoming wedding or trip to the beach. This winter I saw a swimming coach who had to look great in her bathing suit come summer. These younger and healthier individuals were typically referred by their physicians or were informed enough to know that it can be dangerous to crash-diet. My plan is not only a healthful, scientifically designed diet calculated to supply optimal nutrition while losing weight quickly, it also meets the expectations of those desiring superb health and vitality while they find their ideal weight. My formula diet can be combined with an exercise program for astonishing results, but it can also be used effectively by those too ill or too overweight to exercise sufficiently.

In spite of the more than $110 million consumers spend *every day* on diets and "reducing" programs (more than $40 billion per year), Americans are the most obese people in history. To be considered obese, more than one-third of a person's body must be made up of fat. A whopping 34 percent of all Americans are obese, and the problem is getting worse, not better.

Unfortunately, most weight-loss plans either don't work or offer only minor, usually temporary, benefits. There are plenty of "rules and counting" diets, diet drugs, high-protein programs, canned shakes, and other fads that might enable you to lose some weight for a period of time. The problem is that you can't stay on these programs forever. What's worse, many are dangerous.

For example, the Atkins diet (and other diets rich in animal products and low in fruits and unrefined carbohydrates) is likely to significantly increase a person's risk of colon cancer. Scientific studies show a clear and strong relationship between cancers of the digestive tract, bladder, and prostate with low fruit consumption. What good is a diet that lowers your weight but also dramatically increases your chances of developing cancer? Because of such drawbacks, more and more desperate people are turning to drugs and surgical procedures for weight loss.

I have cared for more than ten thousand patients, most of whom first came to my office unhappy, sick, and overweight, having tried every dietary craze without success. After following my health-and-weight-loss formula, they shed the weight they always dreamed of losing, and they kept it off. For the first time in their lives, these patients had a diet plan that didn't require them to be hungry all the time.

Most patients who come to me say that they just can't lose weight, no matter what they do. They are not alone. It is almost universally accepted that obese patients cannot achieve an ideal weight or even an acceptable weight through traditional weight-loss programs. In one study of sixty overweight women who enrolled in a university diet-and-exercise program, none achieved her ideal weight.

My diet plan and recipes are designed for the hardest cases and those who have failed to lose the desired weight on other plans. Following the dietary advice offered in this book, you will achieve remarkable results, regardless of your experience elsewhere. Weight loss averages fifteen pounds the first month and ten pounds each month thereafter. Some people lose as much as a pound a day. There is no hunger, and you can eat as much food as you desire (usually more food than you were eating before). It will work for everyone.

My patients experience other benefits as well. Many of them once suffered from chronic diseases that required multiple medications. A substantial number of my patients have been able to discontinue their medications as they recover from angina, high blood pressure, high cholesterol, diabetes, asthma, fatigue, allergies, and arthritis (to name just a few). More than 90 percent of my diabetic patients who were on insulin at the time of their first visit got off all insulin within the first month.

When I first saw Richard Gross, he had already had angioplasty and bypass surgery, and his doctors were recommending a second bypass operation because his chest pain had recurred and catheterization showed two out of the three bypassed vessels were severely blocked. Because he had suffered brain damage from the first bypass, this man did not want to undergo another operation. Needless to say, he was very motivated to try my noninvasive approach. He followed my recommendations to the letter, and within two months on the plan his chest pains disappeared. His blood pressure normalized, his total cholesterol came down (without drugs) to 135, and he no longer required the six medications he had been taking for angina and hypertension. Now, seven years later, he is still free of any signs of vascular insufficiency.

I see numerous patients whose physicians have advised them to have angioplasty or bypass surgery but who have decided to try my aggressive nutritional management first. Those who follow the formula described in this book invariably find that their health improves and their chest pains gradually disappear. Of hundreds of cardiac patients treated in this manner, all but a few have done exceptionally well, with chest pain resolving in almost every case (only one went to repeat angioplasty because of a recurrence of chest symptoms), and I have had no patient die from cardiac arrest.

With the help of their doctors, most patients can slowly reduce — and eventually cease — their dependency on drugs. This program often enables my patients to avoid open-heart surgery and other invasive procedures. It often saves their lives.

However many details I provide of my patients' success, you are right to be skeptical. Thousands of patients with successful outcomes does not necessarily translate into your individual success. After all, you might point out, weren't these patients motivated by severe illness or the fear of death? Actually, many were relatively healthy people who came to me for routine medical care. They found a hidden benefit, and just decided to "eat to live" longer and healthier and lose the extra weight they did not need to carry, even if it was only ten to twenty pounds. When faced with the information in this book, they simply changed.

These results sound fantastic, and they are — but they are also true and predictable on my program. The key to this extraordinary diet is a simple formula: H = N/C.

Health = Nutrients/Calories

Your health is predicted by
your nutrient intake divided by your intake of calories.

H = N/C is a concept I call the *nutrient-density* of your diet. Food supplies us with both nutrients and calories (energy). All calories come from only three elements: carbohydrates, fats, and proteins. Nutrients are derived from noncaloric food factors — including vitamins, minerals, fibers, and phytochemicals. These noncaloric nutrients are vitally important for health. *Your key to permanent weight loss is to eat predominantly those foods that have a high proportion of nutrients (noncaloric food factors) to calories (carbohydrates, fats, and proteins). In physics a key formula is Einstein's $E = mc^2$. In nutrition the key formula is $H = N/C$.*

Every food can be evaluated using this formula. Once you begin to learn which foods make the grade — by having a high proportion of nutrients to calories — you are on your way to lifelong weight control and improved health.

Eating large quantities of high-nutrient foods is the secret to optimal health and permanent weight control. In fact, eating much larger portions of food is one of the beauties of the Eat to Live diet. You eat more, which effectively blunts your appetite, and you lose weight — permanently.

The Eat to Live diet does not require any deprivation. In fact, you do not have to give up any foods completely. However, as you consume larger and larger portions of health-supporting, high-nutrient foods, your appetite for low-nutrient foods decreases and you gradually lose your addiction to them. You will be able to make a complete commitment to this diet for the rest of your life.

By following my menu plans with great-tasting recipes, you will significantly increase the percentage of high-nutrient foods in your diet and your excess weight will start dropping quickly and dramatically. This will motivate you even more to stick with it. This approach requires no denial or hunger. Patients of mine, such as Joseph Miller, have lost sixty pounds in two months while feeling full and content. You can lose as much weight as you want even if diets have never worked for you in the past.

This book will allow everyone who stays on the program to become slimmer, healthier, and younger looking. You will embark on an adventure that will transform your entire life. Not only will you lose weight, you will sleep better, feel better physically, have more energy, and feel better emotionally. And you will lower your chances of developing serious diseases in the future. You will learn why diets haven't worked for you in the past and why so many popular weight-loss plans simply do not meet the scientific criteria for effectiveness and safety.

My promise is threefold: substantial, healthy weight reduction in a short period of time; prevention or reversal of many chronic and life-threatening medical conditions; and a new understanding of food and health that will continue to pay dividends for the rest of your life.

All the Information That You Need to Succeed

The main principle of this book is that for both optimal health and weight loss, you must consume a diet with a high nutrient-per-calorie ratio. Very few people, including physicians and dietitians, understand the concept of nutrient-per-calorie density. Understanding this key concept and learning to apply it to what you eat is the main focus of the book— but you must read the *entire* book. There are no shortcuts.

I have found that a comprehensive education in the subject is necessary for my patients to achieve the results they are looking for — but once they understand the concepts, they "own" them. They find it much easier to change. So make no mistake: the complete knowledge base of the book is essential if you want to achieve significant success, but I know that after you read this book you will say, "This makes sense." You will be a weight-loss and nutrition expert, and by the end you will have a strong foundation of knowledge that will serve you (and your newly slim self) for the rest of your life.

Why should you wait until you are faced with a life-threatening health crisis to want health excellence? Most people would choose to disease-proof their body and look great now. They just never thought they could do it so easily. Picture yourself in phenomenal health and in excellent physical condition at your ideal body weight. Not only will your waist be free of fat but your heart will be free of plaque.

Still, it is not easy to change: eating has emotional and social overtones. It is especially difficult to break an addiction. Our American diet style is addicting, as you will learn, but not as addictive as smoking cigarettes. Stopping smoking is very hard, but many still succeed. I have heard many excuses over the years, from smokers aiming to quit and sometimes even from failed dieters. Making any change is not easy. Obviously, most people know if they change their diet enough and exercise, they can lose weight — but they still can't do it.

After reading this book, you will have a better understanding of why changing has been so extremely difficult in the past and how to make it happen more easily. You will also find dramatic results available to you that make the change exciting and well worthwhile. However, you still must look deep within yourself and make a firm decision to do it.

I ask you for six weeks of your life to make my case. After the first six weeks, it becomes a lot easier. The first six weeks are definitely the hardest. You might already have strong reasons to make a commitment to the Eat to Live plan, or you would not be reading this.

Even with patients determined to quit smoking, I insist that if they are faced with significant work-related stress, have an argument, get in a car accident, or any other calamity, they should not go back to smoking and use smoking as a stress reliever. I admonish them, "Call me, wake me in the middle of the night if you have to; I will help you, even prescribe medication if necessary, but just don't give yourself that option of self-medicating with cigarettes." It is not so different with your food addictions — accept no excuse to fall off the wagon in the first six weeks. You can break the addiction only if you give your body a fair chance. Do not say you will give it a try. Do not try; instead, make a commitment to do it right.

When you get married, does the religious figure or justice of the peace ask, "Do you swear to give this person a try?" When people tell me they will give it a try, I say don't bother, you have already decided to fail. It takes more than a try to quit addictions; it takes a commitment. A commitment is a promise that you stick with, no matter what.

Without that commitment, you are doomed to fail. Give yourself the chance to really succeed this time. If you commit to just six weeks on this program, you will change your life forever and turning back becomes much more difficult.

Make a clear choice between success and failure. It takes only three simple steps. *One, buy the book; two, read the book; three, make the commitment.*

The third step is the difficult choice, but that is all it is — another choice. Don't go there yet. First, read the entire book. Study this book; then it will become easier and logical to take the third step — making the commitment to follow the plan for at least six weeks. You must have the knowledge carefully and elaborately described in this book before that commitment is meaningful. It is like getting married. Don't commit to marriage unless you know your partner. It is an educated choice, a choice made from both emotion and knowledge. The same is true here.

Let me thank you for beginning the journey to wellness. I take it personally. I sincerely appreciate all people who take an interest in improving themselves and taking better care of their health. I am committed to your success. I realize that every great success is the result of a strong and sustained effort. I have no aspirations to change every person in America, or even a majority of people. But at least people should be given a choice. This book gives everyone who reads it that choice.

A lifetime of compromised health does not have to be your destiny, because this plan works and it works marvelously. If you weren't sure in the past that you could do it, let me repeat that taking that big step makes all the hard work worthwhile, because then you get the results you desire.

You will always have my respect and appreciation for making that choice to help yourself, your family, and even your country by earning back your health.

Let me know how you do. If there is any way I can help you further, I would look forward to that opportunity. I am enthusiastically waiting to hear from many of you.

Put my ideas through this six-week test before evaluating your progress or deciding how healthy you feel. Do the grocery shopping. If you have lots of weight to lose, begin with my most powerful menu plans and instructions, without compromise, for the full six weeks. You will find the physiology of your body changing so significantly that you will never be the same. Your taste buds will become more sensitive, you will lose most of your cravings to overeat, you will feel so much better, and you will see such remarkable weight-loss results that it will be difficult ever to go back to your former way of eating. If you are on medication for diabetes or even for high blood pressure, make sure your physician is aware of your plan at the outset. He or she will need to monitor dosage to avoid overmedication. Read more about this in chapter seven.

Here is how the book works: Chapters one through four, considered together, are designed to be a comprehensive overview of human nutrition. The foundation of your success is based on the scientific information contained in these four chapters. In chapter one, you will see the problems with the standard American diet and learn how our food choices have the power to either cut short or add many years to our life. You may think you know all this, but let me surprise you with all that you don't know. Chapter two explains why obesity and chronic disease are the inevitable consequences of our poor food choices. I explain the link between low-nutrient foods and chronic disease/premature death as well as the connection between superior health/longevity and high-nutrient foods. In chapter three you will learn about those critical phytochemicals and the secret foods for both longevity and weight control. You will also learn why trying to control your weight by eating less food almost never works. The final chapter of this section of the book explains the problem with a diet rich in animal products and puts into perspective all the misleading advertising claims about foods that people have accepted as truth.

The next two chapters apply the concepts learned in the first four chapters by evaluating other diet plans and tackling many of the current controversies in human nutrition. Chapter five considers many popular weight-loss plans, giving you an in-depth understanding of their pros and cons. It is essential to have a thorough understanding of all scientific claims in this field because many people have become thoroughly confused by misinformation. Chapter six deepens your knowledge of the critical issues in order to understand the accurate information that is essential for maintaining your weight loss over the long term — your most important goal.

Chapter seven illustrates the power of the Eat to Live diet to reverse illness and provides instruction on how to apply this plan to remedy your health problems and find your ideal weight. Applying the Eat to Live formula to reverse and prevent heart disease, auto-immune illnesses, and so much more opens your critical eye to a new way of looking at your well-being. Health care becomes self-care, with food your new weapon to prevent and defeat illnesses. This one is a key chapter for everyone, not just for those with chronic medical problems but for all who want to live a longer, healthier life.

Chapters eight, nine, and ten put the advice into action and teach you how to make the healthy eating plan of this book taste great. In Chapter eight I explain the rules for swift and sustained weight loss and give you the tools you need to adjust your diet to achieve the results you desire. It offers guidelines and a set program that allows you to plan your daily menus. Chapter nine contains menu plans and recipes, including the more aggressive six-week plan designed for those who want to lose weight quickly, as well as vegetarian and nonvegetarian options. Frequently asked questions and answers are put forth in chapter ten, and I provide more practical information to aid you in your quest to regain your health.

It is my mission and my hope to give everyone the tools to achieve lifelong slimness and radiant health. Read on and learn how to put my health formula to work for you.

SOME REAL PEOPLE WHO COULD NOT LOSE WEIGHT
UNTIL STARTING DR. FUHRMAN'S EAT TO LIVE PLAN

Richard Acocella, 44 pounds; Jessie Alexander, 15 pounds; John Ambielli, 48 pounds; Florence Aviv, 45 pounds; Priska Baechler, 35 pounds; Shannon Blanding, 40 pounds; Mary Ann Braher, 30 pounds; Roger Braher, 45 pounds; Lynne Bush, 65 pounds; Robert Butkocy, 20 pounds; Vincent Caputo, 80 pounds; John Carbone, 40 pounds; Linda Castagna, 35 pounds; Robert Castagna, 30 pounds; Susan Chami, 25 pounds; Marlane Check, 35 pounds; June Chin, 40 pounds; Lorna Chin, 35 pounds; Lynn Chisolm, 25 pounds; Doris Compton, 25 pounds; Joseph Curci, 65 pounds; Maureen Curci, 38 pounds; Carol Dauch, 57 pounds; Richard Daum, 60 pounds; Dorothy Day, 40 pounds; Ray DeBoer, 110 pounds; Irene DeLengyel, 60 pounds; Jerry Deluca, 55 pounds; Frances DeSantos, 32 pounds; Thomas Deto, 50 pounds; Bernard Dodger, 60 pounds; Josephine Dombrowski, 55 pounds; Leonard Englebrook, 50 pounds; Delphine Fairley, 45 pounds; Meekness Faith, 25 pounds; Cathy Fall, 50 pounds; Craig Fall, 15 pounds; Robert Fanok, 25 pounds; Patti Farley, 60 pounds; Edward Feinberg, 35 pounds; Mary Ellen Fullum, 65 pounds; Judith Fusco, 65 pounds; James Gannon, 32 pounds; Margaret Giger, 36 pounds; Robert Girgus, 50 pounds; Charles Gisewhite, 35 pounds; Robin Gurman, 145 pounds; Verity Hagan, 45 pounds; William Hageman, 45 pounds; Denise Hall, 55 pounds; Theresa Hayth, 30 pounds; William Hayth, 30 pounds; Joseph Hetman, 30 pounds; Aleene Hogue, 40 pounds; Scott Hogue, 30 pounds; Mary Hundley, 40 pounds; David Jansen, 45 pounds; Russel Kamline, 40 pounds; Ben Kendelski, 35 pounds; Lydia Leoncini, 30 pounds; Louis Liotta, 250 pounds; Virginia Mahaffey, 90 pounds; Patricia Malchuk, 42 pounds; Margaret Massey, 42 pounds; Debbie Maulbeck, 33 pounds; Augusta Mexile, 100 pounds; Ron Meyer, 55 pounds; Linda Migliaccio, 150 pounds; Joseph Miller, 65 pounds; Sharon Lee Molnar, 25 pounds; Joan Moody, 45 pounds; Michael Moody, 62 pounds; Pauline Nappo, 45 pounds; Philip Nicastro, Jr., 50 pounds; Maria Olijnyk, 65 pounds; Allen Olsen, 55 pounds; John Pawlikoski, 45 pounds; JoAnne Pendleton, 52 pounds; Anthony Petito, 200 pounds; Gerardo Petito, 66 pounds; Dave Posmonter, 40 pounds; Louis Revesz, 70 pounds; Jean Roberts, 28 pounds; Mark Robinson, 30 pounds; George Sabosik, 65 pounds; Theresa Scavo, 70 pounds; Michael Schemick, 38 pounds; Judith Schwartz, 24 pounds; Diane Sireci, 45 pounds; Jane Slutsker, 45 pounds; Ted Somers, 36 pounds; Hayes Stagner, 55 pounds; Frank Stanski, 40 pounds; Linda Sticco, 20 pounds; Patricia Stroupe, 40 pounds; Richard Taggart, 40 pounds; Charles Taverner, 46 pounds; Frank Toth, 35 pounds; Angelo Verrusio, 35 pounds; Michelle Watson, 30 pounds; Rhonda Wilson, 75 pounds; Jacob Zaletel, 50 pounds; Charles Zilberberg, 25 pounds

Digging Our Graves
with Forks and Knives
THE EFFECTS OF THE AMERICAN DIET, PART I

Americans have been among the first people worldwide to have the luxury of bombarding themselves with nutrient-deficient, high-calorie food, often called *empty-calorie* or *junk food*. By "empty-calorie," I mean food that is deficient in nutrients and fiber. More Americans than ever before are eating these rich, high-calorie foods while remaining inactive — a dangerous combination.

The number one health problem in the United States is obesity, and if the current trend continues, by the year 2230 all adults in the United States will be obese. The National Institutes of Health estimate that obesity is associated with a twofold increase in mortality, costing society more than $100 billion per year.[1] This is especially discouraging for the dieter because after spending so much money attempting to lose weight, 95 percent percent of them gain all the weight back and then add on even more pounds within three years.[2] This incredibly high failure rate holds true for the vast majority of weight-loss schemes, programs, and diets.

Obesity and its sequelae pose a serious challenge to physicians. Both primary-care physicians and obesity-treatment specialists fail to make an impact on the long-term health of most of their patients. Studies show that initial weight loss is followed by weight regain.[3]

Those who genetically store fat more efficiently may have had a survival advantage thousands of years ago when food was scarce, or in a famine, but in today's modern food pantry they are the ones with the survival disadvantage. People whose parents are obese have a tenfold increased risk of being obese. On the other hand, obese families tend to have obese pets, which is obviously not genetic. So it is the *combination* of food choices, inactivity, and genetics that determines obesity.[4] More important, one can't change one's genes, so blaming them doesn't solve the problem. Rather than taking an honest look at what causes obesity, Americans are still looking for a miraculous cure — a magic diet or some other effortless gimmick.

Obesity is not just a cosmetic issue — extra weight leads to an earlier death, as many studies confirm.[5] *Overweight individuals are more likely to die from all causes, including heart disease and cancer.* Two-thirds of those with weight problems also have hypertension, diabetes, heart disease, or another obesity-related condition.[6] It is a major cause of early mortality in the United States.[7] Since dieting almost never works and the health risks of obesity are so life-threatening, more and more people are desperately turning to drugs and surgical procedures to lose weight.

Health Complications of Obesity

- Increased overall premature mortality
- Adult onset diabetes
- Hypertension
- Degenerative arthritis
- Coronary artery disease
- Cancer
- Lipid disorders
- Obstructive sleep apnea
- Gallstones
- Fatty infiltration of liver
- Restrictive lung disease
- Gastrointestinal diseases

The results so many of my patients have achieved utilizing the Eat to Live guidelines over the past ten years rival what can be achieved with surgical weight-reduction techniques, without the associated morbidity and mortality.[8]

Surgery for Weight Reduction and Its Risks

According to the National Institutes of Health (NIH), wound problems and complications from blood clots are common aftereffects of gastric bypass and gastroplasty surgery. The NIH has also reported that those undergoing surgical treatment for obesity have had substantial nutritional and metabolic complications, gastritis, esophagitis, outlet stenosis, and abdominal hernias. More than 10 percent required another operation to fix problems resulting from the first surgery.[9]

Another tempting solution is liposuction. Studies show that lipo-suction begets a plethora of side effects, the main one being death! A recent survey of all 1,200 actively practicing North American board-certified plastic surgeons confirmed that there are about 20 deaths for every 100,000 liposuctions, whereas the generally accept-able mortality rate for elective surgery is 1 in 100,000.[10] Com-pared with the 16.4 per 100,000 mortality rate of U.S. motor vehicle accidents, liposuction is not a benign procedure. Liposuction is dangerous.

GASTRIC BYPASS SURGERY COMPLICATIONS: 14-YEAR FOLLOW UP[11]

Vitamin B_{12} deficiency	239	39.9 percent
Readmit for various reasons	229	38.2 percent
Incisional hernia	143	23.9 percent
Depression	142	23.7 percent
Staple line failure	90	15.0 percent
Gastritis	79	13.2 percent
Cholecystitis	68	11.4 percent
Anastomotic problems	59	9.8 percent
Dehydration, malnutrition	35	5.8 percent
Dilated pouch	19	3.2 percent

Dangerous Dieting

In addition to undergoing extremely risky surgeries, Americans have been bombarded with a battery of gimmicky diets that promise to combat obesity. Almost all diets are ineffective. They don't work, be-cause no matter how much weight you lose when you are on a diet, you put it right back on when you go off. Measuring portions and trying to eat fewer calories, typically called "dieting," almost never results in permanent weight loss and actually worsens the problem over time. Such "dieting" temporarily slows down your metabolic rate, so often more weight comes back than you lost. You wind up heavier than you were before you started dieting. This leads many to claim, "I've tried everything, and nothing works. It must be genetic. Who wouldn't give up?"

You may already know that the conventional "solution" to being overweight — low-calorie dieting — doesn't work. But you may not know why. It is for this simple yet much overlooked reason: for the vast majority of people, being overweight is not caused by *how much* they eat but by *what* they eat. The idea that people get heavy because they consume a high volume of food is a myth. Eating large amounts of the right food is your key to success and is what makes this plan workable for the rest of your life. What makes many people overweight is not that they eat so much more but that they get a higher percentage of their calories from fat and *refined* carbohydrates, or mostly low-nutrient foods. This low-nutrient diet establishes a favorable cellular environment for disease to flourish.

Regardless of your metabolism or genetics, you can achieve a normal weight once you start a high-nutrient diet style. Since the majority of all Americans are overweight, the problem is not primarily genetic. Though genes are an important ingredient, physical activity and food choices play a far more significant role. In studies on identical twins with the tendency to be overweight, scientists found that physical activity is the strongest environmental determinant of total body and central abdominal fat mass.[12] Even those with a strong family history of obesity effectively lose weight with increased physical activity and appropriate dietary modifications.

Most of the time, the reason people are overweight is too little physical activity, in conjunction with a high-calorie, low-nutrient diet. Eating a diet with plenty of low-fiber, calorie-dense food, such as oil and refined carbohydrates, is the main culprit.

As long as you are eating fatty foods and refined carbohydrates, it is impossible to lose weight healthfully. In fact, this vicious combination of a sedentary lifestyle and eating typical "American" food (high-fat, low-fiber) is the primary reason we have such an incredibly overweight population.

Killing the Next Generation

This book may not appeal to many Americans who are in denial about the dangers of their eating habits and those of their children. Many people will do anything to continue their love affair with rich, disease-causing foods and will sacrifice their health in the process. Many American consumers prefer not to know about the dangers of their diet because they don't want to have their pleasures interfered with. This book is not for them.

If you have to give up something you get pleasure from, your subconscious may prefer to ignore solid evidence or defend illogically held views. Many ferociously defend their unhealthy eating practices. Others just claim, "I already eat a healthy diet," when they do not.

There is a general resistance to change. It would be much easier if healthful eating practices and the scientific importance of nutritional excellence were instilled in us as children. Unfortunately, children are eating more poorly today than ever before.

Most Americans are not aware that the diet they feed their children guarantees a high cancer probability down the road.[13] They don't even contemplate that eating fast-food meals may be just as risky (or more so) than letting their children smoke cigarettes.[14]

The 1992 Bogalusa Heart Study confirmed the existence of fatty plaques and streaks (the beginning of atherosclerosis) in most children and teenagers!

You wouldn't let your children sit around the table smoking cigars and drinking whiskey, because it is not socially acceptable, but it is fine to let them consume cola, fries cooked in trans fat, and a cheeseburger regularly. Many children consume doughnuts, cookies, cupcakes, and candy on a daily basis. It is difficult for parents to understand the insidious, slow destruction of their child's genetic potential and the foundation for serious illness that is being built by the consumption of these foods.

It would be unrealistic to feel optimistic about the health and well-being of the next generation when there is an unprecedented increase in the average weight of children in this country and record levels of childhood obesity. Most ominous were the results reported by the 1992 Bogalusa Heart Study, which studied autopsies performed on children killed in accidental deaths. The study confirmed the existence of fatty plaques and streaks (the beginning of atherosclerosis) in most children and teenagers![15] These researchers concluded: "These results emphasize the need for preventive cardiology in early life." I guess "preventive cardiology" is a convoluted term that means eating healthfully.

Another recent autopsy study appearing in the *New England Journal of Medicine* found that more than 85 percent of adults between the ages of twenty-one and thirty-nine already have atherosclerotic changes in their coronary arteries.[16] Fatty streaks and fibrous plaques covered large areas of the coronary arteries. Everyone knows that junk foods are not healthy, but few understand their consequences —

serious life-threatening illness. Clearly, the diets we consume as children have a powerful influence on our future health and eventual premature demise.[17]

There is considerable data to suggest that childhood diet has a greater impact on the later incidence of certain cancers than does a poor diet later in life.[18]

It is estimated that as many as 25 percent of schoolchildren today are obese.[19] *Early obesity sets the stage for adult obesity.* An overweight child develops heart disease earlier in life. Mortality data suggests that being overweight during early adult life is more dangerous than a similar degree of heaviness later in adult life.[20]

Drugs Are Not the Solution

New drugs are continually introduced that attempt to lessen the effects of our nation's self-destructive eating behavior. Most often, our society treats disease after the degenerative illness has appeared, an illness that is the result of from forty to sixty years of nutritional self-abuse.

Drug companies and researchers attempt to develop and market medications to stem the obesity epidemic. This approach will always be doomed to fail. The body will always pay a price for consuming medicines, which usually have toxic effects. The "side" effects are not the only toxic effect of medications. Doctors learn in their introductory pharmacology course in medical school that all medications are toxic to varying degrees, whether side effects are experienced or not. Pharmacology professors stress never to forget that. You cannot escape the immutable biological laws of cause and effect through ingesting medicinal substances.

If we don't make significant changes in the foods we choose to consume, taking drugs prescribed by physicians will not improve our health or extend our lives. If we wish true health protection, we need to remove the cause. We must stop abusing ourselves with disease-causing foods.

Surprise! Lean People Live Longer

In the Nurses Health Study, researchers examined the association between body mass index and overall mortality and mortality from specific causes in more than 100,000 women. After limiting the analysis to nonsmokers, it was very clear that the longest-lived women were the leanest.[21] The researchers concluded that the increasingly permissive U.S. weight guidelines are unjustified and potentially harmful.

Dr. I-Min Lee, of the Harvard School of Public Health, said her twenty-seven-year study of 19,297 men found there was no such thing as being too thin. (Obviously, it *is* possible to be too thin; however, it is uncommon and usually called anorexia, but that is not the subject of this book.) Among men who never smoked, the lowest mortality occurred in the lightest fifth.[22] Those who were in the thinnest 20 percent in the early 1960s were two and a half times less likely to have died of cardiovascular disease by 1988 than those in the heaviest fifth. Overall, the thinnest were two–thirds more likely to be alive in 1988 than the heaviest. Lee stated, "We observed a direct relationship between body weight and mortality. By that I mean that the thinnest fifth of men experienced the lowest mortality, and mortality increased progressively with heavier and heavier weight." The point is not to judge your ideal weight by traditional weight-loss tables, which are based on Americans' overweight averages. After carefully examining the twenty-five major studies available on the subject, I have found that the evidence indicates that optimal weight, as determined by who lives the longest, occurs at weights at least 10 percent below the average body-weight tables.[23] Most weight-guideline charts still place the public at risk by reinforcing an unhealthy overweight standard. By my calculations, it is not merely 75 percent of Americans that are overweight, it is more like 85 percent.

The Longer Your Waistline, the Shorter Your Lifeline

As a good rule of thumb: for optimal health and longevity, a man should not have more than one-half inch of skin that he can pinch near his umbilicus (belly button) and a woman should not have more than one inch. Almost any fat on the body over this minimum is a health risk. If you have gained even as little as ten pounds since the age of eighteen or twenty, then you could be at significant increased risk for health problems such as heart disease, high blood pressure, and diabetes. The truth is that most people who think they are at the right weight still have too much fat on their body.

A commonly used formula for determining ideal body weight follows:

Women: Approximately ninety-five pounds for the first five feet of height and then four pounds for every inch thereafter.

5'4"	95 + 16 = 111
5'6"	95 + 24 = 119

Men: Approximately 105 pounds for the first five feet of height and then five pounds for every inch thereafter. Therefore, a 5'10" male should weigh approximately 155 pounds.

All formulas that approximate ideal weights are only rough guides, since we all have different body types and bone structure.

Body mass index (BMI) is used as a convenient indicator of overweight risk and is often used in medical investigations. BMI is calculated by dividing weight in kilograms by height in meters (squared). Another way to calculate BMI is to use this formula:

$$BMI = \frac{\text{weight in pounds X 703}}{\text{height in inches (squared)}}$$

A BMI over 24 is considered overweight and greater than 30, obese. However, it is just as easy for most of us merely to use waist circumference.

I prefer waist circumference and abdominal fat measurements because BMI can be inaccurately high if the person is athletic and very muscular. Ideally, your BMI should be below 23, unless you lift weights and have considerable muscle mass. As an example, I am of average height and build (5'10" 150 pounds) and my BMI is 21.5. My waist circumference is 30.5 inches. Waist circumference should be measured at the navel.

The traditional view is that men who have a waist circumference over forty inches and women with one over thirty-five inches are significantly overweight with a high risk of health problems and heart attacks. Recent evidence suggests that abdominal fat measurement is a better predictor of risk than overall weight or size.[24] Fat deposits around your waist are a greater health risk than extra fat in other places, such as the hips and thighs.

What if you feel you are too thin? If you have too much *fat* on your body but feel you are too thin, then you should exercise to build *muscle* to gain weight. I often have patients tell me they think they look too thin, or their friends or family members tell them they look too thin, even though they are still clearly overweight. Bear in mind that by their standards you may be too thin, or at least thinner than they are. The question to ask is: Is their standard a healthy one? I doubt it. Either way: *Do not try to force yourself to overeat to gain weight!* Eat only as much food as your hunger drive demands, and no more. If you exercise, your appetite will increase in response. You should not try to put on weight merely by eating, because that will only add more fat to your frame, not muscle. Additional fat, regardless of whether you like the way you look when you are fatter or not, will shorten your life span.

Once you start eating healthfully, you may find you are getting thinner than expected. Most people lose weight until they reach their ideal weight and then they stop losing weight. Ideal weight is an individual thing, but it is harder to lose muscle than fat, so once the fat is off your body, your weight will stabilize. Stabilization at a thin, muscular weight occurs because your body gives you strong signals to eat, signals that I call "true hunger." *True hunger* maintains your muscle reserve, not your fat.

True Hunger

Once your body gets to a certain level of better health, you begin to feel the difference between *true hunger* and just eating due to desire, appetite, or withdrawal symptoms. Your body is healthier at this stage and you won't experience the withdrawal symptoms such as weakness, headaches, lightheadedness, etc., that most people associate with hunger.

It is our unhealthy tendency to eat without experiencing *true hunger* that contributed to our becoming overweight to begin with. In other words, to have become overweight in the first place, appetite, food cravings, and other addictive drives that induce eating have come into play. Poor nutrition induces these cravings (addictive drives), and nutritional excellence helps normalize or remove them. My experience with thousands of patients following my healthful, high-nutrient eating plan is that most of these people no longer get the discomfort that they formerly mistook for hunger. Even when they delay eating and get very hungry, they no longer experience stomach cramps, headaches, or fatigue accompanying their falling blood sugar. They merely get hungry and they enjoy this new sensation of hunger in the mouth and throat, which makes food taste better than ever. Many of my patients have told me they enjoy this new sensation; they like being able to be in touch with true hunger and the pleasure of satisfying it.

The one point I want to emphasize is that it does not require any precise measuring of calories or specific diet to maintain a thin, muscular weight. It only requires that you eat healthy food and that the hunger drive be real.

> Very few Americans have ever experienced true hunger.

The ability to sense *true hunger,* which is a mouth-and-throat sensation, does not occur until after you are eating healthfully and have a high nutrient-per-calorie diet. Then, when the period of withdrawal from excessive eating of unhealthy foods and caffeine is over, you can be in touch with *true hunger.* You will learn more about headaches, hypoglycemia, and hunger in chapter seven.

The Only Way to Significantly Increase Life Span

The evidence for increasing one's life span through dietary restriction is enormous and irrefutable. Reduced caloric intake is the only experimental technique to consistently extend maximum life span. This has been shown in *all* species tested, from insects and fish to rats and cats. There are so many hundreds of studies that only a small number are referenced below.

Scientists have long known that mice that eat fewer calories live longer. Recent research has demonstrated the same effect in primates, (i.e., you). A recent study published in the *Proceedings of the National Academy of Sciences* found that restricting calories by 30 percent significantly increased life span in monkeys. The experimental diet, while still providing *adequate* nourishment, slowed monkeys' metabolism and reduced their body temperatures, changes similar to those in the long-lived thin mice. Decreased levels of triglycerides and increased HDL (the good) cholesterol were also observed.[25] Studies over the years, on many different species of animals, have confirmed that those animals that were fed less lived longest. In fact, allowing an animal to eat as much food as it desires can reduce its life span by as much as one half.

High-nutrient, low-calorie eating results in dramatic increases in life span as well as prevention of chronic illnesses. From rodents to primates we see:

- Resistance to experimentally induced cancers
- Protection from spontaneous and genetically predisposed cancers
- A delay in the onset of late-life diseases
- Nonappearance of atherosclerosis and diabetes
- Lower cholesterol and triglycerides and increased HDL
- Improved insulin sensitivity
- Enhancement of the energy-conservation mechanism, including reduced body temperature
- Reduction in oxidative stress
- Reduction in parameters of cellular aging, including cellular congestion
- Enhancement of cellular repair mechanisms, including DNA repair enzymes
- Reduction in inflammatory response and immune cell proliferation
- Improved defenses against environmental stresses
- Suppression of the genetic alterations associated with aging
- Protection of genes associated with removal of oxygen radicals
- Inhibited production of metabolites that are potent cross-linking agents
- Slowed metabolic rate[26]

The link between thinness and longevity, and obesity and a shorter life span, is concrete. Another important consideration in other animal studies is that fat restriction has an additional effect on lengthening life span.[27] Apparently, higher-fat intake promotes hormone production, speeds up reproductive readiness and other indicators of aging, and promotes the growth of certain tumors.

In the wide field of longevity research there is only one finding that has held up over the years: eating less prolongs life, as long as nutrient intake is adequate. All other longevity ideas are merely conjectural and unproven.[28] Such theories include taking hormones such as estrogen, DHEA, growth hormones, and melatonin, as well as nutritional supplements. So far, there is no solid evidence that supplying the body with any nutritional element over and above the level present in adequate amounts in a nutrient-dense diet will prolong life.

This is in contrast to the overwhelming evidence regarding protein and caloric restriction.

This important and irrefutable finding is a crucial feature of the H = N/C equation. We all must recognize that if we are to reach the limit of human life span, we must not overeat on high-calorie food. Eating empty-calorie food makes it impossible to achieve optimal health and maximize our genetic potential.

To Avoid Overeating on High-Calorie Foods, Fill Up on Nutrient-Rich Ones

An important corollary to the principle of limiting high-calorie food is that the only way for a human being to safely achieve the benefits of caloric restriction while ensuring that the diet is nutritionally adequate is to avoid as much as possible those foods that are nutrient poor.

Indeed, this is the crucial consideration in deciding what to eat. We need to eat foods with adequate nutrients so we won't need to consume excess "empty" calories to reach our nutritional requirements. Eating foods that are rich in nutrients and fiber, and low in calories, "fills us up," so to speak, thus preventing us from overeating.

To grasp why this works, let us look at how the brain controls our dietary drive. A complicated system of chemoreceptors in the nerves lining the digestive tract carefully monitor the calorie and nutrient density of every mouthful and send such information to the hypothalamus in the brain, which controls dietary drive.

There are also stretch receptors in the stomach to signal satiety by detecting the *volume* of food eaten, not the *weight* of the food. If you are not filled up with nutrients and fiber, the brain will send out signals telling you to eat more food, or overeat.

In fact, if you consume sufficient nutrients and fiber, you will become *biochemically* filled (nutrients) and *mechanically* filled (fiber), and your desire to consume calories will be blunted or turned down. One key factor that determines whether you will be overweight is your failure to consume sufficient fiber and nutrients. This has been illustrated in scientific studies.[29]

How does this work in practice? Let's say we conduct a scientific experiment and observe a group of people by measuring the average number of calories they consumed at each dinner. Next, we give them a whole orange and a whole apple prior to dinner. The result would

MORE NUTRIENTS AND FIBER WILL REDUCE YOUR CALORIC DRIVE

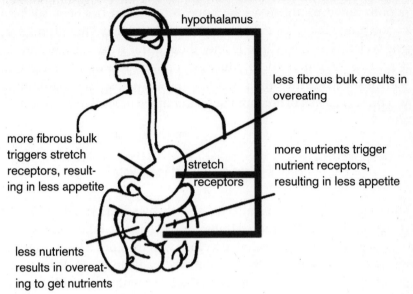

hypothalamus

less fibrous bulk results in overeating

more fibrous bulk triggers stretch receptors, resulting in less appetite

stretch receptors

more nutrients trigger nutrient receptors, resulting in less appetite

less nutrients results in overeating to get nutrients

be that the participants would reduce their caloric intake, on the average, by the amount of calories in the fruit. Now, instead of giving them two fruits, give them the same amount of calories from fruit juice.

What will happen? They will eat the same amount of food as they did when they had nothing at the beginning of their meal. In other words, the juice did not reduce the calories consumed in the meal — instead, the juice became additional calories. This has been shown to occur with beer, soft drinks, and other sources of liquid calories.[30]

Liquid calories, without the fiber present in the whole food, have little effect at blunting our caloric drive. Studies show that fruit juice and other sweet beverages lead to obesity in children as well.[31]

If you are serious about losing weight, don't drink your fruit — eat it. Too much fiber and too many nutrients are removed during juicing, and many of the remaining nutrients are lost through processing, heat, and storage time. If you are not overweight, drinking fresh-prepared juice is acceptable as long as it does not serve as a substitute for eating those fresh fruits and vegetables. There is no substitute for natural whole foods.

There is a tendency for many of us to want to believe in magic. People want to believe that in spite of our indiscretions and excesses, we can still maintain optimal health by taking a pill, powder, or other potion. However, this is a false hope, a hope that has been silenced by too much scientific evidence. There is no magic. There is no miracle weight-loss pill. There is only the natural world of law and order, of cause and effect. If you want optimal health and longevity, you must engage the cause. And if you want to lose fat weight safely, you must eat a diet of predominantly unrefined foods that are nutrient- and fiber-rich.

What if I Have a Slow Metabolic Rate?

Your body weight may be affected slightly by genetics, but that effect is not strong. Furthermore, I am convinced that inheriting a slow metabolic rate with a tendency to gain weight is not a flaw or defect but rather a genetic gift that can be taken advantage of. How is this possible? A slower metabolism is associated with longer life span in all species of animals. It can be speculated that if one lived sixty thousand or just a few hundred years ago, a slower metabolic rate might have increased our survival opportunity, since getting sufficient calories was difficult. For example, the majority of Pilgrims that arrived on our shores on the *Mayflower* died that first winter.[32] They could not make or find enough food to eat, so only those with the genetic gift of a slow metabolic rate survived.

As you can see, it is not always bad to have a slow metabolic rate. It can be good. Sure, it is bad in today's environment of relentless eating and when consuming a high-calorie, low-nutrient diet. Sure, it will increase your risk of diabetes and heart disease and cancer, given today's food-consumption patterns. However, if correct food choices are made to maintain a normal weight, the individual with a slower metabolism may age more slowly.

Our body is like a machine. If we constantly run the machinery at high speed, it will wear out faster. Since animals with slower metabolic rates live longer, eating more calories, which drives up our metabolic rate, will cause us only to age faster. Contrary to what you may have heard and read in the past, our goal should be the opposite: to eat less, only as much as we need to maintain a slim and muscular weight, and no more, so as to keep our metabolic rate relatively slow.

So stop worrying about your slower metabolic rate. A slower metabolic rate from dieting is not the primary cause of your weight problem. Keep these three important points in mind:

1. Resting metabolic rates do decline slightly during periods of lower caloric intake, but not enough to significantly inhibit weight loss.
2. Resting metabolic rates return to normal soon after caloric intake is no longer restricted. The lowered metabolic rate does not stay low permanently and make future dieting more difficult.
3. A sudden lowering of the metabolic rate from dieting does not explain the weight gain/loss cycles experienced by many overweight people. These fluctuations in weight are primarily from going on and getting off diets. It is especially difficult to stay with a reduced-calorie diet when it never truly satisfies the individual's biochemical need for nutrients, fiber, and phytochemicals.[33]

Those with a genetic tendency to overweight may actually have the genetic potential to outlive the rest of us. The key to their successful longevity lies in their choosing a nutrient-rich, fiber-rich, lower-calorie diet, as well as getting adequate physical activity. By adjusting the nutrient-per-calorie density of your diet to your metabolic rate, you can use your slow metabolism to your advantage. When you can maintain a normal weight in spite of a slow metabolism, you will be able to achieve significant longevity.

An Unprecedented Opportunity in Human History

Science and the development of modern refrigeration and transportation methods have given us access to high-quality, nutrient-dense food. In today's modern society, we have available to us the largest variety of fresh and frozen natural foods in human history. Using the foods available to us today, we can devise diets and menus with better nutrient density and nutrient diversity than ever before possible.

This book gives you the information and the motivation you need to take advantage of this opportunity to improve your health and maximize your chances for a disease-free life.

You have a clear choice. You can live longer and healthier than ever before, or you can do what most modern populations do: eat to create disease and a premature death. Since you are reading this book, you have opted to live longer and healthier. "Eat to Live" and you will have achieved the crucial first step.

2

Overfed, Yet Malnourished
THE EFFECTS OF THE AMERICAN DIET, PART II

Now you know the formula for longevity (H = N/C) and that the key to this formula is the nutrient density of your diet. In other words, you must eat a diet rich in nutrients and fiber, with a very low percentage of foods that are not nutrient- and fiber-dense. It is the same formula that will enable your body to achieve slimness.

To help you learn *how* to apply this formula to your life, you first need to understand *why* you must follow it, exploring the relationships between diet, health, and disease. To do so, you need to take a look at how most people eat in reality and what they gain or lose from such eating practices.

The Pros and Cons of Our "Natural Sweet Tooth"

Even though we have many unique human traits, we are genetically closely related to the great apes and other primates. Primates are the only animals on the face of the earth that can taste sweet and see color. We were designed by nature to see, grasp, eat, and enjoy the flavor of colorful, sweet fruits.

Fruit is an essential part of our diets. It is an indispensable requirement for us to maintain a high level of health. Fruit consumption has been shown in numerous studies to offer our strongest protection against certain cancers, especially oral and esophageal, lung, prostate, and pancreatic cancer.[1] Thankfully, our natural sweet tooth directs us to those foods ideally "designed" for our primate heritage — fruit. Fresh fruit offers us powerful health-giving benefits.

Researchers have discovered substances in fruit that have unique effects on preventing aging and deterioration of the brain.[2] Some fruits, especially blueberries, are rich in anthocyanins and other compounds having anti-aging effects.[3] Studies continue to provide evidence that more than any other food, fruit consumption is associated with lowered mortality from all cancers combined.[4] Eating fruit is vital to your health, well-being, and long life.

Regrettably, our human desire for sweets is typically satisfied by the consumption of products containing sugar, such as candy bars and ice cream — not fresh fruit. The U.S. Food and Drug Administration estimates that the typical American now consumes an unbelievable 32 teaspoons of added sugar a day.[5] That's right, in one day.

As we shall see, we need to satisfy our sweet tooth with fresh, natural fruits and other plant substances that supply us not just with carbohydrates for energy but also with the full complement of indispensable substances that prevent illness.

Nutritional Lightweights: Pasta and White Bread

Unlike the fruits found in nature — which have a full ensemble of nutrients — processed carbohydrates (such as bread, pasta, and cake) are deficient in fiber, phytonutrients, vitamins, and minerals, all of which have been lost in processing.

Compared with whole wheat, typical pasta and bread are missing:

- 62 percent of the zinc
- 72 percent of the magnesium
- 95 percent of the vitamin E
- 50 percent of the folic acid
- 72 percent of the chromium
- 78 percent of the vitamin B_6
- 78 percent of the fiber

In a six-year study of 65,000 women, those with diets high in refined carbohydrates from white bread, white rice, and pasta had two and a half times the incidence of Type II diabetes, compared with those who ate high-fiber foods such as whole-wheat bread and brown rice.[6] These findings were replicated in a study of 43,000 men.[7] Diabetes is no trivial problem; it is the fourth-leading cause of death by disease in America, and its incidence is growing.[8]

Walter Willett, M.D., professor of epidemiology and nutrition at the Harvard School of Public Health and co-author of those two studies, finds the results so convincing that he'd like our government to change the Food Guide Pyramid, which recommends six to eleven servings of any kind of carbohydrate. He says, "They should move refined grains, like white bread, up to the sweets category because metabolically they're basically the same."

These starchy (white flour) foods, removed from nature's packaging, are no longer real food. The fiber and the majority of minerals have been removed, so such foods are absorbed too rapidly, resulting in a sharp glucose surge into the bloodstream. The pancreas is then forced to pump out insulin faster to keep up. Excess body fat also causes us to require more insulin from the pancreas. Over time, it is the excessive demand for insulin placed on the pancreas from both refined foods and increased body fat that leads to diabetes. Refined carbohydrates, white flour, sweets, and even fruit juices, because they enter the bloodstream so quickly, can also raise triglycerides, increasing the risk of heart attack in susceptible individuals.

Every time you eat such processed foods, you exclude from your diet not only the essential nutrients that we are aware of but hundreds of other undiscovered phytonutrients that are crucial for normal human function. When the nutrient-rich outer cover is removed from whole wheat to make it into white flour, the most nutritious part of the food is lost. The outer portion of the wheat kernel contains trace minerals, phytoestrogens, lignans, phytic acid, indoles, phenolic compounds, and other phytochemicals, as well as almost all the vitamin E in the food. True whole grain foods, which are associated with longer life, are vastly different from the processed foods that make up the bulk of calories in the modern American diet (MAD).[9]

Medical investigations clearly show the dangers of consuming the quantity of processed foods that we do. And because these refined grains lack the fiber and nutrient density to turn down our appetite, they also cause obesity, diabetes, heart disease, and significantly increased cancer risk.[10]

One recent nine-year study involving 34,492 women between the ages of fifty-five and sixty-nine showed a two-thirds increase in the risk of death from heart disease in those eating refined grains.[11] Summarizing fifteen epidemiological studies, researchers concluded that diets containing refined grains and refined sweets were consistently linked to stomach and colon cancer, and at least twelve breast cancer studies connect low-fiber diets with increased risks.[12] Eating a diet that contains a significant quantity of sugar and refined flour does not just cause weight gain, it also leads to an earlier death.

Refined Foods Are Linked To

- Oral cavity cancer
- Stomach cancer
- Colorectal cancer
- Intestinal cancer
- Breast cancer
- Thyroid cancer
- Respiratory tract cancer
- Diabetes
- Gallbladder disease
- Heart disease[13]

If you want to lose weight, the most important foods to avoid are processed foods: condiments, candy, snacks, and baked goods; fat-free has nothing to do with it. Almost all weight-loss authorities agree on this — you must cut out the refined carbohydrates, including bagels, pasta, and bread. As far as the human body is concerned, low-fiber carbohydrates such as pasta are almost as damaging as white sugar. Pasta is not health food — it is hurt food.

Now I can imagine what many of you are thinking: "But, Dr. Fuhrman! I love pasta. Do I have to give it up?" I enjoy eating pasta, too. Pasta can sometimes be used in small quantities in a recipe that includes lots of green vegetables, onions, mushrooms, and tomatoes. Whole-grain pastas and bean pastas found in health-food stores are better choices than those made from white flour. See chapter nine for tasty ideas. The point to remember is that all refined grains must be placed in that limited category — foods that should constitute only a small percentage of our total caloric intake.

What about bagels? Is the "whole-wheat" bagel you just bought at the bagel store really made from whole grain? No; in most cases, it is primarily white flour. It is hard to tell sometimes. Ninety-nine percent of pastas, breads, cookies, pretzels, and other grain products are made from white flour. Sometimes a little whole wheat or caramel color is added and the product is called whole wheat to make you think it is the real thing. It isn't. Most brown bread is merely white bread with a fake tan. Wheat grown on American soil is not a nutrient-dense food to begin with, but then the food manufacturers remove the most valuable part of the food and then add bleach, preservatives, salt, sugar, and food coloring to make breads, breakfast cereals, and other convenience foods. Yet many Americans consider such food healthy merely because it is low in fat.

Soil Depletion of Nutrients Is Not the Problem — Our Food Choices Are

Contrary to many of the horror stories you hear, our soil is not depleted of nutrients. California, Washington, Oregon, Texas, Florida, and other states still have rich, fertile land that produces most of our fruits, vegetables, beans, nuts, and seeds. America provides some of the most nutrient-rich produce in the world.

Our government publishes nutritional analyses of foods. It takes food from a variety of supermarkets across the country, analyzes it, and publishes the results. Contrary to claims of many health-food and supplement enthusiasts, the produce grown in this country is nutrient-rich and high in trace minerals, especially beans, nuts, seeds, fruits, and vegetables.[14] American-produced grains, however, do not have the mineral density of vegetables. Grains and animal-feed crops grown in the southeastern states are the most deficient, but even in those states only a small percentage of crops are shown to be deficient in minerals.[15]

Thankfully, by eating a diet with a wide variety of natural plant foods, from a variety of soils, the threat of nutritional deficiency merely as a result of soil inadequacy is eliminated. Americans are not nutrient-deficient because of our depleted soil, as some nutritional-supplement proponents claim. Americans are nutrient-deficient because they do not eat a sufficient quantity of fresh produce. Over 90 percent of the calories consumed by Americans come from refined foods or animal products. With such a small percentage of our diet consisting of unrefined plant foods, how could we not become nutrient-deficient?

Since more than 40 percent of the calories in the American diet are derived from sugar or refined grains, both of which are nutrient-depleted, Americans are severely malnourished. Refined sugars cause us to be malnourished in direct proportion to how much we consume them. They are partially to blame for the high cancer and heart attack rates we see in America.

It is not merely dental cavities that should concern us about sugar. If we allow ourselves and our children to utilize sugar, white-flour products, and oil to supply the majority of calories, as most American families do, we shall be condemning ourselves to a lifetime of sickness, medical problems, and a premature death.

Refined sugars include table sugar (sucrose), milk sugar (lactose), honey, brown sugar, high-fructose corn syrup, molasses, corn sweeteners, and fruit juice concentrates. Even the bottled and boxed fruit juices that many children drink are a poor food; with no significant nutrient density, they lead to obesity and disease.[16] Processed apple juice, which is not far from sugar water in its nutrient score, accounts for almost 50 percent of all fruit servings consumed by preschoolers.[17] For example, apple juice contains none of the vitamin C originally present in the whole apple. Oranges make the most nutritious juice, but even orange juice can't compare with the original orange. In citrus fruits, most of the anti-cancer compounds are present in the membranes and pulp, which are removed in processing juice. Those cardboard containers of orange juice contain less than 10 percent of the vitamin C present in an orange and even less of the fiber and phytochemicals. Juice is *not* fruit, and prepackaged juices do not contain even one-tenth of the nutrients present in fresh fruit.

Processed carbohydrates, lacking in fiber, fail to slow sugar absorption, causing wide swings in glucose levels.

Empty calories are empty calories. Cookies, jams, and other processed foods (even those from the health-food store) sweetened with "fruit juice" sound healthier but are just as bad as white-sugar products. When fruit juice is concentrated and used as a sweetener, the healthy nutritional components are stripped away — what's left is plain sugar. To your body, there is not much difference between refined sugar, fruit juice sweeteners, honey, fruit juice concentrate, or any other concentrated sweetener. Our sweet tooth has been put there by nature to have us enjoy and consume real fruit, not some imitation. Fresh-squeezed orange juice and other fresh fruit and vegetable juices are relatively healthy foods that contain the majority of the original vitamins and minerals. But the sweet fruit juices and even carrot juice should still be used only moderately, as they still contain a high concentration of sugar calories and no fiber. Still not an ideal food for those desiring to lose weight. I often use these juices as part of salad dressings and other dishes rather than alone as a drink. Fresh fruits and even dried fruits do contain an assortment of protective nutrients and phytochemicals, so stick with the real thing.

Lester Traband's Yearly Checkup

My patient Les Traband came in for his yearly checkup. He was not overweight and had been following a vegetarian diet for years. I did a dietary review of what he ate regularly. He was eating "healthy" flaxseed waffles for breakfast, lots of pasta, whole-wheat bread, and vegan (no animal products) prepared frozen meals on a regular basis.

I spent about thirty minutes pointing out that he was certainly not following my dietary recommendations for excellent health and presented him with some menu suggestions and an outline of my nutritional prescription for superior health, which he agreed to follow.

Twelve weeks later, he had lost about eight pounds and I rechecked his lipid profile, because I didn't like the results we received from the blood test taken the day of his checkup.

The results speak for themselves:

	2/1/2001	5/2/2001
Cholesterol	230	174
Triglycerides	226	57
HDL	55	78
LDL	130	84
Cholesterol/HDL ratio	4.18	2.23

Enrichment with Nutrients Is a House Made of Straw

White or "enriched" rice is just as bad as white bread and pasta. It is nutritionally bankrupt. You might as well just eat the Uncle Ben's cardboard box it comes in. Refining the rice removes the same important factors: fiber, minerals, phytochemicals, and vitamin E. So, when you eat grains, eat whole grains.

Refining foods removes so much nutrition that our government requires that a few synthetic vitamins and minerals be added back. Such foods are labeled as *enriched* or *fortified*. Whenever you see those words on a package, it means important nutrients are missing. Refining foods lowers the amount of hundreds of known nutrients, yet usually only five to ten are added back by fortification.

As we change food through processing and refining, we rob the food of certain health-supporting substances and often create unhealthy compounds, thus making it a more unfit food for human consumption. As a general rule of thumb: the closer we eat foods to their natural state, the healthier the food.

Not All Whole-Wheat Products Are Equal

Just because a food is called "whole grain" does not make it a good food. Many whole-grain cold cereals are so processed that they do not have a significant fiber per serving ratio and have lost most of their nutritional value.

> Eating fragmented and unbalanced foods causes many problems, especially for those trying to lose weight.

Whole wheat that is finely ground is absorbed into the bloodstream fairly rapidly and should not be considered as wholesome as more coarsely ground and grittier whole grains. The rapid rise of glucose triggers fat storage hormones. Because the more coarsely ground grains are absorbed more slowly, they curtail our appetite better.

Whole-grain hot cereals are less processed than cold cereals and come up with better nutritional scores. They can be soaked in water overnight so you do not have to cook them in the morning. Some hot whole-grain cereals that I recommend are oatmeal (not instant), Roman Meal, Steel Cut Oats, Wheatena, Ralston High Fiber, and Quaker Multigrain.

Unlike eating whole-grain foods, ingesting processed foods can subtract nutrients and actually create nutritional deficiencies, as the body utilizes nutrients to digest and assimilate food. If the mineral demands of digestion and assimilation are greater than the nutrients supplied by the food, we may end up with a deficit — a drain on our nutrient reserve funds.

For most of their lives, the diets of many American adults and children are severely deficient in plant-derived nutrients. I have drawn nutrient levels on thousands of patients and have become shocked at the dismal levels in supposedly "healthy" people. Our bodies are not immune to immutable biological laws that govern cellular function. Given enough time, disease will develop. Even borderline deficiencies can result in various subtle defects in human health, leading to anxiety, autoimmune disorders, cancer, and poor eyesight, to name a few.[18]

Fat and Refined Carbohydrates: Married to Your Waist

The body converts food fat into body fat quickly and easily: 100 calories of ingested fat can be converted to 97 calories of body fat by burning a measly 3 calories. Fat is an *appetite stimulant:* the more you eat, the more you want. If a food could be scientifically engineered to create an obese society, it would have fat, such as butter, mixed with sugar and flour.

The combination of fat and refined carbohydrates has an extremely powerful effect on driving the signals that promote fat accumulation on the body. Refined foods cause a swift and excessive rise in blood sugar, which in turn triggers insulin surges to drive the sugar out of the blood and into our cells. Unfortunately, insulin also promotes the storage of fat on the body and encourages your fat cells to swell.

As more fat is packed away on the body, it interferes with insulin uptake into our muscle tissues. Our pancreas then senses that the glucose level in the bloodstream is still too high and pumps out even more insulin. A little extra fat around our midsection results in so much interference with insulin's effectiveness that two to five times as much insulin may be secreted in an overweight person than in a thin person.

The higher level of insulin in turn promotes more efficient conversion of our caloric intake into body fat, and this vicious cycle continues. People get heavier and heavier as time goes on.

Eating refined carbohydrates — as opposed to complex carbohydrates in their natural state — causes the body's "set point" for body weight to increase. Your "set point" is the weight the body tries to maintain through the brain's control of hormonal messengers. When you eat refined fats (oils) or refined carbohydrates such as white flour and sugar, the fat-storing hormones are produced in excess, raising the set point. To further compound the problem, because so much of the vitamin and mineral content of these foods has been lost

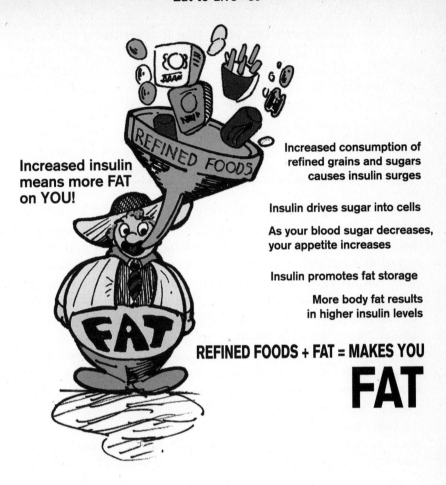

Increased insulin means more FAT on YOU!

Increased consumption of refined grains and sugars causes insulin surges

Insulin drives sugar into cells

As your blood sugar decreases, your appetite increases

Insulin promotes fat storage

More body fat results in higher insulin levels

REFINED FOODS + FAT = MAKES YOU

FAT

during processing, you naturally crave more food to make up for the missing nutrients.

Our Oil-Rich Country, or From Your Lips Right to Your Hips

An effective way to sabotage your weight-loss goal is with high-fat dressings and sauces. Americans consume 60 grams of added fat in the form of oils, which is over five hundred calories a day from this form of no-fiber, empty calories.[19] Refined or extracted oils, including olive oil, are rich in calories and low in nutrients.

Oils are 100 percent fat. Like all other types of fat, they contain nine calories per gram, compared with four calories per gram for carbohydrates. There are lots of calories in just a little bit of oil.

ANALYSIS OF ONE TABLESPOON OF OLIVE OIL

Calories	120
Fiber	none
Protein	none
Fat	13.5 gm
Saturated fat	1.8 gm
Minerals	none (trace, less than .01 mg of every mineral)
Vitamins	none (trace of vitamin E, less than 1 IU)

Fat, such as olive oil, can be stored on your body within minutes, without costing the body any caloric price; it is just packed away (unchanged) on your hips and waist. If we biopsied your waist fat and looked at it under an electron microscope, we could actually see where the fat came from. It is stored there as pig fat, dairy fat, and olive oil fat — just as it was in the original food. It goes from your lips right to your hips. Actually, more fat from your last meal is deposited around your waist than on your hips, for both men and women.[20] Analyzing these body-fat deposits is an accurate way for research scientists to discern food intake over time.[21] Having research subjects remember what they ate (dietary recall analysis) is not as accurate as a tissue biopsy, which reports exactly what was really eaten.

Foods cooked in oil or coated with oils soak up more oil than you think. A low-calorie "healthy" food easily becomes fattening. Most Americans eat negligible amounts of salad vegetables, but when they do eat a small salad, they consume about three leaves of iceberg lettuce in a small bowl and then proceed to pour three or four tablespoons of oily dressing on top. Since oil is about 120 calories per tablespoon, they consume some 400 (empty) calories from dressing and about 18 from lettuce. They might as well forget the lettuce and just drink the dressing straight from the bottle.

One key to your success is to make healthful salad dressings that are low in fat and calories. Some of my favorites are in chapter nine, as well as some commercial dressings with less then twenty calories per tablespoon.

The message Americans are hearing today from the media and health professionals is that you don't need to go on a low-fat diet, you merely need to replace the bad fats (saturated fats mostly from animal products and trans fats in processed foods) with olive oil. Americans are still confused and receive conflicting and incorrect messages.

Olive oil and other salad and cooking oils are not health foods and are certainly not diet foods.

There is considerable evidence to suggest that consuming mono-unsaturated fats such as olive oil is less destructive to your health than the dangerous saturated and trans fats. But a lower-fat diet could be more dangerous than one with a higher level of fat if the lower-fat diet had more saturated and trans fats.

In the 1950s people living in the Mediterranean, especially on the island of Crete, were lean and virtually free of heart disease. Yet over 40 percent of their caloric intake came from fat, primarily olive oil. If we look at the diet they consumed back then, we note that the Cretans ate mostly fruits, vegetables, beans, and some fish. Saturated fat was less than 6 percent of their total fat intake. True, they ate lots of olive oil, but the rest of their diet was exceptionally healthy. They also worked hard in the fields, walking about nine miles a day, often pushing a plow or working other manual farm equipment. Americans didn't take home the message to eat loads of vegetables, beans, and fruits and do loads of exercise; they just accepted that olive oil is a health food.

Today the people of Crete are fat, just like us. They're still eating a lot of olive oil, but their consumption of fruits, vegetables, and beans is down. Meat, cheese, and fish are their new staples, and their physical activity level has plummeted. Today, heart disease has sky-rocketed and more than half the population of both adults and children in Crete is overweight.[22]

Even two of the most enthusiastic proponents of the Mediter-ranean diet, epidemiologist Martin Katan of the Wageningan Agri-cultural University in the Netherlands and Walter Willett of the Harvard School of Public Health, concede that the Mediterranean diet is viable only for people who are close to their ideal weight.[23] That excludes the majority of Americans. How can a diet revolving around a fattening, nutrient-deficient food like oil be healthy?

Ounce for ounce, olive oil is one of the most fattening, calorically dense foods on the planet; it packs even more calories per pound than butter (butter: 3,200 calories; olive oil: 4,020).

The bottom line is that oil will add fat to our already plump waist-lines, heightening the risk of disease, including diabetes and heart at-tacks. Olive oil contains 14 percent saturated fat, so you increase the amount of artery-clogging saturated fat as you consume more of it. I believe consuming more fattening olive oil in your diet will raise your LDL (bad) cholesterol, not lower it. Weight gain raises your cholesterol; unprocessed foods such as nuts, seeds, and vegetables, utilized as a source of fat and calories instead of oil, contain phytosterols and other natural substances that lower cholesterol.[24] Also, keep in mind that in Italy, where they consume all that supposedly healthy olive oil, people have twice the chance of getting breast cancer as in Japan, where they have a significantly lower fat intake.[25]

The Mediterranean Diet looked better than ours because of the increased consumption of vegetation, not because of the oil. People who use olive oil generally put it on vegetables such as salads and tomatoes, so its use is correlated with higher consumption of produce. Their diets were better, in spite of the oil consumption, not because of it.

If you are thin and exercise a lot, one tablespoon of olive oil a day is no big deal, but the best choice for most overweight Americans is no oil at all.

The Popularity of the Mediterranean Diet

Entire books have been written advocating the benefits of the Mediterranean diet. One such book, for those interested in this line of thinking, is *Low-Fat Lies, High-Fat Frauds*, by Kevin Vigilante and Mary Flynn.[26]

They accurately point out that calories *do* matter and explain that the main reason such carbohydrate-restricting, high-fat diets as Atkins and *Sugar Busters* work is that most people can't eat too many calories from high-fat food because they can eat only so much rich, fatty food — so they wind up eating fewer calories. This is only partially true. However, research has shown that weight loss is about the same from any type of food eaten when caloric intake is equally low.[27] Their main message is threefold: first, eat mostly phytochemical-rich plant foods to maximize health and disease prevention; second, caloric restriction and exercise must be maintained for positive results; and third, healthy fats, especially olive oil, should not be restricted, because a diet without these fats is both unhealthy and unpalatable. The diet they recommend, which watches saturated fat intake and avoids trans fats, is a nice improvement over the diet most Americans eat. Certainly it is better to use olive oil than butter or margarine.

I have only a few bones to pick with those advocating this diet style. First, they claim that cooking food in olive oil increases phytochemical absorption and that eating vegetables without a high-fat topping is not as nutritious since the phytochemicals are not absorbed. This is not accurate. When vegetables are cooked, or eaten with fat, some nutrients are more efficiently absorbed and other heat-sensitive nutrients are lost or rendered less absorbable. Many studies show that raw fruits and vegetables offer the highest blood levels of cancer-protective nutrients and the most protection against cancer of any other foods, including cooked vegetation.[28] Any advice not recognizing that raw vegetables and fresh fruits are the two most powerful anti-cancer categories of foods is off the mark.

Paul Talalay, M.D., of the Brassica Chemoprotection Laboratory at the Johns Hopkins School of Medicine is involved with researching the effect of cooking on phytochemicals. He reports "widely different effects on the compounds in vegetables that protect against cancer."[29] These compounds are both activated and destroyed by various cooking methods. Vigilante and Flynn have championed the position that cooking foods in olive oil is the centerpiece of a healthy diet, without adequate scientific evidence. Their interpretation of the scientific literature perpetuates this fallacy. The result is more people unable to lose weight successfully.

My advice is extremely different. I recognize that raw, uncooked vegetables and fruits offer the most powerful protection against disease and I encourage my patients to eat huge salads and at least four fresh fruits per day. Diets with little raw foods are not ideal. As the amount of raw fruits and vegetables are increased in a person's diet, weight loss and blood pressure are lowered effortlessly.[30]

Additionally, raw foods contain enzymes, some of which can survive the digestive process in the stomach and pass into the small intestines. These heat-sensitive elements may offer significant nutritional advantages to protect against disease, according to investigators from the Department of Biochemistry at Wright State University School of Medicine.[31] These researchers concluded that "most foods undergo a decrease in nutritive value in addition to the well-known loss of vitamins when cooked and/or processed." Most vitamins are heat-sensitive, for example 20–60 percent of vitamin C is lost, depending on the cooking method.[32] Thirty to forty percent of minerals are lost in cooking vegetables as well.[33] Consuming a significant quantity of raw foods is essential for superior health.

For the best results, your diet should contain a huge amount of raw foods, a large amount of the less calorically dense cooked vegetation, and a lesser amount of the more calorically rich cooked starchy vegetables and grains. Cooking your food in oil will make your diet less effective and you will not lose weight as easily. You may not even lose any weight at all.

Vigilante and Flynn tested their diet on 120 people, and the average person lost eight pounds in eight weeks. In the same amount of time on my diet, you will lose at least three times that, if you have that much extra weight to lose. Keep in mind, weight loss slows down over time. Most people starting almost any diet after eating haphazardly lose some weight initially. It is easy to drop a few pounds by merely counting calories, but many overweight individuals with a strong genetic tendency to obesity and slow metabolism who need to lose lots of weight may lose very little or none at all. Some may lose an initial five to fifteen pounds, but then when further weight loss becomes even more difficult, they give up.

Another problem with Mediterranean diets is the preponderance of pasta and Italian bread, which not only causes difficulty with weight control but is also an important factor in increasing colon cancer risk in populations with this eating style.[34]

For the very overweight individual, this Mediterranean diet, like other conventional weight-loss programs, is neither restrictive enough nor filling enough to achieve the results desired. Because olive oil adds so many extra calories to their diet, the dieters still have to carefully count calories and eat tiny portions. All those calories supplied by olive oil, almost one-third of the total caloric intake, make the diet significantly lower in nutrients and fiber.

You can always lose weight by exercising more, and I am all for it. However, many very overweight patients are too ill and too heavy to exercise much. As a former athlete, and today as a physician, I am an exercise nut and a fanatic about recommending exercise to my patients, but many patients cannot comply with a substantial exercise program until they are in better health or lose some more weight first. So many people need a diet that will drop weight effectively, *even if they can't do lots of exercise.*

I have tested my recommendation on more than two thousand patients. The average patient loses the most weight in the first four to six weeks, with the average being about twenty pounds. The weight loss continues nicely — those following this program continue to lose about ten pounds the second month and about a pound and a half per week thereafter. The weight loss continues at this comparatively quick rate until they reach their ideal weight.

The bottom line about healthy fats is that raw nuts and seeds, avocados, and unsalted olives (if you can find them) contain healthy fats. However, you should consume a limited amount of these foods, especially if you wish to lose weight. Also remember that oil, including olive oil, does not contain the nutrients and phytonutrients that were in the original olive. The oil has little nutrients (except a little vitamin E) and a negligible amount of phytochemical compounds. If you eat the quantities of oil permitted on the typical Mediterranean diet, where all the vegetables are cooked in oil, you will have difficulty taking off the weight you need to lose.

You can add a little bit of olive oil to your diet if you are thin and exercise a lot. However, the more oil you add, the more you are lowering the nutrient-per-calorie density of your diet — and that is not your objective, as it does not promote health.

The "Magic" of Fiber — A Critical Nutrient

When we think of fiber, we usually think of bran or Metamucil, something that we take to prevent constipation and that tastes like cardboard. Change that thinking. Fiber is a vital nutrient, essential to human health. Unfortunately, the American diet is dangerously deficient in fiber, a deficiency that leads to many health problems (for example, hemorrhoids, constipation, varicose veins, and diabetes) and is a major cause of cancer. As you can see, if you get fiber naturally in your diet from great-tasting food, you get much more than just constipation relief.

When you eat mostly natural plant foods, such as fruits, vegetables, and beans, you get large amounts of various types of fiber. These foods are rich in complex carbohydrates and both insoluble and water-soluble fibers. The fibers slow down glucose absorption and control the rate of digestion. Plant fibers have complex physiological effects in the digestive tract that offer a variety of benefits, such as lowering cholesterol.[35]

Because of fiber, and because precious food components haven't been lost through processing, natural plant foods fill you up and do not cause abnormal physiological cravings or hormonal imbalances.

HOW YOUR BODY BENEFITS
FROM THE FIBER FOUND IN PLANT FOODS

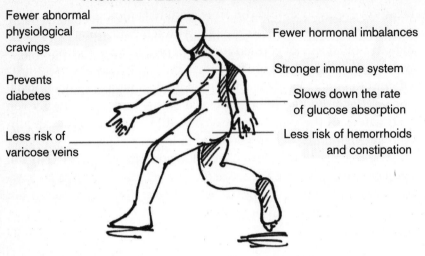

Fewer abnormal physiological cravings

Prevents diabetes

Less risk of varicose veins

Fewer hormonal imbalances

Stronger immune system

Slows down the rate of glucose absorption

Less risk of hemorrhoids and constipation

Confusion in the Marketplace over the Role of Fiber

Some people are so confused that they do not know what to believe anymore. For example, two recent studies about fiber received sensational coverage by the media after appearing in the April 20, 2000, *New England Journal of Medicine*.[36] Newspapers proclaimed the bold headlines HIGH-FIBER DIET DOES NOT PROTECT AGAINST COLON CANCER. No wonder our population is so confused by conflicting messages about nutrition. Some people have actually given up trying to eat healthfully because one day they hear one claim and the next week they hear the opposite. There's a lesson to be learned here: Don't get your health advice from the media.

I am bringing up this issue so you realize not to jump to conclusions on the basis of one study or one news report. You can see how research information is often (mis)reported in the news. I have reviewed more than two thousand nutritional research papers in preparation for this book and many more in prior years, and there is not much conflicting evidence. As in a trial, the evidence has become overwhelming and irrefutable — high-fiber foods offer significant protection against both cancer (including colon cancer) and heart disease. I didn't say *fiber*; I said high-fiber *foods*. We can't just add a high-fiber candy bar or sprinkle a little Metamucil on our doughnut and french fries and expect to reap the benefits of eating high-fiber foods, yet this is practically what the first study did.

The studies mentioned above did *not* show that a diet high in fresh fruits, vegetables, beans, whole grains, and raw nuts and seeds does not protect against colon cancer. It has already been adequately demonstrated in hundreds of observational studies that such a diet *does* offer such protection from cancer at multiple sites, including the colon.

The first study merely added a fiber supplement to the diet. I wouldn't expect adding a 13.5-gram fiber supplement to the disease-causing American diet to do anything. It is surprising that this study was actually conducted. Obviously, adding supplemental fiber does not capture the essence of a diet rich in these protective plant foods.

The second study compared controls against a group of people who were counseled on improving their diet. The participants continued to follow their usual (disease-causing) diet and made only a moderate dietary change — a slight reduction in fat intake, with a modest increase in fruits and vegetables for four years. The number of colorectal adenomas four years later was similar. Colorectal adenomas are not colon cancer; they are benign polyps. Only a very small percentage of these polyps ever advance to become colon cancer, and the clinical significance of small benign adenomas is not clear. In any case, it is a huge leap to claim that a diet high in fruits and vegetables does not protect against cancer. This study did not even attempt to address colon cancer, just benign polyps that rarely progress to cancer.

In both studies, even the groups supposedly consuming a high-fiber intake were on a low-fiber diet by my standards. The group consuming the most fiber only ate 25 grams of fiber a day. The high-fiber intake is merely a marker of many anti-cancer properties of natural foods, especially phytochemicals. The diet plan I recommend is not based on any one study, but on more than two thousand studies and the results I've seen with thousands of my own patients. Following this plan, you will consume between 50 and 100 grams of fiber (from real food, not supplements) per day.

In an editorial, published in the same issue of the *New England Journal of Medicine*, Tim Byers, M.D., M.P.H., basically agreed, stating, "Observational studies around the world continue to find that the risk of colorectal cancer is lower among populations with high intakes of fruits and vegetables and that the risk changes on adoption of a different diet."[37] He further explained that the three- or four-year period assessed by these trials is too brief and cannot assess the effects of long-term dietary patterns that have already been shown to protect against colorectal cancer.

The reality is that healthy, nutritious foods are also very rich in fiber and that those foods associated with disease risk are generally fiber-deficient. Meat and dairy products do not contain any fiber, and foods made from refined grains (such as white bread, white rice, and pasta) have had their fiber removed. Clearly, we must substantially reduce our consumption of these fiber-deficient foods if we expect to lose weight *and* live a long, healthy life.

Fiber intake from food is a good marker of disease risk. The amount of fiber consumed may better predict weight gain, insulin levels, and other cardiovascular risk factors than does the amount of total fat consumed, according to recent studies reported in the October 27, 1999, issue of the *Journal of the American Medical Association*.[38] Again, data show that removing the fiber from food is extremely dangerous.

People who consume the most high-fiber foods are the healthiest, as determined by better waist measurements, lower insulin levels, and other markers of disease risk. Indeed, this is one of the key themes of this book — for anyone to consider his or her diet healthy, it must be predominantly composed of high-fiber, natural foods.

It is not the fiber extracted from the plant package that has miraculous health properties. It is the entire plant package considered as a whole, containing nature's anti-cancer nutrients as well as being rich in fiber.

Phytochemicals:
Nature's "Magic" Pills

There are clear reasons why heart attacks and cancer prevail as our number one and number two killers. Let's examine them.

The American Diet: Designed for Disease

Americans currently consume about 42 percent of their calories from fiberless animal foods and another 51 percent from highly processed refined carbohydrates and extracted oils.[1]

Almost half of all vegetables consumed are potatoes, and half of

U.S. FOOD CONSUMPTION BY CALORIES

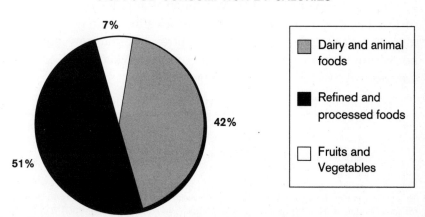

7%

51%

42%

Dairy and animal foods

Refined and processed foods

Fruits and Vegetables

100 CALORIES OF	BAKED POTATO	BAKED SWEET POTATO	FROZEN SPINACH
Protein	2.1 gm	1.7 gm	12.2 gm
Fiber	1.6 gm	3.0 gm	17.36 gm
Calcium	5.4 mg	28 mg	462 mg
Iron	.38 mg	.45 mg	8.5 mg
Magnesium	27 mg	20 mg	242 mg
Zinc	.31 mg	.29 mg	1.8 mg
Selenium	.32 mcg	.7 mcg	5.8 mcg
Vitamin C	13.8 mg	24 mg	100 mg
Vitamin E	.43 mg	.28 mg	4.0 mg
Vitamin A	near zero	21,822 IU	32,324 IU
Volume	one cup	½ cup	three cups

the potatoes consumed are in the form of fries or chips. Furthermore, potatoes are one of the least nutritious vegetables.

The same studies that show the anti-cancer effects of green leafy vegetables and fruits and beans suggest that potato-heavy diets are not healthy and show a positive association with colon cancer.[2] Possibly this association exists because of the way potatoes are consumed — fried or with butter or other dangerous fats. Excluding potatoes, Americans consume a mere 5 percent of their calories from fruits, vegetables, and legumes.

Cheese consumption increased 140 percent between 1970 and 1996, and cheese is the primary source of saturated fat in our diet.[3] Convenience foods have probably been the driving force behind this increase. In fact, two-thirds of our nation's cheese production is for commercially prepared foods, such as pizza, tacos, nachos, fast-food meals, spreads, sauces, and packaged snacks.

From convenience foods to fast-food restaurants, our fast-paced society has divorced itself from healthful eating. It may be convenient to pick up soda, burgers, fries, or pizza, but that convenience is not without its price; the result is that we are sicker than ever, and our medical costs are skyrocketing out of control.

THE MAJOR KILLERS OF AMERICANS

	PERCENT OF ALL DEATHS
Heart attacks, diabetes, and strokes	52
All cancers	38

Source: World Health Organization. 1999. *World Health Statistics Annual*. WHO Statistical Information System (WHOSIS) Table 1: Number of deaths and death rates, ages 55–75 inclusive.

MAJOR FOODS: U.S. PER CAPITA FOOD SUPPLY, 1996

	WEIGHT IN POUNDS	PERCENTAGE BY WEIGHT	PERCENTAGE BY CALORIES
Meats	192	8	12
Eggs	236	9	7
Dairy	576	23	23
Fruits and vegetables	**543**	**22**	**5**
White potatoes	153	6	2
Refined oils	67	3	11
Sweeteners	153	6	13
White flour	198	8	9
Other processed foods	378	15	18

Source: USDA Agriculture Fact Book 98: Chapter 1-A

I insist that our low consumption of unrefined plant foods is largely responsible for our dismal mortality statistics. Most of us perish prematurely as a result of our dietary folly.

Populations with low death rates from the major killer diseases — populations that almost never have overweight members — consume more than 75 percent of their calories from unrefined plant

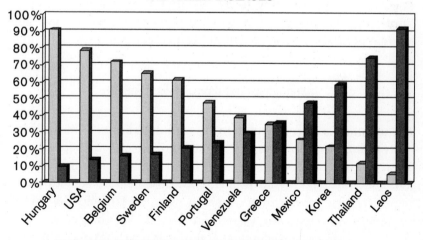

UNREFINED PLANT FOOD CONSUMPTION VS.
THE KILLER DISEASES[4]

☐ Percentage of deaths from heart disease and cancer
■ Percentage of calories from unrefined plant foods

substances. This is at least ten times more than what the average American consumes.

So why is this the case? Why do we see so much heart disease and cancer in wealthier societies? Is it animal products that are so deadly? Are refined carbohydrates solely to blame? Or is it just that plant foods are so miraculously wonderful at protecting us against disease? Or is it all three?

Obviously, the economically poorer regions of the world have significant public health problems: poor sanitation; poverty and malnutrition; high infant-mortality rates; high rates of infectious disease, including AIDS, parasitic diseases, and even tuberculosis. However, in spite of all these things that cause an early death, if we look at the cause-of-death statistics from the World Health Organization (WHO) for people between the ages of fifty-five and seventy-five, we find very few cancer deaths and heart attack deaths in those poor societies.

The diseases of poverty are mostly infectious diseases and are found in areas of the world with compromised nutrition. Heart attacks and the most common cancers (breast, colon, prostate) are found in rich societies where nutritional extravagance is the rule. Nowhere in the world today can we find a society that combines economic wealth with a high intake and variety of unrefined plant foods.

Can you imagine the health potential of a society that would be able to enjoy excellent sanitation, emergency medical care, refrigeration, clean water, flush toilets, and availability of fresh produce year-round and yet avoid nutritional ignorance and nutritional extravagance? We have this opportunity today, an unprecedented opportunity in human history, the opportunity to live a long and healthy life without the fear of disease. This opportunity can be yours.

Nutritional Powerhouses: Plant Foods

Natural plant foods, though usually carbohydrate-rich, also contain protein and fats. On average, 25 percent of the calories in vegetables are from protein. Romaine lettuce, for example, is rich in both protein and essential fatty acids, giving us those healthy fats our bodies require. For more information about essential fats and the protein content of vegetables and various other foods, see chapter six.

Many large-scale epidemiological studies have shown conclusively that certain plant foods play a role in protecting the body against diseases that affect — and *kill* — at least 500,000 Americans each year.

There is no longer any question about the importance of fruits and vegetables in our diet. The greater the quantity and assortment of fruits and vegetables consumed, the lower the incidence of heart attacks, strokes, and cancer.[5] There is still some controversy about which foods cause which cancers and whether certain types of fat are the culprits with certain cancers, but there's one thing we know for sure: raw vegetables and fresh fruits have powerful anti-cancer agents. Studies have repeatedly shown the correlation between consumption of these foods and a lower incidence of various cancers, including those of the breast, colon, rectum, lung, stomach, prostate, and pancreas.[6] This means that your risk of cancer decreases with an increased intake of fruits and vegetables, and the earlier in life you start eating large amounts of these foods, the more protection you get.

Humans are genetically adapted to expect a high intake of natural and unprocessed plant-derived substances. Cancer is a disease of *maladaptation*. It results primarily from a body's lacking critical substances found in different types of vegetation, many of which are still undiscovered, that are metabolically necessary for normal protective function. Natural foods unadulterated by man are highly complex — so complex that the exact structure and the majority of compounds they contain are not precisely known. A tomato, for example, contains more than ten thousand different phytochemicals.

It may never be possible to extract the precise symphony of nutrients found in vegetation and place it in a pill. Isolated nutrients extracted from food may never offer the same level of disease-protective effects of whole natural foods, as nature "designed" them. Fruits and vegetables contain a variety of nutrients, which work in subtle synergies, and many of these nutrients cannot be isolated or extracted. Phytochemicals from a variety of plant foods work together to become much more potent at detoxifying carcinogens and protecting against cancer than when taken individually as isolated compounds.

Authorities Join the Unrefined Plant Food Bandwagon

After years of examining the accumulating evidence, eight top health organizations joined forces and agreed to encourage Americans to eat more unrefined plant food and less food from animal sources, as revealed in the new dietary guidelines published in the July 27, 1999, *Journal of the American Heart Association*. These authorities are the Nutrition Committee of the American Heart Association, the American Cancer Society, the American Academy of Pediatrics, the Council on Cardiovascular Disease in the Young, the Council on Epidemiology and Prevention, the American Dietetic Association, the Division of Nutrition Research of the National Institutes of Health, and the American Society for Clinical Nutrition.

Their unified guidelines are a giant step in the right direction. Their aim is to offer protection against the major chronic diseases in America, including heart disease and cancer. "The emphasis is on eating a variety of foods, mostly fruits and vegetables, with very little simple sugar or high-fat foods, especially animal foods," said Abby Bloch, Ph.D., R.D., chair of the American Cancer Society. Based on a culmination of years of research, these health experts' conclusion was that animal-source foods, with their high levels of saturated fat, are one of the leading causes of heart disease, cancer, strokes, diabetes, obesity, etc. — all the major chronic diseases that cost 1.4 million Americans their lives each year (more than two-thirds of all deaths in the United States).

The Phytochemical Revolution

We are on the verge of a revolution. Substances newly discovered in broccoli and cabbage sprouts sweep toxins out of cells. Substances found in nuts and beans prevent damage to our cells' DNA. Other compounds in beets, peppers, and tomatoes fight cancerous changes in cells. Oranges and apples protect our blood vessels from damage that could lead to heart disease. Nature's chemoprotective army is alert and ready to remove our enemies and shield us from harm.

Hardly a day goes by when some new study doesn't proclaim the health-giving properties of fruits, vegetables, and beans. Unprocessed plant foods contain thousands of compounds, most of which have not yet been discovered, that are essential for maintaining health and maximizing genetic potential. Welcome to the phytochemical revolution.

Phytochemicals, or plant-derived chemicals, occur naturally in plants (*phyto* means "plant"). These nutrients, which scientists are just starting to discover and name, have tremendously beneficial effects on human physiology. The effects of our not consuming sufficient amounts of them are even more astounding — premature death from cancer and atherosclerosis.

Eating a wide variety of raw and conservatively cooked plant foods (such as steamed vegetables) is the only way we can ensure that we get a sufficient amount of these essential health-supporting elements. Taking vitamin and mineral supplements or adding some vitamins to processed foods will not prevent the diseases associated with eating a diet containing a low percentage of calories from whole natural foods.

Scientists cannot formulate into pills nutrients that have not yet been discovered! If the pills did contain sufficient amounts of all the phytonutrients and other essential substances, we would have to swallow a soup bowl full of pills and powders. To date, researchers have discovered more than ten thousand phytochemicals. No supplement can contain a sufficient amount. Thankfully, you can get all these nutrients *today* by eating a wide variety of plant-based foods.

Please bear in mind that I am not against nutritional supplements. In fact, I recommend various supplements to many of my patients with various health problems, and a high-quality multivitamin/multimineral to almost everyone.

I do *not* recommend that most people consume supplements containing vitamin A, isolated beta-carotene, or iron, as there are risks associated with excess consumption of these nutrients. The point to be emphasized is that supplements alone cannot offer optimal protection against disease and that you cannot make an unhealthy diet into a healthy one by consuming supplements.

You Cannot Buy Your Health in a Bottle — You Must Earn It!

When your nutrient intake is out of balance, health problems may result. For example, beta-carotene has been touted as a powerful antioxidant and anti-cancer vitamin. However, in recent years we have discovered that beta-carotene is only one of about five hundred carotenoids. Scientists are finding that taking beta-carotene supplements is not without risk, and supplements are certainly a poor substitute for the real thing — the assortment of various carotenoid compounds found in plants.

The reason researchers believed beta-carotene had such a powerful anti-cancer effect was that populations with high levels of beta-carotene in their bloodstream had exceedingly low rates of cancer. More recently we found out that these people were protected against cancer because of *hundreds* of carotenoids and phytochemicals in the fruits and vegetables they were consuming. It wasn't that beta-carotene was responsible for the low incidence of cancer; it merely served as a flag for those populations with a high fruit and vegetable intake. Unfortunately, many scientists confused the flag for the ship.

Recently, large-scale studies have shown that taking beta-carotene (or vitamin A) in supplemental form may not be such a great idea.[7]

In Finnish trials, taking beta-carotene supplements failed to prevent lung cancer and actually increased its incidence.[8] This study was halted when the researchers discovered that the death rate from lung cancer was 28 percent higher among participants who had taken the high amounts of beta-carotene and vitamin A. Furthermore, the death rate from heart disease was 17 percent higher for those that had taken the supplements than for those just given a placebo.[9]

Another recent study showed a similar correlation between beta-carotene supplementation and increased occurrence of prostate cancer. At this point, as a result of these European studies, as well as similar studies conducted here in the United States,[10] articles in the *Journal of the National Cancer Institute*, the *Lancet*, and the *New England Journal of Medicine* all advise us to avoid taking beta-carotene supplements.[11]

We can learn a lesson from this research. A high intake of isolated beta-carotene may impair the absorption of other carotenoids. Taking beta-carotene or vitamin A may hinder carotenoid anti-cancer activity from zeaxanthin, alpha-carotene, lycopene, lutein, and many other crucial plant-derived carotenoids. When my patients ask what multivitamin they should use, I tell them I'd prefer they take a high-quality multi that does not contain vitamin A or plain beta-carotene. The supplement should contain mixed plant-derived carotenoids, not isolated beta-carotene. (See recommended products at my website, www.drfuhrman.com.)

A high intake of just one nutrient when nature has combined it with many others may make things worse, not better. We humans, especially physicians, are notorious for interfering with nature, thinking we know better. Sometimes we do — all too often we don't. Only later, when it is often too late, do we realize that in fact we have made things worse.

While it still may take decades longer to understand how whole foods promote health, we must accept the fact that the foods found in nature are ideally suited to the biological needs of the species. "The most compelling evidence of the last decade has indicated the importance of protective factors, largely unidentified, in fruits and vegetables," said Walter C. Willett, M.D., Ph.D., chairman of the Department of Nutrition at Harvard's School of Public Health and a speaker at the American Association for Cancer Research.[12]

In other words, a diet in which fruits, vegetables, and other natural plant foods supply the vast majority of calories affords us powerful protection against disease. Phytochemicals in their natural state are potent cancer inhibitors. For example, a recent study published in the *Journal of the National Cancer Institute* reported that men who ate three or more servings of cruciferous vegetables a week had a 41 percent reduced risk of prostate cancer compared with men who ate less than one serving a week.[13] Cruciferous vegetables, such as broccoli and cabbage, are high in isothiocyanates, which activate enzymes present in all cells that detoxify carcinogens. Eating a variety of other vegetation lowered risk even further. Green vegetables, onions, and leeks also contain organosulfur phytonutrients that inhibit abnormal cellular changes that eventually lead to cancer. A wide variety of wholesome plant-based foods is the only real anti-cancer strategy.

SOME ANTI-CANCEROUS SUBSTANCES IN NATURAL PLANT FOOD

Allium compounds	Flavonoids	Phenolic acids
Allyl sulfides	Glucosinolates	Phytoesterols
Anthocyanins	Indoles	Polyacetylenes
Caffeic acid	Isoflavones	Polyphenols
Catechins	Isothiocyanates	Protease inhibitors
Coumarins	Lignans	Saponins
Dithiolthiones	Liminoids	Sulphorophane
Ellagic acid	Pectins	Sterols
Ferulic acid	Perillyl alcohol	Terpenes

The list above is only a small sample of beneficial compounds, and more are being discovered daily. Cancer-prevention studies attempting to dissect the precise ingredients or combination of ingredients in fruits and vegetables are ongoing; but these studies, like the many others before them, are likely to be a huge waste of resources. There are simply too many protective factors that work synergistically to expect significant benefit from taking a few isolated substances. These beneficial compounds have overlapping and complementary mechanisms of action. They inhibit cellular aging, induce detoxification enzymes, bind carcinogens in the digestive tract, and fuel cellular repair mechanisms.[14]

FIVE WAYS PHYTOCHEMICALS PREVENT CANCER

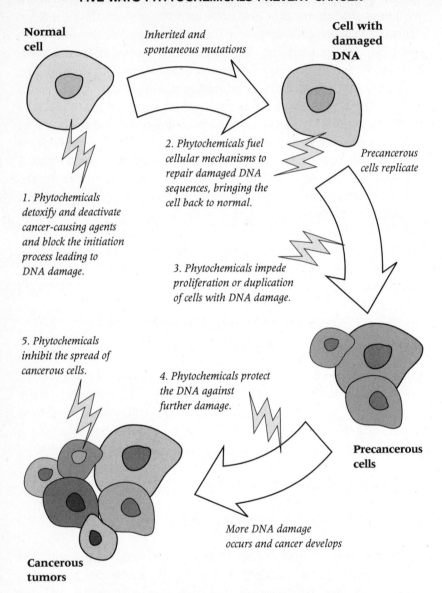

Normal cell

Inherited and spontaneous mutations

Cell with damaged DNA

2. Phytochemicals fuel cellular mechanisms to repair damaged DNA sequences, bringing the cell back to normal.

Precancerous cells replicate

1. Phytochemicals detoxify and deactivate cancer-causing agents and block the initiation process leading to DNA damage.

3. Phytochemicals impede proliferation or duplication of cells with DNA damage.

5. Phytochemicals inhibit the spread of cancerous cells.

4. Phytochemicals protect the DNA against further damage.

Precancerous cells

More DNA damage occurs and cancer develops

Cancerous tumors

Cancer Is Much More Preventable than Treatable

The process of carcinogenesis entails an accumulation of mutations or damage to our DNA (the cellular blueprint) over the course of twenty to forty years. You must start protecting yourself today, not after you find out you have cancer. Cancer is much more preventable than treatable. Instead, many try to dig a well after their house is on fire.

The process of cellular disintegration is extremely prolonged, and we know that many pre-neoplastic lesions (abnormal, but not yet cancer) disappear spontaneously.[15] Studies on both humans and animals have shown that plant-derived nutrients are able to prevent the occurrence of, and even reverse, DNA damage that may later result in cancer.[16] Fortunately, we have the potential to suppress the progression of cancer in its early stages by how we choose to eat. The ability to remove and fix these partially damaged cells is proportional to their exposure to phytochemicals.

When we consume a sufficient variety and quantity of phytochemical substances to maximally arm our immune defenses against cancer, we afford ourselves the ability to repair DNA damage, detoxify cancer-causing agents, and resist disease in general. These same substances also activate other immune-enhancing mechanisms that improve our defenses against viruses and bacteria, making our body disease-resistant in general.

Green Plant Foods vs. Animal Foods

So now you know that it is not merely excess fat that causes disease. It is not merely eating empty-calorie food that causes disease. And it is not merely the high consumption of animal foods such as dairy, meat, chicken, and fish that leads to premature death in America. These factors are important, but most crucial is what we are missing in our diets by not eating enough produce. Let's take a look at some more of the reasons why plant foods are so protective and essential for human health.

To illustrate the powerful nutrient density of green vegetables, let us compare the nutrient density of steak with the nutrient density of broccoli and other greens.

Now, which food has more protein — broccoli or steak? You were wrong if you thought steak.

Steak only has 5.4 grams of protein per 100 calories and broccoli has 11.2 grams, *almost twice as much*.

Keep in mind that most of the calories in meat come from fat; green vegetables are mostly protein (all calories must come from fat, carbohydrate, or protein).

NUTRIENTS PRESENT IN 100-CALORIE PORTIONS OF SELECTED FOODS

	BROCCOLI	SIRLOIN	ROMAINE LETTUCE	KALE
Protein	11.2 g	5.4 g	11.6 g	9.46 g
Calcium	182 mg	2.4 mg	257 mg	455 mg
Iron	2.2 mg	.7 mg	7.9 mg	3.1 mg
Magnesium	71.4 mg	5 mg	43 mg	59 mg
Potassium	643 mg	88 mg	2,071 mg	1,059 mg
Fiber	10.7 g	0	12 g	6.7 g
Phytochemicals	very high	0	very high	very high
Antioxidants	very high	0	very high	very high
Folate	107 mcg	3 mcg	971 mcg	47 mcg
B_2	.29 mg	.04 mg	.71 mg	.38 mg
Niacin	1.64 mg	1.1 mg	3.6 mg	2.2 mg
Zinc	1.1 mg	1.2 mg	1.8 mg	.59 mg
Vitamin C	143 mg	0	171 mg	83 mg
Vitamin A	6,757 IU	24 IU	18,571 IU	21,159 IU
Vitamin E	5 mg	0	3.2 mg	1 mg
Cholesterol	0	55 mg	0	0
Saturated fat	0	1.7 gm	0	0
Weight	357 g	24 g	714 g	333 g
	(12.6 oz)	(.84 oz)	(25.1 oz)	(11.7 oz)

Source: Adams, C. 1986. *Handbook of the Nutritional Value of Foods in Common Units* (New York: Dover Publications).

Popeye Was Right — Greens Pack a Powerful Punch

The biggest animals — elephants, gorillas, rhinoceroses, hippopotamuses, and giraffes — all eat predominantly green vegetation. How did they get the protein to get so big? Obviously, greens pack a powerful protein punch. In fact, all protein on the planet was formed from the effect of sunlight on green plants. The cow didn't eat another cow to form the protein in its muscles, which we call steak. The protein wasn't formed out of thin air — the cow ate grass. Not that protein is such a big deal or some special nutrient to be held in high esteem. I am making this point because most people think animal products are necessary for a diet to include adequate protein. I am merely illustrating how easy it is to consume more than enough protein while at the same time avoiding risky, cancer-promoting substances such as saturated fat. Consuming more plant protein is also the key to achieving safe and successful weight loss.

Now, which has more vitamin E or vitamin C — broccoli or steak? I'm sure you are aware that steak has no vitamin C or vitamin E. It is also almost totally lacking in fiber, folate, vitamin A, beta-carotene, lutein, lycopene, vitamin K, flavonoids, and thousands of other protective phytochemicals. Meat does have certain vitamins and minerals, but even when we consider the nutrients that meat does contain, broccoli has lots more of them. For many important nutrients, broccoli has more than ten times as much as steak. The only exception is vitamin B_{12}, which is not found in plant fare.

When you consider the fiber, phytochemicals, and other essential nutrients, green vegetables win the award for being the most nutrient-dense of all foods. We will give greens a score of 100 and judge all other foods against this criterion.

The Secret of Extreme Longevity

Interestingly, there is one food that scientific research has shown has a strong positive association with increased longevity in humans. So which food do you think that is?

The answer is raw, leafy greens, normally referred to as salad.[17] Leafy greens such as romaine lettuce, kale, collards, Swiss chard, and spinach are the most nutrient-dense of all foods.

Most vegetables contain more nutrients per calorie than any other food and are rich in all necessary amino acids. For example, romaine lettuce, which gets 18 percent of its calories from fat and almost 50 percent of its calories from protein, is a rich powerhouse with hundreds of cancer-fighting phytonutrients that protect us from a variety of threatening illnesses. Being healthy and owning a disease-resistant body is not luck; it is earned.

In a review of 206 human-population studies, raw vegetable consumption showed the strongest protective effect against cancer of any beneficial food.[18] However, less than one in a hundred Americans consumes enough calories from vegetation to ensure this defense.

I tell my patients to put a big sign on their refrigerator that says THE SALAD IS THE MAIN DISH.

The word *salad* here means any *vegetable* eaten raw or uncooked, e.g., a bowl of cold pasta in olive oil with a token vegetable is *not* a salad. I encourage my patients to eat two *huge* salads a day, with the goal of consuming an entire head of romaine or other green lettuce daily. I suggest that you go and make the sign and tape it to your fridge now — and then come back. If you plan on doing it later, you may forget. If you learn but one practical habit from this book, let it be this one.

Green Salad Is Less than 100 Calories per Pound

Did you notice that 100 calories of broccoli is about ten ounces of food, and 100 calories of ground sirloin is less than one ounce of food? With green vegetables you can get filled up, even stuffed, yet you will not be consuming excess calories. Animal products, on the other hand, are calorie-dense and relatively low in nutrients, especially the crucial anti-cancer nutrients.

What would happen if you attempted to eat like a mountain gorilla, which eats about 80 percent of its diet from green leaves and about 15 percent from fruit? Assuming you are a female, who needs about 1,500 calories a day, if you attempted to get 1,200 of those calories from greens, you would need to eat over fifteen pounds of greens. That is quite a big salad! Since your stomach can only hold about one liter of food (or a little over a quart), you would have a problem fitting it all in.

You would surely get lots of protein from this gorilla diet. In fact, with just five pounds of greens you would exceed the RDA for protein and would get loads of other important nutrients. The problem with this gorilla diet is that you would develop a *calorie deficiency*. You would become too thin. Believe it or not, I do not expect you to eat exactly like a gorilla. However, the message to take home is that the more of these healthy green vegetables (both raw and cooked) you eat, the healthier you will be and the thinner you will become.

Now let's contrast this silly and extreme gorilla example to another silly and extreme way of eating, the American diet.

If you attempt to follow the perverted diet that most Americans eat, or even if you follow the precise recommendations of the USDA's pyramid — six to eleven servings of bread, rice, and pasta (consumed as 98 percent refined grains by Americans) with four to six servings of dairy, meat, poultry, or fish — you would be eating a diet rich in calories but extremely low in nutrients, antioxidants, phytochemicals, and vitamins. You would be overfed and malnourished, the precise nutritional profile that causes heart disease and cancer.

Weighing Food and Trying to Eat Smaller Portions Is Futile

Earlier I compared 100 calories of greens with 100 calories of meat. I did not contrast them by weight or by portion size, as is more customary.

I compared equal caloric portions because it is meaningless to compare foods by weight or portion size. Let me provide an example to explain why this is the case. Take one teaspoon of melted butter, which gets 100 percent of its calories from fat. If I take that teaspoon of butter and mix it in a glass of hot water, I can now say that it is 98 percent fat-free, by weight. One hundred percent of its calories are still from fat. It didn't matter how much water or weight was added, did it?

In fact, if a food's weight were important, it would be easy to lose weight, we would just have to drink more water. The water would trigger the weight receptors in the digestive tract and our appetite would diminish. Unfortunately, this is not the way our body's appestat — the brain center in the hypothalamus that controls food intake — is controlled. As explained in chapter one, bulk, calories, and nutrient fulfillment, not the weight of the food, turn off our appestat. Since the foods Americans consume are so calorie-rich, we have all been trying to diet by eating small portions of low-nutrient foods. We not only have to suffer hunger but also wind up with perverted cravings because we are nutrient-deficient to boot.

We must consume a certain level of calories daily to feel satisfied. So now I ask you to completely rethink what you consider a typical portion size. To achieve superior health and a permanently thin physique, you should eat large portions of green foods. When considering any green plant food, remember to make the portion size huge by conventional standards. Eating large portions of these super-healthy foods is the key to your success.

The Nutrient-Weight Conflabulation

Nutrient-weight ratios hide how nutrient-deficient processed food is and make animal-source food not look so fatty. Could this be why the food industry and the USDA chose this method? Could it be a conspiracy to have consumers not realize what they are really eating?

For example, a Burger King bacon double cheeseburger is clearly not a low-fat food. If we calculate its percentage of fat by weight and include the ketchup and the bun, we can accurately state that it is only 18 percent fat (over 80 percent fat-free). However, as a percentage of calories it is 54 percent fat, and the hamburger patty alone is 68 percent fat. McDonald's McLean burger was advertised a few years back as 91 percent fat-free using the same numbers trick, when in fact 49 percent of its calories came from fat.

Likewise, so-called low-fat 2 percent milk is not really 2 percent fat. Thirty-five percent of its calories come from fat. They can call it 98 percent fat-free (by weight) only because of its water content. Low-fat milk is not a low-fat product at all, and neither are low-fat cheeses and other low-fat animal foods when you recalculate their fat on a per calorie percentage basis. This is just a sad trick played on Americans. Incidentally, 49 percent of the calories in whole milk come from fat.

The U.S. Department of Meat, Milk, and Cheese

Using weight instead of calories in nutrient-analysis tables has evolved into a ploy to hide how nutritionally unsound many foods are. The role of the U.S. Department of Agriculture (USDA) was originally to promote the products of the animal agriculture industry.[19] Over fifty years ago, the USDA began promoting the so-called four basic food groups, with meat and dairy products in the number one and two spots on the list. Financed by the meat and dairy industry and backed by nutritional scientists on the payroll of the meat and dairy industry, this promotion ignored science.[20]

This program could be more accurately labeled "the four food myths." It was taught in every classroom in America, with posters

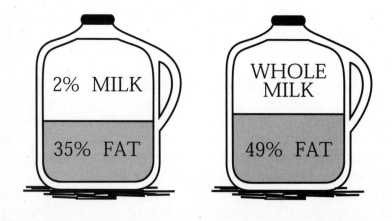

advocating a diet loaded with animal protein, fat, and cholesterol. The results of this fraudulent program were dramatic — in more ways than one. Americans began eating more and more animal foods. The campaign sparked the beginning of the fastest-growing cancer epidemic in history and heart attack rates soared to previously unheard-of levels!

For years and years the USDA resisted lowering cholesterol and dietary fat recommendations in spite of the irrefutable evidence that Americans were committing suicide with food. Heavy political pressure, lobbyists, and money blocked the path to change.[21]

Promoting nutrient analysis of foods by weight instead of by calorie became a great way to keep excess calories, cholesterol, and saturated fat in the diet — a terrific strategy to create a nation with an epidemic of obesity, heart disease, and cancer. Some foreign enemy out to destroy America could not have devised a more effective and insidious plot. How ironic that this was the program designed by our own government, promoted with our own tax dollars, and justified on the ground that it served the public interest.

With all the scientific data available today, including massive investigational studies on human health and diet, you would think that people would know which foods are best to eat and why — but most people are still confused about diet and nutrition. Why?

Part of the problem is that most of us are slow to make changes, especially when they involve personal habits and family traditions. Most people do not embrace change. They are more comfortable with familiarity and cling to long-held but incorrect information. In spite of a vast increase in nutritional information, much of it is contradictory and has led to only more confusion.

Our government spends over $20 billion on price supports that benefit the dairy, beef, and veal industries.[22] This money is given to farmers to artificially reduce the cost of crops used to feed cows, thereby helping to reduce the prices we pay for dairy foods, fowl, and meat. Fruits and vegetables grown primarily for human consumption are specifically excluded from USDA price supports.

Out of one pocket, we pay billions of our tax dollars to support the production of expensive, disease-causing foods. Out of the other pocket, we pay medical bills that are too high because our overweight population consumes too much of these rich, disease-causing foods. Our tax dollars are actually used to make our society sicker and keep our health insurance costs high.

A Food Pyramid that Will Turn You into a Mummy

USDA FOOD GUIDE PYRAMID

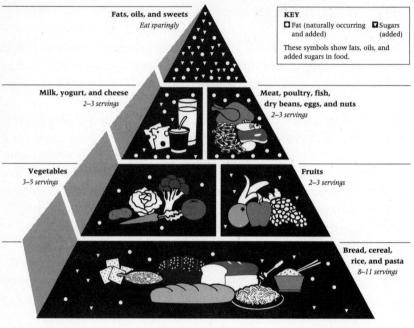

U.S. Department of Agriculture
U.S. Department of Health and Human Services

Since early childhood we have been bombarded with incorrect nutritional dietary advice, and unfortunately the scandal continues today. Even after decades of scientific research refuting its recommendations, the latest USDA recommendation — the Food Guide Pyramid — is only a slight improvement; it still reinforces the dietary errors that people have become accustomed to making.

The food pyramid includes a level of animal food consumption (four to six servings daily) that *causes* the diseases that kill us: heart attacks and cancer. It suggests we should consume a huge quantity of low-nutrient-content foods such as refined cereals, white bread, and pasta.

Foods are grouped in ways that don't make sense anymore. Meat, beans, and nuts are all in the same food group because they are considered protein-rich foods. However, while nuts and beans have been shown to reduce cholesterol levels and heart-disease risk, meat is linked to increased risk. The pyramid offers little help for those really wanting to reduce their health risks.

In light of all the scientific data available, the USDA's recommendations are a disgrace. Our government suggests that people consume five measly servings of fruits and vegetables daily (and even apple juice is considered a serving). The data is overwhelming and conclusive; this dietary recommendation does not allow for enough vegetation to afford people true protection against the killer diseases now epidemic in modern society. Two studies from Harvard Medical School actually put the USDA guidelines to the test in 51,000 men and 67,000 women, and both studies concluded that adherence to these guidelines had no effect on cancer risk.[23] Much higher levels of produce intake are required for significant protection. When intake is truly high, the protection afforded is striking.[24]

After many years of our population being advised to increase its consumption of produce, half of all Americans still don't eat three vegetable servings a day. That total even includes those heart-attack-causing foods that are fried in trans fats — french fries and potato chips. On any given day, no fruit whatsoever passes the lips of half of all Americans.

In 1998 the National Cancer Institute budgeted a million dollars to promote the virtues of fruits and vegetables. Compare that with McDonald's 500 million dollars spent on TV ads alone. The major cause of all diseases afflicting Americans today is a produce-deficient diet.

Based on an exhaustive look at research data from around the world over the past fifteen years, my recommendation is that your diet should contain over 90 percent of calories from unrefined plant foods. This high percentage of nutrient-dense plant foods in the diet allows us to predict freedom from cancer, heart attacks, diabetes, and excess body weight. Fruits, vegetables, and beans must be the base of your food pyramid; otherwise, you will be in a heap of trouble down the road.

The diseases that afflict, and eventually kill, almost all Americans can be avoided. You can live a high-quality, disease-free life and remain physically active and healthy. You can die peacefully and uneventfully at an old age, as nature intended.

To achieve the results in preventing and reversing disease, and attaining permanent healthy body weight, we must be concerned with the *nutritional quality* of our diet.

The picture is becoming crystal clear — the key to what will make you thin will also make you healthy. Once you learn to "eat to live," thinness and health will walk hand in hand, happily ever after.

The Dark Side of Animal Protein

One day we hear that a high-fat diet causes cancer, and the next day a study shows that those on low-fat diets do not have lower cancer rates. The public is so confused and fed up that they just eat anything, and the number of overweight people continues to grow.

How much do you know about nutrition?
True or false?

1. We need milk to get enough calcium to protect us against osteoporosis.
2. A diet high in protein is healthy.
3. The best source of protein is animal foods such as meat, chicken, eggs, fish, and dairy.
4. Plant foods do not have complete protein.
5. To get adequate protein from a plant-based diet, you should combine certain foods to make sure you receive a complete complement of the necessary amino acids at each meal.
6. We can protect ourselves against cancer by switching to low-fat animal foods such as chicken, fish, and skim milk and by omitting red meat.

Answers provided on next page

The China Project

Fortunately, evidence from a massive series of scientific investigations has shed some light on the confusion. The China-Cornell-Oxford Project (also known as the China Project) is the most comprehensive study on the connection between diet and disease in medical history. The *New York Times* called this investigation the "Grand Prix of all epidemiological studies" and "the most comprehensive large study ever undertaken of the relationship between diet and the risk of developing disease."[1]

Spearheaded by T. Colin Campbell, Ph.D., of Cornell University, this study has made discoveries that have turned the nutritional community upside down. To the surprise of many, the China Project has revealed many so-called nutritional facts as demonstrably false. For example, the answer to all the Nutrition Quiz questions above is false.

China was an ideal testing ground for this comprehensive project because the people in one area of China eat a certain diet and the people just a few hundred miles away may eat a completely different diet. Unlike in the West, where we all eat very similarly, rural China is a "living laboratory" for studying the complex relationship between diet and disease.[2]

The China Project was valid because it studied populations with a *full range of dietary possibilities:* from a completely plant-food diet to diets that included a significant amount of animal foods. Adding small quantities of a variable is how scientists can best detect the risk or value of a dietary practice. It's the same principle as comparing nonsmokers with those who smoke half a pack a day, to best observe the dangers of smoking. Comparing a fifty-cigarette per day habit with a sixty-cigarette per day habit may not reveal much more additional damage from those last ten cigarettes.

In China, people live their entire lives in the towns they were born in and rarely migrate, so the dietary effects that researchers looked at were present for the subjects' entire life. Furthermore, as a result of significant regional differences in the way people eat, there were dramatic differences in the prevalence of disease from region to region. Cardiovascular disease rates varied twentyfold from one place to another, and certain cancer rates varied by several hundredfold. In America, there is little difference in the way we eat; therefore, we do not see a hundredfold difference in cancer rates between one town and another.

Fascinating findings were made in this study. The data showed huge differences in disease rates based on the amount of plant foods eaten and the availability of animal products. Researchers found that as the amount of animal foods increased in the diet, even in relatively small increments, so did the emergence of the cancers that are common in the West. Most cancers occurred in direct proportion to the quantity of animal foods consumed.

In other words, as animal food consumption approached zero, cancer rates fell. Areas of the country with an extremely low consumption of animal food were virtually free of heart attacks and cancer. An analysis of the mortality data from 65 counties and 130 villages showed a significant association with animal protein intake (even at relatively low levels) and heart attacks, with a strong protective effect from the consumption of green vegetables.[3]

All animal products are low (or completely lacking) in the nutrients that protect us against cancer and heart attacks — fiber, antioxidants, phytochemicals, folate, vitamin E, and plant proteins. They are rich in substances that scientific investigations have shown to be associated with cancer and heart disease incidence: saturated fat, cholesterol, and arachidonic acid.[4] Diets rich in animal protein are also associated with high blood levels of the hormone IGF-1, which is a known risk factor for several types of cancer.[5]

The China Project showed a strong correlation between cancer and the amount of animal protein, not just animal fat, consumed.[6] Consumption of lean meats and poultry still showed a strong correlation with higher cancer incidence. These findings indicate that even low-fat animal foods such as skinless white-meat chicken are implicated in certain cancers.

Heart Health — It's Not Just Fat and Cholesterol

There was also a relationship between animal protein and heart disease. For example, plasma apolipoprotein B is positively associated with animal-protein intake and inversely associated (lowered) with vegetable-protein intake (e.g., legumes and greens). Apolipoprotein B levels correlate strongly with coronary heart disease.[7] Unknown to many is that animal proteins have a significant effect on raising cholesterol levels as well, while plant protein lowers it.[8]

Scientific studies provide evidence that animal protein's effect on blood cholesterol may be significant. This is one of the reasons those switching to a low-fat diet do not experience the cholesterol lowering they expect unless they also remove the low-fat animal products as well. Surprising to most people is that yes, even low-fat dairy and skinless white-meat chicken raise cholesterol. I see this regularly in my practice. Many individuals do not see the dramatic drop in cholesterol levels unless they go all the way by cutting all animal proteins from their diet.

Red meat is not the only problem. The consumption of chicken and fish is also linked to colon cancer. A large recent study examined the eating habits of 32,000 adults for six years and then watched the incidence of cancer for these subjects over the next six years. Those who avoided red meat but ate white meat regularly had a more than 300 percent increase in colon cancer incidence.[9] The same study showed that eating beans, peas, or lentils at least twice a week was associated with a 50 percent lower risk than never eating these foods.

CHOLESTEROL CONTENT IN	BEEF, TOP SIRLOIN	CHICKEN BREAST, NO SKIN
100 grams	90 mg	85 mg
100 calories	33 mg	51 mg

Source: USDA Food Composition Data[10]

Chicken has about the same amount of cholesterol as beef, and the production of those potent cancer-causing compounds called heterocyclic amines (HCAs) are even more concentrated in grilled chicken than in beef.[11] Another recent study from New Zealand that investigated heterocyclic amines in meat, fish, and chicken found the greatest contributor of HCAs to cancer risk was chicken.[12] Likewise, studies indicate that chicken is almost as dangerous as red meat for the heart. Regarding cholesterol, there is no advantage to eating lean white instead of lean red meat.[13]

The best bet for overall health is to significantly limit or eliminate all types of meat—red and white. Dr. Campbell explains further his view that animal protein (in addition to animal fats) are implicated in disease causation:

I really believe that dietary protein—both the kind and the amount—is more significant, as far as cholesterol levels are concerned, than is saturated fat. Certainly it is more significant than dietary cholesterol. We do know that animal protein has a quick and major impact on enzymes involved in the metabolism of cholesterol. Whether it is the immune system, various enzyme systems, the uptake of carcinogens into the cells, or hormonal activities, animal protein generally only causes mischief.[14]

It may be impossible to extricate which component of animal food causes the most mischief. However, it is clear that while Americans struggle in vain to even marginally reduce the amount of fat in their diet, they still consume high levels of animal products and very little unrefined produce.

> Cholesterol levels can be decreased by reducing both saturated fat and animal protein while eating more plant protein.

Remember, those countries and areas of China with extremely low rates of Western diseases did not achieve them merely because their diets were low in fat. It was because their diets were rich in unrefined plant products — they were not eating fat-free cheesecake and potato chips.

Never forget that coronary artery disease and its end result — heart attacks, the number one killer of all American men and women — is almost 100 percent avoidable. Poring through nation-by-nation mortality data collected by the World Health Organization, I found that most of the poorer countries, which invariably consume little animal products, have less than 5 percent of the adult population dying of heart attacks.[15] The China Project confirmed that there were virtually no heart attacks in populations that consume a life-long vegetarian diet and almost no heart attacks in populations consuming a diet that is rich in natural plant foods and receives less than 10 percent of its calories from animal foods.

My observation of the worldwide data is supported by studies of American vegetarians and nonvegetarians.[16] These studies show that the major risk factors associated with heart disease — smoking, physical inactivity, and animal-product consumption — are avoidable. Every heart attack death is even more of a tragedy because it likely could have been prevented.

Understanding the Conflicting and Confusing Cancer Studies

The China Project data also helps explain findings from the Nurses Study in Boston, which showed that American women who reduced their fat intake surprisingly did not have a decreased risk of breast cancer.[17] First of all, those on the lower-fat diet consumed 29 percent of their calories from fat. This is still a high-fat diet (by my standards) and even higher than the group with the highest fat intake in China. It's like cutting back on smoking from three packs a day to two and expecting to get a significant decrease in lung cancer risk. By the way, the lowest-fat group in China, whose diet was almost entirely composed of plants, was getting 6 percent of their calories from fat, and the high-fat group in China consumed about 24 percent of their calories from fat.

Second, these women who reported eating less fat in the Nurses Study actually consumed just as much or more calories from animal protein than those on the higher-fat diet, and the amount of unrefined plant produce did not increase. The low-fat group in China was not eating anywhere near the quantity of processed foods that we do in America. Their cancer rates were so low not solely because the diet was low in fat and animal protein but also because, unlike Americans, they actually ate lots of vegetables.

Generally speaking, the reason the evidence from the China Project is so compelling is that results from population studies in the West are not very accurate. They generally study adults who have made some moderate dietary change later in life, and all subjects are past the age when dietary influence has the most effect. Certain cancers, such as breast and prostate cancer, are strongly influenced by how we eat earlier in life, especially right before and after puberty.

After studying multiple diseases, not just one type of cancer, the researchers involved in the China Project concluded: "There appears to be no threshold of plant-food enrichment or minimization of animal product intake beyond which further disease prevention does not occur. These findings suggest that even small intakes of foods of animal origin are associated with significant increases in plasma cholesterol concentration, which are associated, in turn, with significant increases in chronic degenerative disease mortality rates."[18] In other words, populations with very low cholesterol levels have not only low heart-disease rates but low cancer rates as well.

The insight provided by the research is simple: As long as Americans continue to practice nutritional indifference, they will suffer the consequences. Don't expect any significant protection from marginal changes.

Cancer Is a Fruit- and Vegetable-Deficiency Disease

Not surprisingly, fruits and vegetables are the two foods with the best correlation with longevity in humans. Not whole-wheat bread, not bran, not even a vegetarian diet shows as powerful a correlation as a high level of fresh fruit and raw green salad consumption.[19] The National Cancer Institute recently reported on 337 different studies that all showed the same basic information:

1. Vegetables and fruits protect against all types of cancers if consumed in large enough quantities. Hundreds of scientific studies document this. The most prevalent cancers in our country are mostly plant-food-deficiency diseases.
2. Raw vegetables have the most powerful anti-cancer properties of all foods.
3. Studies on the cancer-reducing effects of vitamin pills containing various nutrients (such as folate, vitamin C and E) get mixed reviews; sometimes they show a slight benefit, but most show no benefit. Occasionally studies show that taking isolated nutrients is harmful, as was discussed earlier regarding beta-carotene.
4. Beans, in general, not just soy, have additional anti-cancer benefits against reproductive cancers, such as breast and prostate cancer.[20]

Though Americans would prefer to take a pill so they could continue eating what they are accustomed to, it won't give you the protection you are looking for. You can close the cover of this book and put it away right now as long as you can incorporate this crucial dietary change into your life: consume high levels of fruits, green vegetables, and beans. This is the key to both weight loss and better health. Exactly how much veggies and beans you need to eat and how to incorporate them into your diet and make them taste great is covered in chapter eight.

A Vegetarian Diet Is No Guarantee of Good Health

People who omit meat, fowl, and dairy but fill up on bread, pasta, pretzels, bagels, rice cakes, and crackers may be on a low-fat diet, but because their diet is also low in vitamins, minerals, phytochemicals, important essential fatty acids, and fiber, it is conspicuously inadequate and should not be expected to protect against cancer. Additionally, because these refined grains are low in fiber, they do not make you feel full until after you have taken in too many calories from them. In other words, both their nutrient-to-calorie and nutrient-to-fiber ratios are extremely low.

Let me repeat this again to be clear: Following a strict vegetarian diet is not as important as eating a diet rich in fruits and vegetables. A vegetarian whose diet is mainly refined grains, cold breakfast cereals, processed health-food-store products, vegetarian fast foods, white rice, and pasta will be worse off than a person who eats a little chicken or eggs, for example, but consumes a large amount of fruits, vegetables, and beans.

Studies have confirmed this. Multiple studies have shown that vegetarians live quite a bit longer than nonvegetarians do.[21] But when we take a close look at the data, it appears that those who weren't as strict had longevity statistics that were equally impressive as long as they consumed a high volume of a variety of unrefined plant foods.

Remember, long-term vegans (strict vegetarians who consume no dairy or other foods of animal origin) almost never get heart attacks. If you have heart disease or a strong family history of heart disease, you should consider avoiding all animal-based products. To quote a respected authority, William Castelli, M.D., director of the famed Framingham Heart Study in Massachusetts:

> We tend to scoff at vegetarians, but they're doing much better than we are. Vegans have cholesterol levels so low, they almost never get heart attacks. Their average blood cholesterol is about 125 and we've never seen anyone in the Framingham study have a heart attack with a level below 150.

The research shows that those who avoid meat and dairy have lower rates of heart disease, cancer, high blood pressure, diabetes, and obesity.[22] The data is conclusive: vegetarians live longer in America, probably a lot longer.

How Much Longer Do Vegetarians Live?

This is a difficult question to answer accurately, as there are few studies on lifelong vegetarians in countries with electricity, refrigeration, good sanitation, and adequate nutrition. American studies done in 1984 on Seventh-Day Adventists, a religious group that provides dietary and lifestyle advice to its members, sheds some light on this issue. Adventist leadership discourages the consumption of meat, fowl, and eggs; pork is prohibited. Because eating animal products is only discouraged and not necessarily prohibited, there is a large range in animal-product consumption. Some Adventists never eat meat and eggs, whereas others consume them daily. When we take a careful look at the Seventh-Day Adventist data, those who lived the longest were those following the vegetarian diet the longest, and when we look at the subset who had followed a vegetarian diet for at least half their life, it appears they lived about thirteen years longer than their average, non-smoking Californian counterparts.[23] Most of the participants in this study were converted to the religion, not born into it. There was no data on those following such a diet since childhood. However, the data from this carefully constructed study was compelling; and what is of considerable interest to me is the association of green salad consumption and longer life.[24] Leafy greens, the most nutrient-rich foods on the planet, were the best predictor of extreme longevity.

Some nutritional experts would argue that a strict vegetarian who follows a diet rich in natural vegetation, not refined grains, has the longest longevity potential, as indicated by evaluating the China Project data together with hundreds of the smaller food-consumption studies—but, of course, this is still educated speculation. Let's not argue whether it is all right to eat a little bit of animal foods or not, and thereby miss the point that cannot be contradicted or disagreed with:

> Whether you eat a vegetarian diet or include a small amount of animal foods, for optimal health you must receive the majority of your calories from unrefined plant food. It is the large quantity of unrefined plant food that grants the greatest protection against developing serious disease.

The Breast and Prostate Cancer Mystery Unraveled

So much has been written about the causes of breast cancer (there are entire books devoted to the subject), yet women are still confused. This section should not be skipped over by men. Men have mothers, daughters, sisters, and wives they must help protect, and the same factors that cause breast cancer cause prostate cancer. Men with a family history of breast cancer have an increased risk of prostate cancer, and women with a family history of prostate cancer have an increased risk of breast cancer.[25] So there is a strong link between these two hormonally sensitive cancers.

American women are now twice as likely to develop breast cancer as they were a century ago, and most of this increase has occurred in the past fifty years. In spite of all the fear and publicity, American women are still in the dark about what they can do to protect themselves, and researchers looking for a simple cause have met with frustration. The reason is that breast cancer, like most cancers, is multicausal. Considering a number of contributing factors simultaneously is essential to understand the rapid climb in the incidence of breast cancer in recent decades. We know much today about the causes of breast cancer, and the good news is that genetics plays a minor role and the disease does not strike at random. The war against breast cancer can be won.

Understanding the Factors Involved in the Development of Cancer

Carcinogenesis, the process that leads to cancer, is believed to occur in a series of steps. It is a multistage process that begins with precancerous cellular damage that gradually proceeds to more malignant changes. The first step is the development of cellular abnormalities, which eventually leads to cancer. This usually occurs during adolescence, and soon after puberty.[26] Remember that unhealthy childhood nutritional practices cause excessive sex hormone production and early pathologic changes in the breast tissue that set the stage for cancer many years later.

We know that puberty at an earlier age is a significant marker of increased risk, and we know that there is overwhelming evidence that ovarian hormones play a crucial role, at all stages, in the development of breast cancer.[27] It is common knowledge among physicians that the earlier a woman matures, as measured by the age of her first menstrual period, the higher her risk for breast cancer.[28] Both early menarche and greater body weight are markers of increased risk of breast cancer.[29]

Women are not the only sex affected; the same increased risk as a result of early maturation is seen with both prostate cancer and testicular cancer.[30] If we grow and mature more rapidly, we increase our cancer risk and age faster. We see the same thing in lab animals; if we feed them so they grow faster, they die younger.[31]

Ominously, the onset of menstruation has been occurring at a younger and younger age in Western societies during this century.[32] The average age in the United States is now about twelve years. According to the World Health Organization, the average age at which puberty began in 1840 was seventeen.[33]

During the time period that the age of menarche (the onset of menstruation) has decreased from seventeen to about twelve in Western Europe and the United States, there has been a concomitant change in Western eating habits. There has been an increased con-

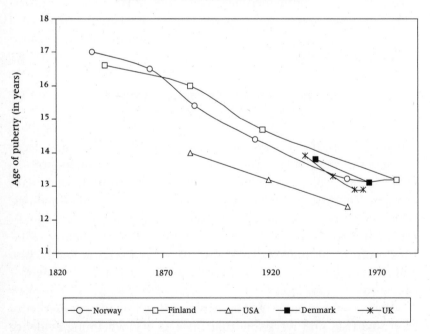

AGE OF PUBERTY OVER TIME

Source: Tanner, J. M. 1973. Trend toward earlier menarche in London, Oslo, Copenhagen, the Netherlands and Hungary. *Nature* 243: 75–76.

sumption of fat, refined carbohydrates, cheese, and meat and a huge decrease in the consumption of complex carbohydrates such as starchy plants. Modern studies of girls on vegetarian diets characterized by more complex carbohydrates and no meat show a later age of menarche and as one would expect, a significant reduction of acne as well.[34] A greater consumption of animal foods leads to a higher level of hormones related to early reproductive function and growth.[35] These hormonal abnormalities persist into adulthood.[36] Uterine fibroids also develop from a diet deficient in fruits and vegetables and heavy in meat. As the consumption of meat increases and vegetation decreases, one's risk of fibroids increases proportionately.[37] In other words, the stage is set by our poor dietary habits early in life. Breast and prostate cancer are strongly affected by our dietary practices when we are young.

First European and then American studies have indicated that the protein richness of one's diet is a more sensitive marker of early menarche than increased body weight.[38] This conclusion is consistent with the data relating earlier menarche with increased animal protein use in South African girls.[39] Then in the 1990s, when the data from the massive China-Oxford-Cornell Project was dissected, we again saw the high correlation between breast-cancer incidence and the consumption of animal products.[40]

In China, animal-food consumption correlated well with early menarche and increasing levels of sex hormones. Serum testosterone levels had the best correlation with breast cancer, even better than estrogen. Of note is that increasing levels of testosterone significantly increases the risk of both breast cancer and prostate cancer. Testosterone rises as well with increasing levels of obesity, and being overweight is another consistent risk factor.[41]

What makes the data from the China Project so intriguing is that breast cancer incidence is so low in China compared with Western countries and that animal-food consumption is so much lower than in America. Even those consuming the most animal products in China consume less than half the amount Americans do. As animal-food intake increased from about once a week in the lowest third to about four times a week in the highest third, breast cancer rates increased by 70 percent. Of note is that the only difference among the diets was the addition of meat in varying amounts. Consumption of fresh vegetables in all groups was about the same, offering little chance of confounding variables. There was a strong increase in the occurrence of breast cancer mortality with increasing animal-product consumption.

In this country, we consume an enormous amount of cheese. Our record-high increase in cheese consumption is alarming: a 193 percent increase in the past twenty-five years.[42] Cheese has more saturated fat and more hormone-containing and -promoting substances than any other food, and the incidence of our hormonally sensitive cancers has skyrocketed.

In spite of studies that do not show an impressive association with small differences in fat consumption later in life, large changes early in life have huge repercussions.[43] When we consider the diet consumed throughout our life, meat and dairy continue to be implicated as a strong causal factor in breast cancer.[44] There is almost no breast cancer at all in populations that consume less than 10 percent of their calories from fat.[45] After reviewing many studies on this issue for the *Journal of the National Cancer Institute*, a group of prominent scientists concluded that the studies that failed to show the relationship between animal-product consumption and breast cancer suffered from methodological problems.[46]

Unraveling the Protein Myth

We have been indoctrinated since early childhood to believe that animal protein is a nutrient to be held in high esteem. We have been brought up with the idea that foods are good for us if they help us grow bigger and faster. Nothing could be further from the truth.

The public as well as the media are confused about this issue. They continue to associate the term *better nutrition* with earlier maturity and larger stature resulting from our greater consumption of animal protein and animal fats. These unfavorable trends are repeatedly reported as positive events. Earlier writers and nutritionists have mistakenly equated rapid growth with health. I believe an increased rate of growth is not a good thing. The slower a child grows, the slower he or she is aging. Slower growth, taking longer to reach maturity, is predictive of a longer life in animal studies.[47] We are finding the same thing in humans: an unnaturally rapid growth and premature puberty are risk factors for cancers and other diseases later in life. Evidence continues to mount that these same factors leading to early maturity and excessive growth in childhood increase the occurrence of cancer in general, not just breast and prostate cancer.[48] Excluding malnutrition or serious disease, the slower we grow and mature, the longer we live.

The other side of the story is that in the past ten years it is not just the fat in animal foods that causes cancer and heart disease. Animal protein is also getting a bad rap by legitimate nutritional researchers and scientists in studies. Scientists have discovered a link between animal protein and cancer in both laboratory and human epidemiological studies, and reducing one's consumption of animal protein slows the aging process.[49]

Animal-product consumption in general is proportionally associated with multiple types of cancer. A massive international study that amassed data from fifty-nine different countries showed that men who ate the most meat, poultry, and dairy products were the most likely to die from prostate cancer, while those who ate the most unrefined plant foods and nuts were the least likely to succumb to this disease.[50]

Another recent study from Germany found colon cancer and rectal cancer decreased by about 50 percent in adult vegetarians. However, a significantly greater reduction of cancer and all-cause mortality (about a 75 percent reduction) was related to being on a vegetarian diet for more than twenty years.[51] The degree of protection correlated well with number of years on a vegetarian diet. Other studies on vegetarian diet in different countries show almost the same thing.[52] The causes start accumulating early.

There is considerable evidence that exposure to certain outlawed pesticides, especially PCBs and DDT, may promote further pathologic changes. Women who have breast cancer have a higher concentration of these chemicals in their breast tissue than do women who do not have cancer.[53] This has also been noted in Long Island, where there is a particularly high rate of breast cancer. Researchers hypothesize that the increased exposure to these chemicals, still in our environment, is the result of eating coastal fish. Added to all of

---

Cancers Associated with Increased Consumption of Animal Products [54]

Bladder cancer	Lung cancer
Brain cancer	Lymphoma
Breast cancer	Oralpharyngeal cancer
Colon cancer	Ovarian cancer
Endometrial cancer	Pancreatic cancer
Intestinal cancer	Prostate cancer
Kidney cancer	Skin cancer
Leukemia	Stomach cancer

this is the exposure to trans fats and cancer-causing compounds that are released when meat, fish, or fowl is grilled, fried, or barbecued.[55] Clearly, cancer causation is a complicated, multifactorial issue.

Exercise Powerfully Reduces Cancer Risk

Researchers at the University of Tromsø in Norway report that women who exercise regularly reduce their risk of developing breast cancer substantially. Their study involved more than 25,000 women age twenty to fifty-four at the time of their entry into the study. The researchers found that younger, premenopausal women (under forty-five years old) who exercised regularly had 62 percent less risk than sedentary women. The risk reduction was highest for lean women who exercised more than four hours per week; these women had a 72 percent reduction in risk.

Diet and exercise have a much more important role to play in cancer prevention than mammograms and other detection methods. Keep in mind that mammograms merely detect, not prevent, cancer; they show disease only after the cancerous cells have been proliferating for many years.[56] By that time the majority of cancers have already spread from their local site and surgically removing the tumor is not curative. Only a minority of women who have their breast cancers detected by a mammogram have their survival increased because of the earlier detection.[57] The majority would have done just as well to find it later. I am not aiming to discourage women ages fifty to sixty-five from having mammograms; rather, my message is that this alone is insufficient. Mammograms, which do nothing to prevent breast cancer, are heavily publicized, while women hear nothing else about what they can do to prevent and protect themselves against breast cancer in the first place.

Do not underestimate the effect of a superior diet on gradually removing and repairing damage caused by years of self-abuse. Do not be discouraged just because you cannot bring your risk down to zero because of your mistakes in the past. The same thing could be said for cigarette smokers. Should they not quit smoking, merely because their risk of lung cancer can't be brought down to zero when they quit? Actually, lung cancer rates are considerably lower (about one-fifth) in countries that have a high vegetable consumption, even though they may smoke like crazy.[58] Raw fruits and vegetables offer powerful protection; leafy greens are the most protective.[59]

My main point is that our population has been ignoring those interventions that can most effectively save lives. We search for more answers because the ones we have found are not to our liking. Our most powerful artillery on the war against breast cancer, and cancer in general, is to follow the overall advice presented in this book and begin at as young an age as possible.

Increasing the Survival of Cancer Patients

It would be difficult for anyone to disagree that superior nutrition has a protective effect against cancer. The question that remains is: Can optimal nutrition or nutritional intervention be an effective therapeutic approach for patients who already have cancer? Can the diet you eat make a difference if you have cancer? Scientific data indicates that the answer is yes.

Researchers looking for answers to these questions studied women with cancer and found that saturated fat in the diet promoted a more rapid spread of the cancer.[60] Other researchers found similar results. For a woman who already has cancer, her risk of dying increased 40 percent for every 1,000 grams of fat consumed monthly.[61] Studies also indicate that high fruit and vegetable intake improved survival, and fat on the body increases the risk of a premature death.[62]

Similar findings are found in the scientific literature regarding prostate cancer and diet, indicating that diet has a powerful effect on survival for those with prostate cancer.[63] *For humans, too much animal food is toxic.*

ANIMAL PROTEIN	PLANT PROTEIN
Raises cholesterol	Lowers cholesterol
Cancer promoter	Cancer protector
Promotes bone loss	Promotes bone strength
Promotes kidney disease	No effect
Accelerates aging	No effect
Packaged with	*Packaged with*
Saturated fat	Fiber
Cholesterol	Phytochemicals
Arachidonic acid	Antioxidants

When it is consumed in significant volume, animal protein, not only animal fat, is earning a reputation as a toxic nutrient to humans. More books are touting the benefits of high-protein diets for weight loss and are getting much publicity. Many Americans desire to protect their addiction to high-fat, nutrient-inadequate animal foods. These consumers form a huge market for such topsy-turvy scientific-sounding quackery.

Today the link between animal products and many different diseases is as strongly supported in the scientific literature as the link between cigarette smoking and lung cancer. For example, subjects who ate meat, including poultry and fish, were found to be twice as likely to develop dementia (loss of intellectual function with aging) than their vegetarian counterparts in a carefully designed study.[64] The discrepancy was further widened when past meat consumption was taken into account. The same diet, loaded with animal products, that causes heart disease and cancer also causes most every other disease prevalent in America including kidney stones, renal insufficiency and renal failure, osteoporosis, uterine fibroids, hypertension, appendicitis, diverticulosis, and thrombosis.[65]

Are Dairy Foods Protecting Us from Osteoporosis?

Dairy products are held in high esteem in America. Most people consider a diet without dairy unhealthy. Without dairy foods, how could we obtain sufficient calcium for our bones? Let's examine this accepted wisdom: is it true, or have we been brainwashed by years and years of misinformation and advertising?

Hip fractures and osteoporosis are more frequent in populations in which dairy products are commonly consumed and calcium intakes are commonly high. For example, American women drink thirty to thirty-two times as much cow's milk as the New Guineans, yet suffer forty-seven times as many broken hips. A multicountry analysis of hip-fracture incidence and dairy-product consumption found that milk consumption has a high statistical association with higher rates of hip fractures.[66]

Does this suggest that drinking cow's milk causes osteoporosis? Certainly, it brings into question the continual advertising message from the National Dairy Council that drinking cow's milk prevents osteoporosis. The major finding from the Nurses Health Study, which included 121,701 women ages thirty to fifty-five at enrollment in 1976, was that the data does not support the hypothesis that the consumption of milk protects against hip or forearm fractures.[67] In fact, those who drank three or more servings of milk a day had a slightly higher rate of fractures than women who drank little or no milk.

This does not mean that dairy causes osteoporosis. However, it does suggest that dairy products are not protecting us from osteoporosis as we have been indoctrinated to believe since childhood. On the contrary, studies show fruits and vegetables are protective against osteoporosis.[68]

Osteoporosis has a complex etiology that involves other factors such as dietary acid-alkaline balance, trace minerals, phytochemicals in plants, exercise, exposure to sunlight, and more. Dr. Campbell, head of nutritional research at Cornell and of the China Project, reported, "Ironically, osteoporosis tends to occur in countries where calcium intake is highest and most of it comes from protein-rich dairy products. The Chinese data indicate that people need less calcium than we think and can get adequate amounts from vegetable source plant food." He told the *New York Times* that there was basically no osteoporosis in China, yet the calcium intake ranged from 241 to 943 mg per day (average, 544). The comparable U.S. calcium intake is 841 to 1,435 mg per day (average, 1,143), mostly from dairy sources, and, of course, osteoporosis is a major public health problem here.

To understand the causes of osteoporosis, one must comprehend the concept of negative calcium balance. Let's say you consume about 1,000 mg of calcium a day. About a third of the calcium ingested gets absorbed. So if you absorb about 300 mg, the remaining 700 mg remains in the digestive tract and passes out with your stool. If, in this same twenty-four-hour period, you excreted 350 mg of calcium in your urine, would you be in a negative or positive calcium balance?

	NEGATIVE BALANCE	POSITIVE BALANCE
Ingested	1,000 mg	500 mg
Absorbed	300 mg	200 mg
Excreted	350 mg	100 mg
Retained	− 50 mg	+100 mg

A negative calcium balance means more calcium is excreted in the urine than is absorbed through digestion. A positive calcium balance means more calcium is absorbed than is excreted. A negative balance over time results in bone loss, as the additional calcium must come from our primary calcium storehouse, our bones.

Epidemiologic studies have linked osteoporosis not to low calcium intake but to various nutritional factors that cause excessive calcium loss in the urine. The continual depletion of our calcium reserves over time, from excessive calcium excretion in the urine, is the primary cause of osteoporosis. Now, let us consider the factors that contribute to this excessive urinary calcium excretion.

Dietary Factors That Induce Calcium Loss in the Urine[69]

animal protein
salt
caffeine
refined sugar
alcohol
nicotine
aluminum-containing antacids
drugs such as antibiotics, steroids, thyroid hormone
vitamin A supplements

Published data clearly links increased urinary excretion of calcium with animal-protein intake but not with vegetable-protein intake.[70] Plant foods, though some may be high in protein, are not acid-forming. Animal-protein ingestion results in a heavy acid load in the blood. This sets off a series of reactions whereby calcium is released from the bones to help neutralize the acid. The sulfur-based amino acids in animal products contribute significantly to urinary acid production and the resulting calcium loss.[71] The Nurses Health Study found that women who consumed 95 grams of protein a day had a 22 percent greater risk of forearm fracture than those who consumed less than 68 grams.[72]

The most comprehensive epidemiological survey involving hip fractures and food was done in 1992.[73] The authors sought out every peer-reviewed geographical report ever done on hip-fracture incidence. They located thirty-four published studies of women in sixteen countries. Their analysis showed that diets high in animal protein had the highest correlation with hip-fracture rates, with an 81 percent correlation between eating animal protein and fractures.

The extra calcium contained in dairy foods simply cannot counteract the powerful effect of all the factors listed in the table above. The average American diet is not only high in protein but high in salt, sugar, and caffeine and low in fruits and vegetables. Fruits and

COUNTRY	ANIMAL PROTEIN INTAKE (APPROXIMATE G/DAY)	HIP FRACTURE RATE (PER 100,000 PEOPLE)
South Africa (blacks)	10.4	6.8
New Guinea	16.4	3.1
Singapore	24.7	21.6
Yugoslavia	27.3	27.6
Hong Kong	34.6	45.6
Israel	42.5	93.2
Spain	47.6	42.4
Netherlands	54.3	87.7
United Kingdom	56.6	118.2
Demark	58	165.3
Sweden	59.4	187.8
Finland	60.5	111.2
Ireland	61.4	76
Norway	66.6	190.4
United States	72	144.9
New Zealand	77.8	119

vegetables can help buffer the acid load from all the animal protein and reduce calcium loss.[74] So we need to consume a lot more calcium to make up for the powerful combination of factors that induce calcium loss in the urine.

Some researchers believe it is possible to compensate for our high protein intake just by consuming more calcium.[75] This might be the case if the only thing we did to excess was consume a little too much animal protein, but in the context of everything else we do wrong in the American diet and lifestyle, it just doesn't fly.

Drinking more milk is simply not protective. Taking extra calcium supplements may help trim the calcium loss a little and slow the rate of bone loss, but not enough. We need to reduce the other causes, too. We even add vitamin A to milk, and many women take vitamin A supplements, which contributes further to more calcium loss.[76]

All these factors help explain why calcium intake does not correlate well with reduced hip-facture rates around the globe. The Eskimos are a perfect example. They consume a huge amount of calcium, over 2,000 mg a day, from all the soft fish bones they eat, yet they have the highest hip-fracture rate in the world because they consume so much animal protein from fish.[77]

The Best Food for Bones: Fruits and Vegetables

Green vegetables, beans, tofu, sesame seeds, and even oranges contain lots of usable calcium, without the problems associated with dairy. Keep in mind that you retain the calcium better and just do not need as much when you don't consume a diet heavy in animal products and sodium, sugar, and caffeine.

Many green vegetables have calcium-absorption rates of over 50 percent, compared with about 32 percent for milk.[78] Additionally, since animal protein induces calcium excretion in the urine, the calcium retention from vegetables is higher. All green vegetables are high in calcium.

The American "chicken and pasta" diet style is significantly low in calcium, so adding dairy as a calcium source to this mineral-poor diet makes superficial sense — it is certainly better than no calcium in the diet. However, much more than just calcium is missing. The only reason cow's milk is considered such an important source of calcium, is that the American diet is centered on animal foods, refined grains, and sugar, all of which are devoid of calcium. Any healthy diet containing a reasonable amount of unrefined plant foods will have sufficient calcium without milk. Fruits and vegetables strengthen bones. Researchers have found that those who eat the most fruits and vegetables have denser bones.[79] These researchers concluded that not only are fruits and vegetables rich in potassium, magnesium, calcium, and other nutrients essential for bone health, but, because they are alkaline, not acid-producing, they do not induce urinary calcium loss. Green vegetables in particular have a powerful effect on reducing hip fractures, for they are rich not only in calcium but in other nutrients, such as vitamin K, which is crucial for bone health.[80]

Got Milk — Or Leave It?

Dairy is best kept to a minimum. There are many good reasons not to consume dairy. For example, there is a strong association between dairy lactose and ischemic heart disease.[81] There is also a clear association between high-growth-promoting foods such as dairy products and cancer. There is a clear association between milk consumption and testicular cancer.[82] Dairy fat is also loaded with various toxins and is the primary source of our nation's high exposure to dioxin.[83] Dioxin is a highly toxic chemical compound that even the U.S. Environmental Protection Agency admits is a prominent cause of many types of cancer in those consuming dairy fat, such as butter and cheese.[84] Cheese is also a power inducer of acid load, which increases calcium loss further.[85] Considering that cheese and butter are the foods with the highest saturated-fat content and the major source of our dioxin exposure, cheese is a particularly foolish choice for obtaining calcium.

Cow's milk is "designed" to be the perfect food for the rapidly growing calf, but as mentioned above, foods that promote rapid growth promote cancer. There is ample evidence implicating dairy consumption as a causative factor in both prostate and ovarian cancer.[86] In April 2000 a Harvard study reported that having 2.5 servings of dairy each day boosted prostate cancer risk by more than 30 percent.[87] Another recent controlled study conducted in Greece has shown a strong association between dairy products and prostate cancer.[88] By analyzing the data, the authors calculated that if the population of Greece were to increase its consumption of tomatoes and decrease its consumption of dairy products, prostate cancer incidence could be reduced by 41 percent, and an even greater reduction would be possible in America, where the dietary risk is even higher.

Investigating the link between lactose (milk sugar) and ovarian cancer among the 80,326 women enrolled in the Nurses Health Study, Dr. Kathleen Fairfield and her associates reported that women who consumed the highest amount of lactose (one or more servings of dairy per day) had a 44 percent greater risk for all types of invasive ovarian cancer than those who ate the lowest amount (three or fewer servings monthly). Skim and low-fat milk were the largest contributors to lactose consumption.[89] Dairy products are just not the healthiest source of calcium.

Perhaps the strongest argument against dairy products in our diet: lots of us are lactose-intolerant. Those lactose-intolerant folks, who don't digest dairy well, are continually barraged with information that makes them believe they will lose their bones if they don't consume dairy products in some way. They may be better off without it.

If you choose to consume dairy, use only fat-free dairy products and minimize your intake to small amounts. Remember the 90 percent rule: eat 90 percent health-giving whole-plant foods. Dairy may be a part of that 10 percent; however, it is not essential for good health and carries potential health risks, especially products containing dairy fat such as butter and cheese.

You do not need dairy products to get sufficient calcium if you eat a healthy diet. All unprocessed natural foods are calcium-rich; even a whole orange (not orange juice) has about 60 mg of calcium.

CALCIUM IN 100 CALORIES OF

bok choy	1,055
turnip greens	921
collard greens	559
kale	455
romaine lettuce	257
tofu	236
milk	194
broccoli	182
sesame seeds	170
soybeans	134
cucumber	108
cauliflower	88
carrots	63
fish	38
eggs	32
T-bone steak	5
pork chop	2

Government health authorities advise us to consume 1,500 mg of calcium daily. This is a tremendous amount of calcium. So much is recommended because of all the factors mentioned above. Even this high level of calcium will not prevent osteoporosis, but in a population with so many factors that cause osteoporosis, the extra calcium will make the negative balance less negative and partially slow the rate of osteoporosis. However, the only way to prevent osteoporosis and have strong bones is to exercise and to stop the causes of high urinary calcium excretion. *Eat to Live* describes a diet that protects against osteoporosis.

Are You Dying to Lose Weight?

A Closer Look at the Atkins Plan, The Zone, and Eating for Your Blood Type

Since it is estimated that more than 75 percent of all Americans are overweight, it is not surprising that diet and weight-loss books abound.[1] Recent investigations report such a sweeping and rapid increase of obesity globally that it is considered a serious medical epidemic, affecting a significant portion of our world's population.[2] Because overweight and obesity dramatically increase the risk of all the major causes of death, it may be the most serious health issue facing the world. Each new book promises advice on how to become the new, thinner you.

The success of diet books can be measured in a number of ways. You can measure the success of a book by its popularity, by how well the program it describes works, or by how many pounds you can reasonably expect to lose. However, there are more important considerations.

Weight loss and overall health are inseparable. A weight-loss program can be considered successful only if the weight loss is permanent, safe, and promotes overall health. Temporary weight loss is of little or no benefit, especially if it compromises your health.

Dangerous Weight-Loss Schemes

Unfortunately, some of the most heavily promoted and bestselling books are also among the most dangerous. Some of the more popular books are *Dr. Atkins' Health Revolution* and *New Diet Revolution; The Zone,* by Barry Sears; and *Protein Power,* by Michael and Mary Eades.

The popularity of these books is evidence that people are looking for a quick, effortless way to lose weight without having to curtail their dangerous love affair with rich, unhealthful foods. People are desperate to lose weight, and these books preach what people want to hear: that you can eat lots of fat, cholesterol, and saturated fat and still lose weight. This illicit romance can lead to tragic consequences, with some people literally dying to lose weight.

High-protein-diet gurus usually claim that they hold the truth and that all other doctors and scientists are wrong. They promote the idea that their recommended diet is the healthiest. They would have their devotees believe there is a worldwide conspiracy of more than 3,500 scientific studies involving more than 15,000 research scientists reporting a relationship between the consumption of meats, poultry, eggs, and dairy products and the incidence of heart disease, cancer, kidney failure, constipation, gallstones, diverticulosis, and hemorrhoids, just to name a few health problems.

Reviewing and understanding both the positive and negative aspects of various popular diets will aid in your understanding of nutritional science in general. It is a worthwhile exercise to reinforce and expand the information gained from prior chapters and to look at some of the scientific studies to help us understand the perpetuated myths and controversies. My patients have a high success rate in not just losing but also keeping off the weight permanently because they receive such a comprehensive and scientific edification in human nutrition. It will help you give up believing in magical diets.

The Atkins Cancer Revolution

Robert Atkins's books, as well as other authors advocating high-protein weight-loss plans, recommend diets for health and weight loss with significantly more animal protein than is typically consumed by the average American. Americans already eat approximately 40 percent of their calories from animal products; we have seen a tragic sky-rocketing in cancer and heart-disease rates in the past fifty years as a result of such nutritional extravagance.[3] You can lose some weight on the Atkins Diet, but you run the risk of losing your health at the same time.

Atkins recommends that you eat primarily high-fat, high-protein, fiberless animal foods and attempt to eliminate carbohydrates from your diet. Atkins's menus average 60–75 percent of calories from fat and contain no whole grains and no fruit. Analyses of the proposed menus show animal products make up more than 90 percent of the calories in the diet.

Hundreds of scientific studies have documented the link between animal products and various cancers. Though it would be wrong to say that animal foods are the sole cause of cancer, it is now clear that increased consumption of animal products combined with the decreased consumption of fresh produce has the most powerful effect on increasing one's risk for various kinds of cancer. Atkins convinces his followers that he knows better than leading nutritional research scientists who proclaim that "meat consumption is an important factor in the etiology of human cancer."[4]

Dr. Atkins's books actually recommend such foods as fried pork rinds, heavy cream, and bacon cheeseburgers. The first page of *Dr. Atkins' Health Revolution* states:

> Imagine losing weight with a diet that lets you have bacon and eggs for breakfast, heavy cream in your coffee, plenty of meat and even salad with dressing for lunch and dinner! No wonder Dr. Atkins calls it a "diet revolution."

A meat-based, low-fiber diet, like the one Atkins advocates, includes little or no fruit, no starchy vegetables, and no whole grains. Following Atkins's recommendations could more than double your risk of certain cancers, especially meat-sensitive cancers, such as epithelial cancers of the respiratory tract.[5] For example, a study conducted by the National Cancer Institute looked at lung cancer in nonsmoking women so that smoking would not be a major variable. Researchers found that the relative risk of lung cancer was six times greater in women in the highest fifth of saturated-fat consumption than those in the lowest fifth.

It is not only that his menu plans are incredibly high in saturated fat, it is that Atkins's menus prohibit and restrict the foods known to offer powerful protection against cancer. Even his more permissive diets, supposedly for maintenance, are dangerously low in these anti-cancer foods. Atkins's devotees adopt a dietary pattern completely opposite of what is recommended by the leading research scientists studying the link between diet and cancer.[6]

Specifically, fruit exclusion alone is a significant cancer marker. Stomach and esophageal cancer are linked to populations that do not consume a sufficient amount of fruit.[7] Scientific studies show a clear and strong dose-response relationship between cancers of the digestive tract, bladder, and prostate with low fruit consumption.[8] To the surprise of many investigators, fruit consumption shows a powerful dose-response association with a reduction in heart-disease, cancer, and all-cause mortality.[9] There is also a striking consistency in many scientific investigations that show a reduction in incidence of colorectal and stomach cancer with the intake of whole grains.[10] Colon cancer is strongly associated with the consumption of animal products.[11] And these researchers have concluded that the varying level of colon cancer in the low-incidence population compared with the high-incidence population could not be explained by "protective" factors such as fiber, vitamins, and minerals; rather, it was influenced almost totally by the consumption of animal products and fat.

More saturated fat Less fruit	=	Higher cancer risk
Less saturated fat More fruit	=	Lower cancer risk

There are numerous ways to lose weight. However "effective" they may be, some are just not safe. We wouldn't advocate smoking cigarettes or snorting cocaine simply because doing so would be effective in promoting weight loss. Advocating a weight-loss program based on severe carbohydrate restriction is irresponsible. You may pay a substantial price — your life!

Short-Term Benefits? Long-Term Dangers!

An argument can be made for the usefulness of diets like the one advocated by Atkins because they often do result in weight loss. Being overweight is such a health risk that there are some real health benefits one receives from losing weight, even if the mode of weight loss places the person at increased cancer risk. Losing weight — even by a high-protein, high-fat, low-fiber diet — will lower triglycerides, decrease insulin resistance, and lower blood pressure.

These high-protein diets strongly forbid refined carbohydrates, junk food, and the nutritionally depleted white pasta, white rice, and bread that most Americans consume in large quantities. That is the good part. They also frequently recommend that the dieter consume hundreds of dollars of nutritional supplements each month. Sure, the supplements are better than nothing on such an unbalanced diet, but they do not make it safe.

The conventional American diet is so unhealthy and fattening that an obese individual following the Atkins diet may derive some marginal benefit if he or she can use it successfully to keep his or her weight down, because of all the various adverse medical complications associated with obesity and because the added supplements add some missing micronutrients. However, the reality is that no matter how many supplements are taken and how much psyllium fiber is prescribed, it is simply impossible to make up for so many important substances that are lacking in the diet. There are too many essential nutrients that have never met the inside of a vitamin jar, and no supplemental gymnastics can ever offset the destructive effects of so much animal food and so little fibrous produce. Plus, on his plan, consuming even a moderate amount of the healthy carbohydrate foods such as fruits and starchy vegetables stops ketosis and you regain your weight.

High-fat diets are unquestionably associated with obesity, and eating meat actually correlates with weight gain, not weight loss, unless you radically cut carbs from your diet to maintain a chronic ketosis.[12] Researchers from the American Cancer Society followed 79,236 individuals over ten years and found that those who ate meat more than three times per week were much more likely to gain weight as the years went by than those who tended to avoid meat.[13] The more vegetables the participants ate, the more resistant they were to weight gain.

The Atkins diet, along with other similar plans, is virtually the opposite of the one dictated by our primate heritage. It has almost no fiber, utilizing instead the precise foods that science has established as the primary causes of cancer and heart attacks, and specifically excludes the foods that have been shown to have a powerful anti-cancer effect. Then you are told to take hundreds of dollars of supplements each month to make up for the deficiencies. Does this make sense to you?

	ATKINS (FROM HIS BOOK)	FUHRMAN EAT TO LIVE (SAMPLE)
Total calories	2,550	1,600
Fiber	5.4 gm	77 gm
Protein	188 gm	60 gm
Fat	167 gm	19 gm
Carbohydrate	67 gm	314 gm
Saturated fat	60 gm	2 gm
Sodium	5,920 mg	592 mg
B-carotene	212 mcg	8,260 mcg
Vitamin C	30 mg	625 mg
Calcium	543 mg	877 mg
Magnesium	187 mg	593 mg
Iron	18 mg	22 mg
Manganese	1.5 mg	8.1 mg
Vitamin E	10 IU	22 IU
Folate	316 mcg	1,242 mcg
Chromium	0.034 mg	0.168 mg

The Atkins menu above, like most of his meal plans, averages 60 percent of calories from fat. Obviously, the Eat to Live menu has fewer calories and almost no saturated fat and is much higher in fiber and other (anti-cancer) plant-derived nutrients.

Remember, the grams of fiber consumed, when acquired from natural foods, mark the level of other phytochemicals — which may make the difference between a long life and a premature death.

It is difficult to imagine a physician, practicing as a nutritional expert, selling millions of books while recommending 60 grams of disease-promoting saturated fat a day.[14]

Telling people what they want to hear sells books, products, and services. Atkins continues to make irresponsible statements in support of his dangerous advice. Take, for example, statements from his winter 2001 *Health Revelations Special Report* (an advertisement brochure for his newsletter):

> *Reverse heart disease with filet mignon!*
> *Stop strokes with cheese!*
> *Prevent breast cancer with butter!*

The worst part is that most people do not have a comprehensive knowledge of the world's nutritional literature and research and therefore are not in a position to evaluate his fraudulent claims.

Ketone Metabolism — Fundamental to the Survival
of Our Species

So how do these high-protein diets work? How can you eat all the fat and grease that you want and still lose weight?

Humans are primates; genetically and structurally, we closely resemble the gorilla. We are designed, just like the other large primates, to survive predominantly on plant foods rich in carbohydrates. When the human body finds that it does not have enough carbohydrates to run its "machinery" properly, it produces *ketones,* an emergency fuel that can be utilized in times of crisis.

At rest, the brain consumes about 80 percent of our energy needs. Under normal conditions, the brain can utilize only glucose as fuel. However, the human organism has evolved a remarkable adaptation that enables it to survive for long periods of time without food.

In the first few days of no carbohydrate fuel (food), the body's glucose reserves dwindle and the only way we can produce enough fuel for our hungry brain is by breaking down muscle tissue to manufacture glucose. Glucose cannot be manufactured from fat. Fortunately, our body has a built-in mechanism that allows us to conserve our muscle tissue by metabolizing a more efficient energy source — our fat supply.

After a day or two of not eating, the body dips into its fat reserves to produce ketones as an emergency fuel. As the level of ketones rise in our bloodstream, the brain accepts ketones as an alternative fuel. In this manner, we conserve muscle and increase survival during periods of food deprivation, such as fasting. For those interested in more information about the biochemistry of fasting and its effect on human health, I recommend my book *Fasting and Eating for Health, A Medical Doctor's Guide for Conquering Disease.*

Atkins's dietary recommendations prey on this survival mechanism. When we restrict carbohydrates so markedly, the body thinks we are calorically deprived and ketosis results. The body begins to lose fat, even if we are consuming plenty of high-fat foods, as Atkins recommends. Once you stop the diet, you'll gain all the weight back and more; if you stay on the diet, you risk a premature death. Take your pick. Once you start consuming carbohydrate-containing fruits, vegetables, or beans, the ketosis ends and the meat and fat become fattening again. Meat consumption leads to weight gain, unless you have caused a carbohydrate-deficiency ketosis.

To make matters even worse, you pay an extra penalty from a diet so high in fat and protein to generate a chronic ketosis. Besides the increased cancer risk, your kidneys are placed under greater stress and will age more rapidly. It can take many, many years for such damage to be detected by blood tests. By the time the blood reflects the abnormality, irreversible damage may have already occurred. Blood tests that monitor kidney function typically do not begin to detect problems until more than 90 percent of the kidneys have been destroyed.

Protein is metabolized by the liver, and the nitrogenous wastes generated are broken down and then excreted by the kidney. These wastes must be eliminated for the body to maintain normal purity and a stable state of equilibrium. Most doctors are taught in medical school that a high-protein diet ages the kidney.[15] What has been accepted as the normal age-related loss in renal function may really be a cumulative injury secondary to the heavy pressure imposed on the kidney by our high-protein eating habits.[16]

By the eighth decade of life, Americans lose about 30 percent of their kidney function.[17] Many people develop kidney problems at young ages under the high-protein stress. Low-protein diets are routinely used to treat patients with liver and kidney failure.[18] A recent multitrial analysis showed that reducing protein intake for patients with kidney disease decreased kidney-related death by about 40 percent.[19]

Diabetics, who are at increased risk of kidney disease, are extremely sensitive to the stress a high-protein diet places on the kidney.[20] In a large, multicentered study involving 1,521 patients, most of the diabetics who ate too much animal protein had lost over half of their kidney function, and almost all the damage was irreversible.[21] In my practice, I have seen numerous patients who have experienced significant worsening of their kidney function after attempting weight loss and diabetic control with high-protein diets. Coincidence? I think not. Damage from such lopsided nutritional advice can be very serious.

Ketogenic diets, like Atkins's, have been used to treat children with seizure disorders when medication alone is unresponsive. Medical studies reveal that these diets can result in serious health consequences. Investigators report a greater potential for adverse events than had ever been anticipated. The dangers of these high-protein diets include hemolytic anemia, abnormal liver function, renal tubular acidosis, and spontaneous bone fractures (despite calcium supplementation).[22] Kidney stones are another risk of high-protein diets.[23]

These studies point out that there are many subtle adverse outcomes not being attributed to this dangerous way of eating.

Enter the Barry Sears Danger Zone

The Zone, by Barry Sears, Ph.D., is another weight-loss book that has attracted much attention. Sears promises permanent weight loss and improved health and energy by eating more protein and fat. Miraculously, this can be accomplished without caloric restriction because, according to him, he has a greater understanding of human physiology and the importance of eicosanoids than anyone else. Are his extraordinary claims true, or just more scientific-sounding silliness? Unfortunately, most people do not have the scientific background to see through Sears's false claims and inaccurate pseudoscience.

Sears's menu plans are less dangerous than Atkins's because he permits small amounts of fruit and starchy vegetables. But his gimmick of narrowly focusing on eicosanoid production (while ignoring the many other biochemical causes of disease) gives his book a failing grade with legitimate nutritional scientists.

Sears advocates eating a measured portion of concentrated protein, starch, and fat at every meal and snack. His theory is that doing so will ease glucose more gently into the blood, avoiding swings in insulin secretion. He considers these swings the critical factor in driving the production of the bad inflammatory hormones, called eicosanoids.

Throughout his book, he portrays carbohydrates as the cause of the increasing girth of Americans. Sears and Atkins, as well as other high-protein advocates, argue that the continual growth in the abdominal girth of Americans is the result of misguided nutritional advice advocating lower fat consumption. They claim that low-fat diets are the cause of obesity and are actually dangerous. As Sears stated:

> *Americans were told to eat less fat and more carbohydrates. That, said the experts, is how you get skinnier. We're now fifteen years into the experiment, and one doesn't have to be a rocket scientist to see that it isn't working. In fact, all data analysis during the last fifteen years of this experiment shows that in spite of the fact that the American public has dramatically cut back on the amount of fat consumed, the country has experienced an epidemic rise in obesity.*

One could write an entire book describing and explaining Sears's inaccuracies, which is not the purpose here, so I will merely highlight a few of his major errors.

Sears's claim that Americans have dramatically cut their fat intake is incorrect. In fact, nationally recognized food surveys, such as the National Food Consumption Survey and the National Health and Nutrition Survey, indicate that Americans consume somewhere between 34 and 37 percent of their calories from fat.[24] Americans are still eating a very high fat diet. The reason for the rise in obesity in America is no mystery: we eat a high-calorie, high-fat diet. We are eating more meals outside the home, relying more heavily on convenience foods, and consuming larger food portions. Consistent with trends in weight, caloric intake rose 15 percent between 1970 and 1994.[25] The data actually shows increased consumption of junk food, fat, and calories in recent years.[26]

Weight has increased in America simply because total calorie consumption has risen and activity or exercise has fallen. Our diets are more nutrient-deficient than ever. Precisely balancing your protein and fat intake to enter some hypothetical zone will not make you lose weight, unless you have reduced calorie consumption.

Numerous epidemiological and clinical trials have shown that diets low in fat and high in complex carbohydrates correlate with lower body weights worldwide. High-fat diets always show a direct response relationship not only to obesity but also to heart attacks and cancer.[27]

How Important Is the Glycemic Index?

According to Sears, the rate at which carbohydrates enter the bloodstream (a food's glycemic index) determines whether or not we maintain good health and optimal weight. Yet scientific evidence indicates that the glycemic index of a food is not a reliable predictor of the effect food has on blood glucose levels, cholesterol, and insulin levels.[28]

In his book, Sears warns that eating bananas, carrots, lima beans, and potatoes could be dangerous to your health merely because they have a higher glycemic index. Obviously, the glycemic index is not the major factor in deciding whether we should consider a food healthful.

We wouldn't want to recommend a diet of all high-glycemic foods; however, the addition of nutrient-dense foods such as bananas, papayas, apricots, carrots, and lima beans is healthy and conducive to weight loss. Just because the glycemic index of these healthy plant foods is a little higher than some other plant foods does not mean they should be eliminated. The studies on the negative effects of high-glycemic foods always analyze diets that contain refined flour and simple sugar and are low in micronutrients and fiber. I agree that low-glycemic diets can reduce the risk of cardiovascular disease, diabetes, and obesity. However, it is the poor quality of the high-glycemic diet in general that promotes weight gain and disease — not merely because of the high glycemic index. You need not be concerned about the glycemic index of a particular natural food if it is otherwise nutrient- and fiber-rich and is part of a healthful diet.

In fact, the presence or lack of fiber is a much more reliable predictor of blood glucose control.[29] Plant fibers — the indigestible and unabsorbed part of the plant foods — are now looked at in a completely different way than in the past. We now understand that it is not merely the amount but the variety of fiber in the diet that protects against cancer. Our digestive tract is teeming with many species of bacteria that convert these fibers into numerous essential fatty acids and other nutritive substances with strong immune-enhancing and anti-cancer properties.[30] These bacterial degradation products are essential for optimal health and protection against various cancers, especially colon cancer.

The fiber content of the food or meal is more important than the glycemic index. All these high-protein gurus are forced to neglect the hottest area of nutritional research today — phytochemicals and plant fibers — because it would make their diets look dangerous. And the fiber content parallels the level of phytochemicals, which have powerful effects on preventing many diseases, including cancer.

And you can't just add psyllium fiber supplement to an American diet and think your fiber needs will be met. You must eat a variety of soluble and insoluble plant fibers from a wide assortment of natural foods to achieve optimal health. The low quantity of numerous plant fibers and other plant-derived nutrients becomes an insurmountable health risk in all diets that include animal-based foods in substantial quantity.

The glycemic index is a complicated issue, but not a major concern.

It is not true that a higher insulin level after meals is the main cause of weight gain, as Sears claims. This is a complicated subject. Absorbing excess calories more slowly, with the resultant more gradually increased glucose level and insulin response, will still cause the same amount of weight gain. A flatter insulin response curve does not lead to fewer calories converted to fat.[31] Balancing fat, carbohydrate, and protein intake, even if it could modify the insulin response, would have little or no effect on one's weight. All excess calories will still be stored as fat.

Furthermore, there is evidence to implicate dietary animal protein as an important factor in raising insulin levels. Although dietary protein itself provokes relatively little insulin release, it can markedly increase the insulin response to carbohydrates when consumed in the same meal.[32] Thus, avoiding animal protein or segregating it so it is not consumed along with high-carbohydrate foods may reduce mealtime insulin secretion — completely the opposite of Sears's half-baked theory.

So the glycemic index need not be a major concern. The only way a glucose surge and the resulting insulin surge can cause weight gain is by causing us to get hungry more quickly and eat more calories later and more often. This will occur only if you are eating a low-nutrient, high-calorie diet. The factors that control appetite and hunger are affected by more than the glycemic index.

This is just one more reason not to eat refined grains and sweets and to structure an eating plan around natural high-fiber plant foods. These processed, high-glycemic foods promote overeating. When the glycemic index is used as a rationale to eat more high-protein and high-fat animal products, it will have no beneficial effect on weight and can create serious health risks.

A Zone of Contention — Dozens of Erroneous Claims

In addition to overstating the importance of the postprandial glycemic index, Sears makes other faulty claims to support his unhealthful recommendations. Sears ignores the wealth of information showing a vast biochemical difference between plant and animal proteins. It doesn't matter whether this difference is due to amino acid patterns or the packaging. Plant proteins lower cholesterol and cancer risk, while animal proteins cause them to rise.[33]

Second, Sears even goes so far as to claim that vegetarian diets are bad for the heart and that patients on Dean Ornish's vegetarian diet will have more heart attacks and die sooner than the patients on the American Heart Association diet. Sears states, "My guess is that the people who stay on his program will ultimately have more heart attacks, more strokes, and a higher cardiovascular death rate than the dropouts. . . . For these people, a high-carbohydrate diet will induce an overproduction of bad eicosanoids, thus greatly increasing their risk of cardiovascular disease." Dr. Ornish has been popular since his "Lifestyle Heart Trial" was published in the *Lancet* in 1991. This study documented the reversal of coronary blockages in heart disease patients eating vegetarian diets. Sears is wrong again — this time, with deadly advice for the heart patient. There are at least seventeen studies to date, including Ornish's follow-up study, that have proved Sears wrong.[34] The patients who have continued the Ornish program have improved their condition over time.

Even more ridiculous is his claim that Ornish's patients developed more insulin resistance because of their high-carbohydrate diet, in spite of an average weight loss of twenty-four pounds. Probably every nutritional scientist and physician in America knows that insulin levels and insulin resistance parallel body weight.[35] That is basic Physiology 101.

Sears goes on to state that eicosanoids are the body's super hormones that control the appearance of every disease, from heart disease and cancer to autoimmune illnesses and obesity. Furthermore, to keep these eicosanoids in proper balance, you need a precise ratio of protein to carbohydrate — three grams of protein to every four of carbohydrate. There is no scientific evidence to back these bold claims. There are no studies to suggest his assertions, and Sears has never measured the eicosanoid levels of people on his diet.

In fact, we now have studies that look at insulin response and insulin resistance and the ability to lose weight. In these studies, Sears's views do not hold up to scientific scrutiny. When overweight individuals with varying degrees of insulin resistance and high insulin levels were put on weight-loss diets, it was found in spite of a wide discrepancy in insulin responses, there was no relationship between insulin levels and the ability to lose weight.[36] Insulin levels, insulin resistance, and the insulin response to meals did not hinder the ability to lose weight — not in the short run, not in the long run.[37] The nutritional quality of the diet makes the difference in controlling appetite, not choosing foods based on insulin response.

Sears makes dozens of other ridiculous claims that contradict the scientific literature. Everything from athletes performing better on high-fat diets to the effect of eating rice on heart attack rates in Japan and China.

	SEARS'S ZONE MENU	FUHRMAN'S EAT TO LIVE MENU
Total calories	1,409	1,600
Fiber	17.2 gm	77 gm
Protein	96 gm	60 gm
Fat	58 gm	19 gm
Carbohydrate	132 gm	314 gm
Saturated fat	20 gm	2 gm
Sodium	4,130 mg	592 mg
B-carotene	**274 mcg**	**8,260 mcg**
Vitamin C	160 mg	625 mg
Calcium	742 mg	877 mg
Magnesium	227 mg	593 mg
Iron	9 mg	22 mg
Manganese	1.5 mg	8.1 mg
Vitamin E	7.6 IU	22 IU
Folate	**211 mcg**	**1,242 mcg**
Chromium	.067 mg	.168 mg

The low levels of beta-carotene and folate on the Sears Zone menu is a good marker of the low level of other plant-derived anti-cancer phytonutrients.

Just a Second-Rate Low-Calorie Diet

The final death blow to Sears's diet is that it is based on extreme calorie restriction and is not maintainable by anyone, not even him. John McDougall, M.D., and others have correctly pointed out that nobody could follow a Zone diet for long.[38]

According to his book, Barry Sears weighs 210 pounds and is 6 feet 5 inches. He says he eats 100 grams of protein a day, as that is what he calculates is best for him. Based on the 30:30:40 ratio that he insists is the key to good health, his Zone diet consists of:

100 grams protein	= 400 calories
44 grams fat	= 400 calories
133 grams carbohydrates	= 530 calories
TOTAL	1,330 calories

Like all extreme calorie-restricted diets, how long could an active six-foot-five male eat this way? Clearly, Sears could not have followed his own diet for long; he admits to losing only thirty-five pounds over the past four years.

If Sears consumed only 1,330 calories daily and was six-five, and his caloric needs, even with no exercise, were about 2,400 calories daily, he would be over 1,000 calories short every day. One pound of fat amounts to 3,500 calories, so Sears would have been losing two pounds a week on his diet. Since he says he has been on his diet for over four years, he should have lost over four hundred pounds! In a debate with Sears, McDougall asked him: Did you start your diet at over six hundred pounds? Do you defy the laws of nature? Or is it that you cannot and do not follow your own diet?

Since he did not lose more than nine pounds per year, he must have consumed at least 2,300 calories daily. If he is following his own rules — that to be in the Zone, you must adhere to a 30:30:40 ratio — he must be eating 173 grams of protein and 77 grams of fat. Therefore, he must be in the extremely high-protein, high-fat zone. Sears denies eating more than 44 grams of fat a day; if he is telling the truth, then he is on only 100 grams of protein and 44 grams of fat — so he must consume 1,500 calories a day from carbohydrates. That would place him out of his Zone, with 17 percent protein, 17 percent fat, and 66 percent carbohydrate. Sears most likely eats a high-carbohydrate diet himself, closer to the one recommended in this book than to his own diet. Sears couldn't answer these questions and changed the subject.

Many of the Zone followers have become disenchanted, gained all their weight back, and given up hope.

Unfortunately, any person entering his Zone with a daily consumption of twelve ounces of animal products is entering the high cancer zone as well!

There is a clear, linear relationship between animal-food consumption and both heart disease and cancer. Sears's goal of about 60 percent of total caloric intake from fat and protein a day places his devotees at the highest worldwide consumption of animal products. Accordingly, they should expect to experience a similarly high incidence of the killer diseases that afflict Americans.

In contrast, I repeat my recommendation regarding animal foods, to make sure my message is absolutely clear: excess consumption of animal foods has repeatedly been shown to be dangerous. No more than 10 percent of one's total calorie consumption should come from animal foods. There is insufficient data at this point to suggest that there is a clear longevity advantage from adhering to a pure vegan diet (one entirely free of animal foods). However, the scientific literature suggests that there is a longevity advantage to dropping your animal-food consumption to as little as one or two servings per week. The most consistent finding in the nutritional literature throughout every epidemiological study is that as fruit and vegetable consumption increases in the diet, chronic diseases and premature deaths decrease.

Elevated Insulin Levels — A True Measure of Cardiac Risk

An elevated (fasting) insulin level may be as powerful a predictor of future heart disease as a high blood cholesterol level. As stated earlier, insulin level parallels excess abdominal fat stores. The thicker your waist, the more insulin is pumped out by the pancreas.

Insulin is a hormone that is secreted by the pancreas and transports sugar from the blood into your cells. High levels of blood sugars drive up insulin in order to help "clear" the blood of the excess sugars. Fat on our body makes our cells resistant to the effects of insulin, and the pancreas must respond with higher production.

A Finnish study that started in 1971 tracked 970 policemen for twenty-two years. Their ages ranged from thirty-four to sixty-five years old. All participants showed no sign of heart disease, diabetes, or other cardiovascular disease when the study started. During the twenty-two years of follow-up, the men with the highest insulin levels had more than double the heart attack occurrence of those with lower levels. The researchers have suggested that the predictive power of insulin levels was of the same magnitude as that of cholesterol levels.[39] A tape measure around the waist would have shown the same results.

So, it certainly is true — as the advocates of animal-food-rich diets, such as Atkins, Heller, Sears, and others proclaim — carbohydrates drive up insulin levels temporarily. These writers, however, have not presented the data in an accurate fashion.

A diet revolving around unrefined carbohydrates (fruits, vegetables, whole grains, and legumes) will not raise blood sugars or insulin levels. Studies have shown that such a diet can reduce fasting insulin levels 30–40 percent in just three weeks.[40] Obviously, a low-fat diet that is high in refined sugars and refined carbohydrates and low in fiber is *not* a healthy diet. To lump refined and unrefined carbohydrates together is inaccurate and misleading.

Center your diet on "whole," unrefined, unprocessed carbohydrates — fruits, vegetables, and legumes — and you will be doing your heart and your health a "whole" lot of good!

A Different Diet for Each Blood Type?

Another bestseller, *Eat Right for Your Type,* by Peter D'Adamo, teaches us that the four different blood types require four very different eating plans. He explains:

1. Type O blood people (the Hunters) are designed for a lot of meat and will hurt themselves with wheat and beans. He asserts that "the gluten lectins inhibit your insulin metabolism, interfering with the efficient use of calories for energy. . . . Certain beans and legumes, especially lentils and kidney beans, contain lectins that deposit in your muscle tissues, making them more alkaline and less 'charged' for physical activity. Type O's have a tendency to low thyroid function."
2. People with type A blood (the Cultivators) should eat a vegetarian diet, as they are biologically predisposed to heart disease, cancer, and diabetes. D'Adamo interestingly lists vegetable oil as a food that encourages weight loss for this blood type.
3. Type B blood people (the Nomads) do well with a varied diet and extra dairy products. They are resistant to heart disease and cancer, but more prone to immune system disorders like multiple sclerosis and lupus. Meat and liver encourage weight loss in type B blood individuals, according to D'Adamo, and he recommends that Caucasians and African individuals with blood type B consume six to ten ounces of cheese weekly.
4. People with type AB blood require a mixed diet, some meat, but not chicken. D'Adamo writes: "So, although you are genetically programmed for the consumption of meats, you lack enough stomach acid to metabolize them efficiently, and the meat you eat tends to get stored as fat."

I tried hard to be fair to D'Adamo because I know there is some evidence in the scientific literature that genetics and even blood type can predispose one to certain illnesses, such as heart attacks and some cancers, but his claims are so ridiculous that it leaves me with no choice but to be amazed that he could actually make such mind-boggling claims without supporting documentation or scientific studies. Furthermore, in reviewing the references mentioned in his book, he did not include even a small fraction of the hundreds of studies performed on this subject by scientists in the past thirty years. All the major studies I found documenting the relationship between blood type and disease were surprisingly missing.

Since D'Adamo did not supply the scientific references to back up his claims, I first did a complete Medline search for all articles in the scientific literature over the past thirty years on the association between ABO blood type and various diseases, as well as all the available literature on lectins. I read more than two hundred scientific articles to see if D'Adamo has any scientific support for his claims. I figured this was more research than most readers would do before evaluating his far-fetched opinions.

What I found was that the scientific literature does support a slight increased risk of coronary heart disease in blood type A, about average risk in type B and AB, and a slightly decreased risk of early cardiac death in type O.[41] One study showed that type AB had the highest risk of fatal cardiac events, and another larger study that examined 7,662 men in twenty-four British towns found a slightly higher incidence of ischemic heart disease in people with type A blood.[42] Of course, they did find quite a large percentage of heart patients with type O blood, and many towns with the largest number of type O people had the most heart disease.

In another study that looked at a consecutive series of 191 patients undergoing coronary bypass surgery, there was a disproportionately large number of patients with type O blood undergoing bypass.[43] The conclusion of these researchers was that ABO-related factors have had an insignificant impact on the evolution of coronary artery disease. Obviously, type Os are not immune to the damage from eating a diet rich in animal products, saturated fat, and cholesterol.

Over 95 percent of Americans develop atherosclerotic heart disease or cancer, not just the type As. We are all susceptible to the nutritional inadequacy present in our diet. In spite of the fact that those with type O blood are a touch more resistant to certain cancers and coronary thrombosis, they still need to eat less animal food and more fruits and vegetables if they hope to obtain a long, disease-free life.

Encouraging animal-product consumption in any blood group is detrimental to their long-term health.

All of us, of every blood type, will develop atherosclerosis — and most of us will die of it — if we eat the American diet. And your risk of a premature cardiac death might be even greater if you follow the diets recommended by D'Adamo for type Os and type Bs.

Heart disease and certain illnesses do have genetic factors that place some of us at higher risk than others. Heart disease or atherosclerosis is genetically heterogeneous. This means that there are many genes that affect your risk. Blood type is only one of many genetic markers involved and represents only a small percentage of genetic susceptibility on the human genome. That blood groups show a slight tendency to increased risk is consistent with the accepted view that genetics plays a role in determining risk. For example, the genetic influence on HDL cholesterol levels has a strong influence on longevity, independent of blood type.[44]

When considering all the genetic risk factors together, we must conclude that environmental influences on atherosclerosis are much stronger than the genetic ones. Even if we combined all the genetic influences and stratified the risk of heart disease or cancer in individuals in a more accurate way than blood type alone, we would still find that environmental factors are more important. Cholesterol levels, body weight, smoking, physical activity, food choices, and blood pressure have been shown to have a much stronger influence on disease risk than blood grouping.[45]

4 Blood Types, 4 Diets, 4 Get It!

D'Adamo's book mixes some interesting factual information about blood types with a whole lot of far-fetched assertions that have no basis in fact. Most of them are just plain wrong.

He makes many unscientific and incorrect claims that show a poor understanding of human physiology. Do fattening, calorie-rich foods such as vegetable oils become weight-loss-promoting foods when consumed by a blood type A? Do these individuals not obey the first law of thermodynamics, as do the other blood types? Does meat cause weight gain when we don't secrete enough acid to digest it properly, as D'Adamo asserts? Many of his claims run contrary to established concepts in human physiology, and he suggests wild theories without supporting evidence. For example, is the amount of acid secreted by the stomach linked to blood type? Was this ever scientifically investigated? He produces no study that illustrates this.

D'Adamo needs to review a little basic physiology; for one thing, acid doesn't digest protein anyway. Pepsin does.

Glands in the mucous membrane lining of the stomach store pepsinogen, an inactive protein. The hormones gastrin and secretin stimulate the release of pepsinogen into the stomach, where it is mixed with hydrochloric acid and converted into its active enzyme, pepsin. Acid merely creates the optimal pH (between 2 to 4) to activate pepsinogen and change it into its active form, pepsin.[46] If it were true, as D'Adamo claims, that a certain blood type could secrete a little more or less acid, it would have little or no effect on the ability to digest animal protein. Except in the elderly, low acid levels in the stomach are exceedingly rare.[47] It is almost unheard-of that individuals can't secrete enough acid to effectively lower stomach pH to convert pepsinogen to pepsin. One concerned about having insufficient stomach acid could always draw a serum gastrin, a fairly reliable method of detecting bona fide hypochlorhydria, or low stomach acid.[48]

Having AB blood type with lower gastric acid secretion wouldn't make eating meat more fattening anyway, contrary to what D'Adamo claims. The incompletely digested proteins would pass on down and get degraded by intestinal bacteria, reducing the absorption of amino acids and contributing to caloric loss and weight loss, not weight gain.

Do blood type Os have a tendency toward low thyroid function because, as D'Adamo states, "type Os tend not to produce enough iodine"? First of all, our bodies do not produce any minerals, such as iodine. Iodine, as well as other minerals, can be absorbed only from what we consume in our diet. And if that is not bad enough, the only medical study I could find regarding the claim that type Os have a tendency to low thyroid function illustrated the exact opposite. Excessive thyroid function was found to be more common in type O individuals, and low thyroid function was more common in type As.[49] Then D'Adamo states that foods such as salt and liver encourage weight loss in these type Os. Is he serious?

One could go on and on explaining his errors and omissions, but the main point is that the book is too inaccurate to take seriously, and despite the real relationship of certain blood types and genetic risks, we all need to minimize our risk of heart attack and cancer by eating the most nutritionally dense and phytochemically strong diet as possible. D'Adamo's dietary recommendations are simply not based on solid science.

We Are All Genetically Different

The concept that sometimes people need to adjust their diet in order to accommodate genetic individuality is not without merit. For example, darker-skinned people of African descent clearly do not tolerate dairy products well and have a higher incidence of lactose intolerance than those of Scandinavian descent. After thousands of years of their northern European ancestors consuming a dairy-rich diet, they are better equipped to digest milk products. Scandinavian countries, where people consume lots of dairy, also have the highest heart attack and cancer rates in the world. This means that the ability to digest and consume a certain food does not make the body impervious to the damage caused by that food. Scandinavians are still humans and they still kill themselves prematurely with their high consumption of dairy and other animal-based foods, just as most of you will if you continue to eat significant quantities of these foods.

The Attack of the Lectins — Great Science Fiction

D'Adamo doesn't just paint a picture of genetic predisposition to disease; he prescribes certain good foods and bad foods for each blood type merely on the basis of his own questionable observations, which he considers scientific. He claims that certain high-calorie foods cause weight loss in certain blood types and that other low-calorie, nutrient-dense foods cause weight gain, depending on blood type. He offers food choices, herbal remedies, supplemental plans, exercise programs, antibiotic preferences, and all types of specific advice based merely on a person's blood type. He is right that we are all different to a degree; however, our differences are complex and involve more than just a few glycoproteins in our red blood cells.

He does not produce a single scientific reference to establish his basic premise that sensitivity to plant lectins on hundreds of foods is governed by blood type. His theory hinges on the action of lectins, proteins found on and in certain foods, which can cause serious illness and even death if consumed by the wrong blood type. He claims that when the wrong food is consumed by the wrong blood type, red blood cell agglutination (clumping) occurs, along with other serious and cancer-causing changes. Patients come into my office after reading his book fearing for their lives if they eat a food that D'Adamo claims is dangerous for their type. But when we compare the information presented by D'Adamo with the information that is available in the scientific literature, the picture just doesn't match.

Again, part of what D'Adamo says is true, but his interpretation is so exaggerated and distorted as to make his assertions almost valueless. Not all lectins are toxic; most are even nutritious, with significant beneficial effects. Only some lectins are truly toxic, such as in red kidney beans, and need to be destroyed by cooking prior to eating. But most other lectins, such as tomato lectins, have been shown to be harmless. The beneficial effects of plant lectins include anti-tumor and anti-cancer activity, meaning they inhibit the induction of cancer by carcinogens.[50] Some of the most fascinating and consistently observed biochemical effects of plant lectins are their inhibitory effect on protein synthesis in abnormal or malignant cells, but not in normal cells. They may prove to be a useful tool in treating cancer in the future.

D'Adamo states on page 27 of his book that "the effects of lectins on different blood types are not just a theory. They're based on science." His conclusion, he explains, has been made on the basis of urinary indican readings in his patients. However, indican in the urine does not register antibody-antigen reaction or agglutination.[51] This outmoded test is notoriously unpredictable and is also affected by unabsorbed protein. D'Adamo also claims that his conclusions have been based on the agglutination he saw in blood exposed to food-derived lectins. Don't think agglutination on a microscopic slide means much — our blood is supposed to agglutinate when removed from the body and exposed to air. To call his unjustified conclusions and his wild claims scientific is an insult to every legitimate scientist.

On a positive note, D'Adamo's book raises the awareness of the potential problems of lectins in certain foods and the likelihood that some of us may be genetically sensitive to specific food lectins. It is controversial whether lectins are a significant contributor to disease, but the evidence is suggestive. This is a valuable subject to pursue, and possibly D'Adamo's work will lead to more research on this subject.

Many lectins are powerful allergens in susceptible people and may partially explain food sensitivities that do not correspond with IgE (the typical allergy) blood testing. Of particular interest is the implication for autoimmune disease, such as rheumatoid arthritis, and true to the suspicion, many rheumatoid arthritis patients note worsening reactions after eating various foods.[52]

For many rheumatoid arthritis patients who are diet-sensitive, one of the most common food triggers is wheat. The wheat lectin is attracted to n-acetyl glucosamine, a molecule exposed in the joints of rheumatoid arthritis patients.[53] Wheat, corn, soy, and dairy are typical pain triggers for patients with rheumatoid arthritis.[54]

Many people are sensitive to wheat and dairy. They feel better and have fewer allergic reactions, regardless of blood type, when they reduce or remove wheat and dairy from their diet. We just can't credit D'Adamo's blood-type theory as the reason for their feeling better when they restrict wheat and dairy.

A Confusing Array of Weight-Loss and Health Opinions

What is truly astonishing is that D'Adamo's book, without scientific support or even scientific plausibility, can become a bestseller. The popularity of his book hammers home the point that Americans are totally confused and misinformed about nutrition. Scientific-sounding, attention-grabbing gimmicks can impress the average consumer, who is attracted to ideas and books that have a trick or a hook, such as food combinations or magic healing foods.

Just so you don't think I am against every diet program that is not my own, there are other weight-loss programs that are based on science. They differ somewhat in their interpretation of the scientific literature and are generally not as nutritionally aggressive as my plan. The main drawback to some of these other worthwhile books is that they may not be effective enough for the individual with a serious metabolic hindrance to weight loss. Here is a suggested reading list for those interested in other viewpoints:

> *The McDougall Program for Maximum Weight Loss,* by John McDougall, M.D.
> *Turn Off the Fat Genes,* by Neal Barnard, M.D.
> *The Volumetrics Weight-Control Plan,* by Barbara Rolls, Ph.D., and Robert Barnett
> *The New Pritikin Program,* by Robert Pritikin
> *Eat More, Weigh Less,* by Dean Ornish, M.D.
> *The Anti-Aging Plan,* by Roy Walford, M.D.

Most Weight Loss Plans Are a Waste of Your Money

What is wrong with every single commercial weight-loss program? They are all too high in fat and too low in fiber because they cater to the American love affair with rich, high-fat food.

Weight Watchers' brand foods contain 24 percent of calories from fat. Lean Cuisine contains 25 percent of calories from fat. The Jenny Craig program requires the purchase of packaged meals with entreés such as cheese soufflé and Salisbury steak, meals that are almost as bad as what most Americans eat at home. These commercial diet plans, since they are not very low in fat, must restrict portion sizes to offer "low calorie" meals. These "skimpy" portions represent an obsolete approach with a dismal track record.

It is merely a matter of time before those trying to keep their portions small increase the amount of food they are eating. The amount of fiber is insufficient and the nutrient density of the diet is poor. These diets restrict calories, but because the food choices and meal plans are so calorie-dense, the dieters must eat tiny portions in order to lose weight. These choices don't satisfy our desire to eat, and we wind up craving food and becoming frustrated. When dieters can't stand eating thimble-size portions anymore and finally eat until satisfied, they put weight on with a vengeance. You may be able to hold your breath under water for a short period, but when you resurface you will be hungry for air and will be forced to speed up your respiratory rate. In a similar manner, if you cannot eat small portions forever, it just isn't likely to work for long.

You can't eat out of boxes and consume powdered drinks forever, either. If you do lose some weight, you will always gain it back. Instead, *permanent* changes in your eating habits must be made. Learning new recipes and adopting different ways of eating that you can live with will maintain your weight loss and protect your health for the rest of your life.

You will be amazed how easily and effortlessly you will lose weight when you adopt a diet that consists primarily of fresh fruits, vegetables, whole grains, and beans. This is a diet with less than 15 percent of calories from fat. I can assure you that the fat will effortlessly melt away from your body. I know how often you have heard that promise. This time it is true.

The result of denying yourself food is that when you go back to eating normally, fat accumulates even more easily than before be-

cause of a low metabolic rate. This leads to the familiar yo-yo phenomenon in which dieters lose some weight, only to rebound to a
heavier weight than when they started.

In contrast, I tell my patients to eat as much food as they can. In
fact, when they are eating foods that are rich in water-soluble fiber
and have high nutrient-per-calorie density, they can literally "stuff
themselves to health" and still enjoy substantial weight loss. You get
the best results by keeping the micronutrients high and the macronutrients moderate. The caloric intake is comparatively low to the
American norm, on this healthiest of all diets, but there is no metabolic rebound, because it is exceedingly rare for someone to gain all
this knowledge and then go back to unhealthy eating again. They are
too informed, and too impressed with their health improvements, to
go back and gamble away their newfound health. On top of that, my
patients have been weaned from their desire for rich, fatty food.

So, instead of searching for weight-loss gimmicks and tricks, try
to adopt a resolution to be healthy first. Focusing on your health,
and not your weight, will eventually result in achieving successful
long-term weight loss. Eating a healthy diet, one that is rich in an assortment of natural plant fibers, will help you crave less and feel satisfied without overeating. All diet plans fail because they cater to
modern American tastes, which include too much processed foods or
animal products to be healthy.

Stop measuring portions and trying to follow complicated formulas. Instead, eat as many vegetables, beans, and fresh fruits as possible, and less of everything else. Any other program is an insult to
your intelligence.

Nutritional Wisdom Makes You Thin

N ow that we've cleared up some of the misinformation crowding the bookshelves in the diet and nutrition section at bookstores, we can go on to analyze food components. After reading this chapter, you will understand *how* eating lots of nutrient-dense foods will make you lose weight.

Unrefined Carbohydrates Encourage Weight Loss

Our bodies need carbohydrates more than any other substance. Our muscle cells and brains are designed to run on carbohydrates. Carbohydrate-rich foods, when consumed in their *natural state*, are low in calories and high in fiber compared with fatty foods, processed foods, or animal products.

Fat contains about nine calories per gram, but protein and carbohydrates contain approximately four calories per gram. So when you eat high-carbohydrate foods, such as fresh fruits and beans, you can eat *more* food and still keep your caloric intake relatively low. The high fiber content of (unrefined) carbohydrate-rich food is another crucial reason you will feel more satisfied and not crave more food when you make unrefined carbohydrates the main source of calories in your diet.

It is usually the small amount of added refined fat or oils that makes natural carbohydrates so fattening. For example, one cup of mashed potatoes is only 130 calories. Put just one tablespoon of butter on top and you have added another 100 calories.

Protein, fat, and carbohydrates are called *macronutrients*. Vitamins and minerals are referred to as *micronutrients*. All plant foods are a mixture of protein, fat, and carbohydrate (the macronutrients). Even a banana contains about 3.5 percent protein, almost the same as mother's milk. Fruit and starchy vegetables, such as sweet potatoes, corn, carrots, and butternut squash, are predominantly carbohydrate but also contain some fat and protein. Green vegetables are about half protein, a quarter carbohydrate, and a quarter fat. Legumes and beans are about half carbohydrate, a quarter protein, and a quarter fat.

One of the principles behind the health and weight-loss formula in this book is not to be overly concerned about the macronutrient balance; if you eat healthful foods, you will automatically get enough of all three macronutrients as long as you do not consume too many calories from white flour, sugar, and oil. So don't fear eating foods rich in carbohydrates and don't be afraid of eating fruit because it contains sugar. Even the plant foods that are high in carbohydrate contain sufficient fiber and nutrients and are low enough in calories to be considered nutritious. As long as they are unrefined, they should not be excluded from your diet. In fact, it is impossible to glean all the nutrients needed for *optimal* health if your diet does not contain lots of carbohydrate-rich food.

Fresh fruits, beans and legumes, whole grains, and root vegetables are all examples of foods whose calories come mainly from carbohydrate. It is the nutrient-per-calorie ratio of these foods that determines their food value. There is nothing wrong with carbohydrates; it is the empty-calorie, or refined, carbohydrates that are responsible for the bad reputation of carbs.

Understanding the Concept of Caloric Density

Because meats, dairy, and oils are so dense in calories, it is practically impossible for us to eat them without consuming an excess of calories. These calorie-rich foods can pile up a huge number of calories way before our stomachs are full and our hunger satisfied. However, eating foods higher in nutrients and fiber and lower in calories allows us to become satiated without consuming excess calories.

MORE BULK MEANS FEWER CALORIES

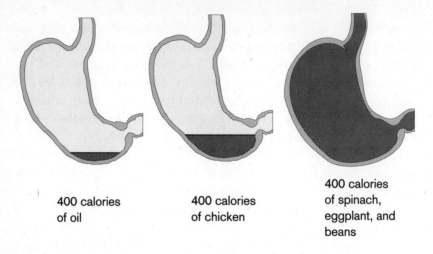

400 calories
of oil

400 calories
of chicken

400 calories
of spinach,
eggplant, and
beans

When subjects eating foods low in caloric density, such as fruits and vegetables, are compared with those consuming foods richer in calories, those on meal plans with higher calorie concentrations were found to consume twice as many calories per day in order to satisfy their hunger.[1]

Interestingly, the Chinese, who on average consume more calories, are thinner than Americans.[2] In China the calorie intake per kilogram of body weight is 30 percent higher than in the United States. The Chinese eat about 270 more calories per day than Americans, yet they are invariably thin. Exercise cannot fully explain this difference, as researchers discovered the same thing with Chinese office workers as well.

This may be because calories from carbohydrates are not as likely to increase body fat as the same number of calories from high-fat foods such as oils and meats, which make up such a high proportion of the American diet. The data suggests that when a very low fat diet is consumed (15 percent average dietary fat in rural China), as compared to the typical Western diet (30–45 percent of calories from fat), more calories are burned to convert carbohydrate into fat, so the body cannot store fat easily.

Your body must burn about 23 percent of the calories consumed from carbohydrates to make the conversion from glucose into fat, but it converts food fat into body fat quickly and easily. One hundred calories of ingested fat can be converted to ninety-seven calories of body fat, burning a measly three calories. So the fat you eat is easily and rapidly stored by the body.

Converting food fat into body fat is easy; the process doesn't even modify the molecules. Research scientists can actually take fat biopsies off your hips or waist and tell you where it came from — pig fat, dairy fat, chicken fat, or olive oil; the fat is still the same as it was on your plate, but now it is under your skin. The saying "from your lips to your hips" is literally true. Fat is also an appetite stimulant — the more you eat, the more you want.

Foods That Make You Thin

Appetite is not controlled by the weight of the food but by fiber, nutrient density, and caloric density. It is even useful to approximate the amount of calories per volume. Since the stomach can hold about one liter of food, let's look at how many calories are in a whole stomachful of a particular food.

It's pretty clear which foods will let you feel full with the least amount of calories — fruits and green vegetables. Green vegetables, fresh fruits, and legumes again take the gold, silver, and bronze medals. Nothing else in the field is even close.

CALORIC RATIOS OF COMMON FOODS

	CALORIES PER POUND	CALORIES PER LITER	FIBER GRAMS PER POUND
Oils	3,900	4,100	0
Potato chips or french fries	2,600	3,000	0
Meat	2,000	3,000	0
Cheese	1,600	3,400	0
White bread	1,300	1,500	0
Chicken and turkey (white meat)	900	1,600	0
Fish	800	1,400	0
Eggs	700	1,350	0
Whole grains (wheat and rice)	600	1,000	3
Starchy vegetables (potatoes and corn)	350	600	4
Beans	**350**	**500**	**5**
Fruits	**250**	**300**	**9**
Green vegetables	**100**	**200**	**5**

Green vegetables are so incredibly low in calories and rich in nutrients and fiber that the more you eat of them, the more weight you will lose. One of my secrets to nutritional excellence and superior health is the one pound–one pound rule. That is, try to eat at least one pound of raw green vegetables a day and one pound of cooked/steamed or frozen green vegetables a day as well. One pound raw and one pound cooked — keep this goal in mind as you design and eat every meal. This may be too ambitious a goal for some of us to reach, but by working toward it, you will ensure the dietary balance and results you want. The more greens you eat, the more weight you will lose. The high volume of greens not only will be your secret to a thin waistline but will simultaneously protect you against life-threatening illnesses.

THE NUTRIENT-DENSITY LINE

The nutrient-density scores below are based on identified phytochemicals, antioxidant activity, and total vitamin and mineral content.

Highest nutrient density   Lowest nutrient density
= 100 points   = 0

100   Raw leafy green vegetables (darker green has more nutrients)
      romaine lettuce, leaf lettuces, kale, collards, spinach, Swiss chard, parsley, daikon

97   Solid green vegetables (raw, steamed, or frozen)
      artichokes, asparagus, bok choy, broccoli, Brussels sprouts, cabbage, celery, cucumber, kohlrabi, okra, peas, peppers, snow peas, string beans, zucchini

50   Non-green, non-starchy vegetables
      beets, eggplant, mushrooms, onions, tomatoes, yellow and red peppers, bamboo shoots, water chestnuts, cauliflower

48   Beans/legumes (cooked, canned, or sprouted)
      red kidney beans, chickpeas, pinto beans, cowpeas, navy beans, cannellini beans, soybeans, lentils, white beans, lima beans, pigeon peas, black-eyed peas, black beans

45	Fresh fruits
	apples, apricots, bananas, blackberries, blueberries, cantaloupes, grapefruits, grapes, kiwis, mangoes, nectarines, all melons, oranges, peaches, pears, persimmons, pineapples, plums, raspberries, strawberries, tangerines, watermelons
35	Starchy vegetables
	white potatoes, sweet potatoes, butternut squash, acorn squash, winter squash, parsnips, pumpkins, turnips, corn, carrots, chestnuts
22	Whole grains
	barley, buckwheat, millet, oats, brown rice, wild rice, quinoa
20	Raw nuts and seeds
	almonds, cashews, filberts, macadamias, pecans, pine nuts, pistachios, pumpkin seeds, sunflower seeds
15	Fish
13	Fat-free dairy
11	Wild meats and fowl
11	Eggs
8	Red meat
4	Full-fat dairy
3	Cheese
2	Refined grains (white flour)
1	Refined oils
0	Refined sweets

Vegetables have powerful levels of carotenoids and other nutrients that prevent age-related diseases. For example, the leading cause of age-related blindness in America is macular degeneration. If you eat greens at least five times per week, your risk drops by more than 86 percent.[3] Lutein and zeaxanthin are carotenoids with powerful disease-prevention properties. Researchers have found that those with the highest blood levels of lutein had the healthiest blood vessels, with little or no atherosclerosis.[4]

LUTEIN AND/OR ZEAXANTHIN IN FOODS[5] (in micrograms)

1 cup cooked kale	28,470
1 cup cooked collard greens	27,710
1 cup cooked spinach	23,940
1 cup cooked Swiss chard	19,360
1 cup cooked mustard greens	14,850
1 cup chopped red pepper	13,600
1 cup cooked beet greens	11,090
1 cup cooked okra	10,880
4 cups romaine lettuce	12,770

Nutrient: Weight Ratios Are Misleading

William Harris, M.D., performed an analysis of major food groups, though he didn't assign phytochemical activity, titled "Less Grains, More Greens."[6] Dr. Harris explains in detail why ranking and analyzing foods by nutrient:weight ratios, the nutritional establishment's usual method, is ill advised and misleading.[7]

People do not eat until a certain weight of food is consumed but rather until they are calorically and nutritively fulfilled. He compares an analysis of spinach with that of spinach with water added (spinach soup) and shows how the weight (added water) does not change the nutrients received. If we analyze the nutrients by weight, we incorrectly think spinach with water added is much less nutritious.

Furthermore, Harris explains why the food industry, especially the producers of animal products, is opposed to nutrient:calorie analysis. It is because nutrient-per-weight sorting hides how deficient animal foods are in nutrients, especially the crucial anti-cancer nutrients. As Dr. Harris states, nutrient weight sorting is "a great way to keep excess calories, cholesterol and saturated fat in the diet, which is a splendid way to grow an arteriosclerotic, obese, cancer-ridden nation, which is what we have."

Fats Are Essential

It is true that most of us eat too much fat, but scientific research is revealing that too little fat can be a problem, too. We have learned that not merely are we consuming too much fat but, more important, we are consuming the wrong fats. Americans consume too much of some bad fats and not enough of other fats that we need to maximize health.

Essential fatty acids (EFAs) are polyunsaturated dietary fats that the body cannot manufacture, so they are required for health. EFAs are important for the structure and function of cell membranes and serve as precursors to hormones, which play an important role in our health. These fats are essential, not only in growth and development but also in the prevention and treatment of chronic diseases.[8]

The two primary essential fatty acids are linoleic acid, an omega-6 fat, and alpha-linolenic acid, an omega-3 fat. The body can make other fatty acids, called nonessential fats, from these two basic fats. Linoleic acid's first double bond is at the location of its sixth carbon, so it is called an omega-6 fatty acid, and alpha-linolenic acid's first double bond is on its third carbon, so it is called an omega-3 fatty acid.

OMEGA-6 FAT	OMEGA-3 FAT
Linoleic acid	**Linolenic acid**
▼	▼
GLA (gamma linolenic acid)	EPA (eicospentainoic acid)
▼	▼
AA (arachidonic acid)	DHA (docosahexainoic acid)
▼	▼
pro-inflammatory prostaglandins and leukotrienes	**anti-inflammatory prostaglandins and leukotrienes**

Optimal health depends on the proper balance of fatty acids in the diet. The modern diet that most of us eat supplies an excessive amount of omega-6 fat, but often too little omega-3 fat. This relative deficiency of omega-3 fats has potentially serious implications. Also, the consumption of too much omega-6 fat leads to high levels of arachidonic acid (AA). Higher levels of arachidonic acid can promote inflammation.

When we have insufficient omega-3 fat, we do not produce enough DHA, a long-chain omega-3 fat with anti-inflammatory effects. High levels of arachidonic acid and low levels of omega-3 fats can be a contributory cause of heart disease, stroke, autoimmune diseases, skin diseases, depression, and possibly increased cancer incidence.[9]

Most Americans would improve their health if they consumed more omega-3 fats and less omega-6 fats. I recommend that both vegetarians and nonvegetarians make an effort to consume one to two grams of omega-3 fat daily.

ADD A FEW GRAMS OF OMEGA-3 FAT TO YOUR DIET

Flaxseed	1 tablespoon	1.7 grams
Flax oil	1 teaspoon	2.2 grams
Walnuts, English (12 walnut halves)	4 tablespoons	2 grams
Soybeans (green, frozen, or raw)	1½ cup	2 grams
Tofu	1½ cup	2 grams

A diet very high in omega-6 fat makes matters worse; your body makes even less DHA fat. We need enough DHA fat to ensure optimum health. The high level of omega-6 fat competes for the enzymes involved in fatty acid desaturation (conversion to longer-chain fats) and interferes with the conversion of alpha-linolenic acid (omega-3) to EPA and DHA. Therefore, our high fat intake contributes to our DHA fat deficiency.

Our modern diet, full of vegetable oils and animal products, is very high in omega-6 fat and very low in omega-3 fat; the higher the omega-6 to omega-3 ratio, the higher the risk of heart disease, diabetes, and inflammatory illnesses.[10]

Saturated fat, cholesterol, and trans fat also interfere with conversion to DHA. Much of the beneficial effects of a diet rich in plant foods are the low level of saturated fat and trans fat (harmful fats), and the relatively high level of essential fatty acids (beneficial fats). Both meat-based diets and vegetarian diets can be deficient in these healthy fats if they do not contain sufficient green leaves, beans, nuts, seeds, or fish. So, eat less of the fatty foods you usually consume and eat more walnuts, flaxseed, soybeans, and leafy green vegetables.

The Fat Dictionary

All fats are equally fattening — containing nine calories per gram, compared with four calories per gram for carbohydrates and protein.

SATURATED FAT Some naturally occurring fats are called *saturated* because all the carbon are single bonds. These fats are solid at room temperature and are generally recognized as a significant cause of both heart disease and cancer. Saturated fats are found mainly in meat, fowl, eggs, and dairy. Coconut and palm oil are largely saturated and are also not desirable. The foods with the most saturated fat are butter, cream, and cheese.

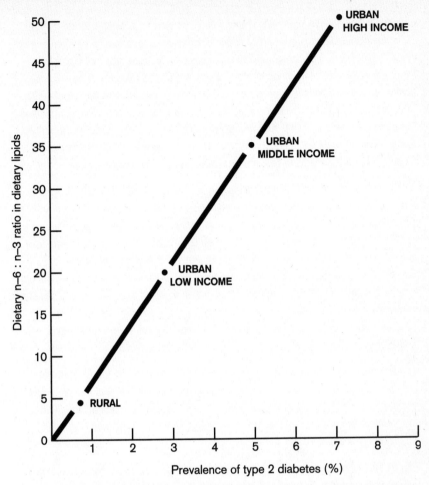

Diabetes is only one of many diseases linked to excessive omega-6 fats. From A. P. Simopoulos, "Essential Fatty Acids in Health and Chronic Disease," *American Journal of Clinical Nutrition* (September 1999).

UNSATURATED FAT These fats are a mix of monounsaturated and polyunsaturated fat. Eating unsaturated fats lowers cholesterol when substituted for saturated fats, but excessive amounts may promote cancer.

POLYUNSATURATED FAT These fatty acids have more than one double bond in their chain. These fats include corn oil, soybean oil, safflower oil, and sunflower oil. They are soft at room temperature. These fats promote the growth of cancer in lab animals more than olive oil (a monounsaturated fat) does.

MONOUNSATURATED FAT These fats have only one double bond in their carbon chain. They are liquid at room temperature and thought to have health benefits. The supposed health benefits of these fats appear when these fats are used in place of dangerous saturated fats. Even polyunsaturated oils will lower cholesterol if used in place of saturated fat. Monounsaturated fat is found in avocados, almonds, peanuts, and most other nuts and seeds. Keep in mind that no isolated or refined fat, even these monounsaturated fats, should be considered health food. Oils with the highest percentage of monounsaturated fats include olive, canola, and peanut oils.

HYDROGENATED FAT Hydrogenation is a process of adding hydrogen molecules to unsaturated fats, thereby turning these oils, which are liquid at room temperature, into harder, more saturated fats such as margarine. Hardening the fat extends its shelf life so the oil can be used over and over again to fry potatoes in a fast-food restaurant or be added to such processed food as crackers and cookies. While hydrogenation does not make the fat completely saturated, it creates *trans fatty acids,* which act like saturated fats. Evidence is accumulating to implicate the harmful nature of these man-made fats in both cancer and heart disease. Avoid all foods whose ingredients contain partially hydrogenated or hydrogenated oils.

CHOLESTEROL is a waxy fat produced by the body and found in animal foods such as meat, fowl, dairy, and eggs. Eating cholesterol raises blood cholesterol, but not as much as eating saturated fats and trans fats. The amount of cholesterol in plants is so negligible that you should consider them cholesterol-free.

DHA FAT is a long-chain omega-3 fat that is made by the body, but it can also be found in fish, such as salmon and sardines. DHA is used in the production of anti-inflammatory mediators that inhibit abnormal immune function and prevents excessive blood clotting. DHA is not considered an essential fat, because the body can manufacture sufficient amounts if adequate short-chain omega-3 fats are consumed (flax, walnuts, soybeans, leafy green vegetables). However, because of genetic differences in the enzyme activity and because of excess omega-6 fats, many people who do not consume fish regularly are deficient in this important fat.

ARACHIDONIC ACID is a long-chain omega-6 fat produced by the body, but it is also found in meat, fowl, dairy, and eggs. Products formed from excessive amounts of this fatty acid have the potential to increase inflammation and are disease-causing. They may increase high blood pressure, thrombosis, vasospasm, and allergic reaction. They are linked to arthritis, depression, and other common illnesses.

There's Something Fishy about Fish Oils

Most of the publicity about the beneficial effects of essential fats has focused on fish oils, which are rich in EPA, an omega-3 fat. One problem with fish oils is that much of the fat has already turned rancid. If you have ever cut open a capsule of fish oil and tasted it, you will find it tastes like gasoline. Not only are many people intolerant of the burping, indigestion, and smelling like a fish, but it is also possible that the rancidity of the fat places a stress on the liver. I have noted abnormal liver function on the blood tests of a few patients who were taking fish oil tablets. These few patients had their liver function return to normal when they stopped taking the fish oils.

Large amounts of fish oils inhibit immune function.[11] Lowering the function of natural killer cells is not a good thing, as our defenses against infection and cancer diminish. Because of this immune suppression, as well as the toxicity issues, I do not routinely recommend that my patients take fish oil capsules — though there are a few exceptions.

This ability of fish oils to decrease the activity of the immune system makes them useful for some patients with autoimmune illness, such as rheumatoid arthritis or inflammatory bowel disease. Some rheumatoid arthritis patients are "fish oil responsive," and many others are not. I often perform a three-month trial of fish oil supplementation to determine a patient's responsiveness. With such patients, the risks of the added oil are minimal compared with the potential benefits, especially if they can avoid toxic drugs.

Another case in which fish oils may be useful is the rare individual who does not convert omega-3 fats into DHA sufficiently. These people may be more prone to depression, allergies, and inflammatory skin disease such as eczema. There are blood tests available for a physician to analyze the fatty acid balance on red blood cell membranes and thereby determine a deficiency of DHA or omega-3 fat. These people often benefit from the addition of fish oils or plant-derived DHA. Laboratory-cultivated DHA made from microalgae is a pure form of DHA without rancidity, mercury, or other toxins. It is well tolerated and does not have a rancid taste or odor.

Does Fish Prevent Heart Disease?

There are two components to a heart attack or stroke. First, you must develop atherosclerotic plaque. This plaque builds up over many years from eating a diet deficient in unrefined plant foods. Almost all Americans have such plaque. Autopsy studies demonstrate athero-sclerosis even in the vast majority of American children.[12]

Once these fatty plaques accumulate and partially block a coro-nary artery, a clot can develop in a defect or crack in the surface of the plaque. This clot is called a thrombus, which can enlarge and completely block the vessel, causing a heart attack, or break off and travel upstream, obstructing a more distal coronary site. A traveling thrombus is called an embolus. Emboli and thrombi are the cause of almost all heart attacks and strokes.

Fish contains omega-3 fatty acids (EPA and DHA) that interfere with blood clotting much the same way aspirin does. Once you have significant atherosclerosis, it is helpful to take such anti-clotting agents, especially if you continue a dangerous diet. These fish-derived fats also have some effect on protecting the arterial walls from dam-age from other fats. For people eating saturated fat containing animal products, it is advisable to consume one or two weekly portions of fatty fish, such as sardines, salmon, trout, halibut, or mackerel, and reduce the consumption of other animal products accordingly. In-creasing fish intake beyond one or two servings per week has not been shown to offer additional protection.[13]

However, the best way to prevent a heart attack or stroke is to follow a high-nutrient diet with little or no animal products, thereby ensuring that such blockages don't develop in the first place. Then eating fish won't matter. It is true that increasing blood levels of these important fish-derived fats reduces the incidence of heart attacks sig-nificantly.[14] However, contrary to popular belief, not only vegetarians but most others eating diets with adequate plant material get most of their long-chain omega-3 fatty acids from non-fish sources.[15] In fact, the reason the fish-derived fats, EPA and DHA, are not considered es-sential fats is that almost all people have enzymes to convert the plant-derived omega-3 fat rapidly into EPA and DHA.[16]

Fish is a double-edged sword, especially because fish has been shown to increase heart attack risk if it is polluted with mercury.[17] Keep in mind that even though men in Finland consume lots of fish, their mortality from coronary heart disease is one of the highest in the world.[18] It seems that the cardioprotective effects of eating a little fish is lost when you eat lots of fish, most likely because lots of fish exposes you to high mercury levels, which can promote lipid peroxidation.[19] Lipid peroxidation occurs when body lipids react with oxygen to cause a compound that plays a major role in the development of diseases such as heart disease, diabetes, and arthritis.

In addition, those who consume fish in the hope of reducing their cardiac risk may be getting more than they bargained for — namely, toxic contaminants, including some that carry a cancer risk.

Fish is one of the most polluted foods we eat, and it may place consumers at high risk for various cancers. Scientists have linked tumors in fish directly to the pollutants ingested along the aquatic food chain, a finding confirmed by the National Marine Fisheries Service Laboratory. In some instances, such as with the PCBs in Great Lakes trout and salmon, it can be shown that a person would have to drink the lake water for 100 years to accumulate the same quantity of PCB present in a single half-pound portion of these fish, reported John J. Black, Ph.D., senior cancer research scientist for the Roswell Park Memorial Institute to the American Cancer Society.[20] From the flounder in Boston Harbor to English sole in Puget Sound, scientists report that hydrocarbon pollution from habitat concentrate in fish. There are high cancer rates around New Orleans, where fresh fish and shellfish are a staple of the local cuisine.

FISH WITH HIGHEST AND LOWEST MERCURY LEVELS

HIGHEST	LOWEST
tilefish	salmon
swordfish	flounder
mackerel	sole
shark	tilapia
white snapper	trout
tuna	

Source: Mercury levels in seafood species. U.S. Food and Drug Administration, Center for Food Safety and Applied Nutrition. Office of Seafood, May 2001.

Higher levels of mercury found in mothers who eat more fish have been associated with birth defects, seizures, mental retardation, developmental disabilities, and cerebral palsy.[21] This is mostly the result of women having eaten fish when they were pregnant. Scientists believe that fetuses are much more sensitive to mercury exposure than are adults, although adults do suffer from varying degrees of brain damage from fish consumption.[22] Even the FDA, which normally ignores reports on the dangers of our dangerous food practices, acknowledges that large fish such as shark, swordfish, and yellowfin and bluefin tuna, are potentially dangerous. Researchers are also concerned about other toxins concentrated in fish that can cause brain damage way before the cancers caused by chemical-carrying fish appear.

Fish may also lower the effectiveness of our immune system. Those on high fish diets have lower blood markers of immune system function, representing a lowered defense against infection and cancer.[23] Another problem with fish is that because these fish oils inhibit blood clotting, they increase the likelihood that the delicate vessels in the brain can bleed, causing a hemorrhagic stroke. At the same time fish reduces the risk of heart attacks, it may be increasing the risk of a bleeding problem. Regular fish consumption or fish oils should be avoided if a person has a family history or is at risk of hemorrhagic stroke or other bleeding disorders.

The bottom line: Choose fish over other animal products, but be aware that the place where it was caught, and the type of fish, matters. Don't accept recreational fish from questionable waters. Farmed fish is safer. Never eat high-mercury-content fish. Don't eat fish more than twice a week, and if you have a family history of hemorrhagic stroke, limit it further to only once a month.

Extracted Oils, One Slick Customer

Americans consume large quantities of oil, a refined food, processed at high temperatures. When oils are subject to heat, the chemical structure of the essential fatty acids are changed to toxic derivatives known as lipid peroxides and other toxic and potentially cancer-causing by-products.[24] Clearly, it is best to avoid fried foods and heated oils, not only because they will destroy your chances to achieve a normal weight but because they are also potentially cancer-causing.

Get your fats as nature packaged them. It is best to consume the little fats we need in their original unprocessed, unheated, and natural packages: whole food. Ground flaxseed is healthier than flaxseed oil, as it contains valuable fiber, lignans, and other phytonutrients, not just omega-3 fat. Raw sunflower seeds, pumpkin seeds, corn, olives, and avocados are healthy, but their extracted oils may not be. Even cold-pressed oils are subject to the damaging effects of heat and contain lipid peroxides. So I usually recommend to my patients that instead of consuming the oils, they consume a tablespoon of ground flaxseed daily, or some walnuts, to ensure adequate omega-3 fat intake.

Remember, when you extract the oil from the whole food it was packaged in, you remove it from its antioxidant- and phytochemical-rich protective environment. You turn a moderate nutrient-to-calorie food into a low nutrient-to-calorie food, and at the same time damage the quality of the fat with heat. Romaine lettuce, kale, collards, and Swiss chard are rich in fiber, vitamins, minerals, phytochemicals, vegetable protein, and essential fats — again, another reason I consider leafy green vegetables the king of all foods.

Your diet should not be fat-free. Indeed, it would be nearly impossible to make this diet fat-deficient, because even green vegetables and beans contain beneficial fats. The focus should be on reducing (or removing) the harmful and processed fats, and instead consuming the healthy fats that are naturally contained in whole natural foods. Nonprocessed fats contained in avocados, sunflower seeds, and almonds, to name just a couple of sources, can be healthy additions to a wholesome diet of natural foods. Even though these foods have lots of calories, they pack a significant nutritive punch; they are rich in vitamin E and other antioxidants and are not nutrient-depleted the way the oil is when it is extracted, processed, and put in a bottle.

Be aware, however, that unless you are physically very active and slim, you should watch the amount of these relatively fat-rich plant products, as they obviously will interfere with reaching your ideal weight. If you are slim and exercise regularly, you can consume three to four ounces of raw nuts or seeds daily, an avocado, or a little olive oil. Growing children, or an individual who is having difficulty gaining weight, can eat a little more dietary fat, but it still should mostly be fat from the wholesome foods described above.

When you are overweight, you have a good store of fat on your body, so you don't need to worry about not ingesting enough fat. You are not going to become fat-deficient, even if your diet is low in fat. As you lose weight, you will actually be on a "high-fat diet," as you will be utilizing the fat you have around your midsection for energy. The only concern is to maintain a healthy fatty acid ratio, so I advise ingesting one tablespoon of ground flaxseed every day, if possible. Many like to sprinkle it over fruit or add it to a salad.

Is There an Increased Risk of Stroke from Low-Fat Diets?

There is considerable evidence that while animal fats are definitely associated with an increase in heart disease, more fat *may* offer protection against hemorrhagic stroke at the same time.[25] Of course, recent investigations have shown the strong protective effects of fruits and vegetables, but apparently some data suggests that fat, even animal fat, offers some protection to the smaller intracerebral vessels that cause hemorrhagic strokes.[26]

There are two main types of strokes: ischemic and hemorrhagic. Almost all heart attacks and the vast majority of strokes are associated with ischemia (lack of blood flow) from blood clots. The small percentage of strokes that are hemorrhagic (approximately 8 percent) result not from a cholesterol-laden vessel leading to a clot but from a rupture of a small artery in the brain as a result of years and years of high blood pressure.[27] Some of these small, fragile blood vessels in the brain possibly become more resistant to rupture when they are more diseased with fat. It is entirely possible that in certain cases, the same diet that leads to abnormal clot formation and causes 99 percent of heart attacks and over 90 percent of strokes may help the small intracerebral vessels resist the tendency to rupture from years of uncontrolled hypertension that results from a high-salt diet. This is in no way a legitimate excuse to eat more saturated fat. It makes more sense to eat the healthful anti–heart attack diet and keep your blood pressure down by not consuming much added salt.

The data is so confusing because many of the studies group all types of strokes together, when they are in fact very different diseases with completely different causes. Considering embolic strokes, the data from both human and rat studies illustrates the importance of adequate essential omega-3 fat intake, including an increased omega-3: omega-6 ratio.[28] These omega-3 fats are the same ones that protect against heart attacks, which are also of an embolic nature. Keep in mind, *saturated fat intake has consistently been associated with an increase in strokes in general* because most strokes are of the ischemic (embolic) variety.[29]

Finally, to make things even more confusing, some monounsaturated fat intake offers a degree of protection against strokes and does not have the cholesterol-raising and other negative effects of saturated fats.[30] The studies showing the nutritional value of mono-unsaturated fats lend support to the Mediterranean diet and those advocating a diet rich in olive oil. Obviously, some omega-6 fat is still essential and necessary for normal disease resistance.

My view is that thin individuals should consume more monoun-saturated fats from wholesome high-fat vegetation such as avocados, raw nuts, and seeds. Heavier people, because of their higher risk of heart disease, diabetes, and cancer as well as the very limited occur-rence of hemorrhagic stroke in the overweight, should limit their in-take of these fats. Since heavier people have more stored fat on their body, they do not benefit from a higher intake of dietary fat the same way thin individuals do. As the overweight lose weight, they are al-ready on a high-fat diet, consuming their stored body fat.

Let me remind you that the best fats are the monounsaturated fats and essential fats (omega-3 and omega-6) present in whole, nat-ural plant foods, including avocados, olives, and raw nuts and seeds. Studies continue to show that consumption of raw nuts protects against both heart attack and stroke, without the risks of increasing heart disease and cancer, as is the case with the high consumption of animal-origin fats.[31] When the fats you consume are from whole food, rather than oil, you gain nature's protective package: a balance of vitamins, minerals, fibers, and phytonutrients.

Trans Fat: A Wolf in Sheep's Clothing

Which is worse for your heart and your waistline — a McDonald's Quarter Pounder, a large order of fries, Dunkin' Donuts, or a Häagen-Dazs ice cream?

The answer is that it doesn't matter; they all contain significant disease-promoting substances such as saturated fat or trans fat. Dough-nuts and french fries are fried in partially hydrogenated oil, rich in trans fats. A doughnut could be worse for you than eating eight strips of bacon. Even Oreo cookies, Wheat Thins, and other cholesterol-free foods are deceptively dangerous.

Trans fats do not exist in nature. They are laboratory-designed and have adverse health consequences. They interfere with the body's production of beneficial fatty acids and promote heart disease.[32] As trans fatty acids offer no benefits and only clear adverse metabolic consequences, when you see the words *partially hydrogenated* on the side of a box, consider it poisonous and throw it in the trash.

The government doesn't require manufacturers to disclose how much trans fat is in their products. Trans fats are surely cancer-promoting and raise your cholesterol as much as saturated fat.[33] Considering that they also reduce HDL (the good cholesterol), trans fats may be even more atherogenic than even saturated fatty acids.[34] Convincing evidence from the Nurses Health Study and others indicate that trans fats are as closely associated with heart attacks as the fats in animal products.[35]

In a press release in 1990, McDonald's announced, "McDonald's french fries to be cooked in cholesterol-free 100 percent vegetable oil." The switch was to partially hydrogenated vegetable shortening. Now all the fast-food giants — McDonald's, Burger King, Wendy's, Arby's, and Hardee's, as well as almost every brand of french fries in the freezer case of your supermarket — are just as bad for your heart as if they were fried in pig fat.

Trans fats are found ubiquitously in processed food: crackers, cookies, cakes, frozen foods, and snacks. Most of these enticing desserts, fried foods, and convenience foods are deadly, heart-attack-causing foods, even if they contain no animal products and no cholesterol, because of the trans fats they contain. Even Orville Redenbacher's natural microwavable popcorn contains artery-clogging trans fats.

More than two years ago, the Center for Science in the Public Interest petitioned the FDA to count trans fat as saturated fat on labels and to ban claims like "low cholesterol" or "low saturated fat" on foods that are high in trans fats. The FDA may eventually move forward; meanwhile, those in the nutritional know are outraged by the FDA's political catering to the food manufacturers, when we know these fats are responsible for as much as 25 percent of all heart attacks.

The Fatty Conclusion

There is no question that a high-fat diet increases the risk of many cancers. This has been demonstrated in hundreds of animal and human studies. An extensive overview of the fat-diet link recently published in the *American Journal of Clinical Nutrition* concludes that it's not only the *amount* of fat but the *type* of fat that is linked to increased risk (just like the type of protein). It gets complicated, so here are the main points:

1. Any extracted oil (fat) can promote cancer because consuming even the healthiest fats, such as olive oil, in excess adds too many empty calories. Excess calories have toxic effects, contributing to obesity, premature aging, and cancer.
2. Excess omega-6 fatty acids promote cancer risk, while omega-3 fats, which are harder to come by, tend to lower risk. Omega-6 fats are found in polyunsaturated oils like corn oil and safflower, whereas the omega-3 fatty acids are rich in seeds, greens, and some fish.
3. The most dangerous fats for both heart disease and cancer are saturated fats and trans fatty acids. You would be foolish not to carefully avoid these. Trans fats may raise breast cancer risk by as much as 40 percent.[36] They are the fats listed as partially hydrogenated on the food labels.
4. Whole natural plant foods (whole grains, greens, nuts, and seeds) supply adequate fat. If you eat an assortment of natural foods, you will not be deficient in fat. We do not need to take fish oil, evening primrose oil, or any other oil when we eat healthy foods.

Remember, a low-fat diet can be worse than a higher-fat diet if it has more saturated fat or trans fat and if it contains an excessive amount of refined carbohydrates. The type of fat is more important than the amount of fat. Data from the Nurses Study also found that nurses eating more monounsaturated fats and polyunsaturated fats were less likely to suffer from heart disease than nurses on a lower-fat diet.[37]

Taking a careful look at the data, it appears that it was the percentage of calories from animal foods and the amount of saturated fat in the diet that correlated with heart attack risk, rather than the total amount of fat. Animal products, dairy, eggs, chicken, turkey, and red meat contain the most dangerous type of fat.

Note that lean meat or fowl, which contains two to five grams of fat per ounce, contains less fat, less saturated fat, and fewer calories per ounce than cheese, which has eight to nine grams of fat per ounce. And cheese has much more saturated fat (the most dangerous fat), about ten times as much saturated fat as chicken breast.

Cheese is the food that contributes the most saturated fat to the

	PERCENTAGE OF CALORIES FROM FAT	PERCENTAGE OF FAT THAT IS SATURATED FAT
Cream cheese	89	63
Gouda cheese	69	64
Cheddar cheese	74	64
Mozzarella cheese	69	61
Mozzarella cheese, part skim	56	64
Kraft Velveeta Spread	65	66
Kraft Velveeta Light	43	67
Ricotta, whole milk	68	64
Ricotta, part skim	51	62

American diet and is one of the most dangerous foods in the world to consume. Though it tastes good, it should be used very rarely, if at all. Most cheeses are more than 50 percent of calories from fat, and even low-fat cheeses are very high-fat foods.

Americans have this fetish with watching fat and forgetting everything else we know about nutrition. Fat is not everything. If the fats you consume are those healthy fats found in raw seeds, nuts, and avocados, and if your diet is rich in unrefined foods, you needn't worry so much about the fat — unless you are overweight.

The take-home message regarding fat is this: Avoid saturated fats and trans fats (hydrogenated fats) and try to include some foods that contain omega-3 fat in your diet.

Giving Up the Myths about Protein — Like Changing Your Religion

Remember those four basic food group charts we all saw in every classroom in elementary school? Protein had its own box, designated by a thick steak, a whole fish, and an entire chicken. Dairy foods had their own special box as well. A healthy diet, we were taught, supposedly centered on meat and milk. Protein was thought to be the most favorable of all nutrients, and lots of protein was thought to be the key to strength, health, and vigor. Unfortunately, cancer rates soared. As a result of scientific investigations into the causes of disease, we have had to rethink what we were taught. Old habits die hard; most Americans still cling to what they were taught as children. There are very few subjects that are more distorted in modern culture than that of protein.

Keep in mind that we do need protein. We can't be healthy without protein in our diet. On the other hand, plant foods have plenty of protein, and you do not have to be a nutritional scientist or dietitian to figure out what to eat and you don't need to mix and match foods to achieve protein completeness. Any combination of natural foods will supply you with adequate protein, including all eight essential amino acids as well as unessential amino acids.

It is unnecessary to combine foods to achieve protein completeness at each meal. The body stores and releases the amino acids needed over a twenty-four-hour period. About one-sixth of our daily protein utilization comes from recycling our own body tissue. This recycling, or digesting our own cells lining the digestive tract, evens out any variation from meal to meal in amino acid "incompleteness." It requires no level of nutritional sophistication to get sufficient protein, even if you eat only plant foods.

It is only when a vegetarian diet revolves around white bread and other processed foods that the protein content falls to low levels. However, the minute you include unprocessed foods such as vegetables, whole grains, beans, or nuts, the diet becomes protein-rich.

Green Grass Made the Lion

Which has more protein — oatmeal, ham, or a tomato? The answer is that they all have about the same amount of protein per calorie. The difference is, the tomato and the oatmeal are packaged with fiber and other disease-fighting nutrients, and the ham is packaged with cholesterol and saturated fat.

Some people believe that only animal products contain all the essential amino acids and that plant proteins are incomplete. False. They were taught that animal protein is superior to plant protein. False. They accept the outdated notion that plant protein must be mixed and matched in some complicated way that takes the planning of a nuclear physicist for a vegetarian diet to be adequate. False.

I guess they never thought too hard about how a rhinoceros, hippopotamus, gorilla, giraffe, or elephant became so big eating only vegetables. Animals do not make amino acids from thin air; all the amino acids originally came from plants. Even the nonessential amino acids that are fabricated by the body are just the basic amino acids that are modified slightly in some way by the body. So the lion's muscles can be composed of only the protein precursors and amino acids that the zebra and the gazelle ate. Green grasses made the lion.

PROTEIN CONTENT OF COMMON FOODS
IN INCREASING ORDER OF PROTEIN PER CALORIE

	PROTEIN (GRAMS)	CALORIES	PROTEIN PER CALORIE	PERCENT PROTEIN
One banana	1.2	105	0.01	5
One cup of cooked brown rice	4.8	220	0.02	9
One corn on the cob	4.2	150	0.03	11
One baked potato	3.9	120	0.03	13
One cup of regular pasta	7.3	216	0.03	14
One 6-oz. fruit yogurt	7.0	190	0.04	15
Two slices of whole-wheat bread	4.8	120	0.04	16
One Burger King cheeseburger	18.0	350	0.05	21
Meatloaf with gravy (Campbell's)	14.0	230	0.06	24
One cup of frozen peas	9.0	120	0.08	30
One cup of lentils (cooked)	16.0	175	0.09	36
One cup of tofu	18.0	165	0.11	44
One cup of frozen broccoli	5.8	52	0.11	45
One cup of cooked spinach	5.4	42	0.13	51

Note that green vegetables have the most protein per calorie of all the above.

I see about twenty to thirty new patients per week, and I always ask them, "Which has more protein — one hundred calories of sirloin steak or one hundred calories of broccoli?" When I tell them it's broccoli, the most frequent response I get is "I didn't know broccoli had protein in it." I then ask them, "So where did you think the calories in broccoli come from? Did you think it was mostly fat, like an avocado, or mostly carbohydrate, like a potato?"

People know less about nutrition than any other subject. Even the physicians and dietitians who attend my lectures quickly volunteer the answer, "Steak!" They are surprised to learn that broccoli has about twice as much protein as steak.

When you eat large quantities of green vegetables, you receive a considerable amount of protein. Remember, one 10-ounce box of frozen broccoli contains more than ten grams of protein.

How Much Protein Do We Need?

Over the years the amount of protein recommended by authorities has bounced up and down like a yo-yo. It wasn't until nitrogen-balance studies became available that we could actually measure protein requirements.

Today the recommended daily allowance (RDA) is 0.8 mg/kg body weight, or about 44 grams for a 120-pound woman and 55 grams for a 150-pound male. This is a recommended amount, not a minimum requirement. The assumption is that about .5 mg/kg is needed, and then a large safety factor was built into the RDA to almost double the minimum requirement determined by nitrogen-balance studies. Still, the average American consumes over 100 grams of protein daily — an unhealthy amount.

Health authorities such as the World Health Organization recommend only 5 percent of calories from protein. In fact, as little as 2.5 percent of calories from protein may be all that is necessary for normal people.[38] Regardless of the many opinions on adequate or optimal protein intake, most plant foods, except fruit, supply at least 10 percent of calories from protein, with green vegetables averaging about 50 percent. The high-nutrient diets that are plant food predominant, like I recommend, supply approximately 40–70 grams of protein daily in the range of 1,200 to 1,800 calories per day. That is plenty of protein.

Furthermore, the outdated notion of "high biological value" protein is based on essential amino acid profiles that grant eggs a 100 percent score based on the nutritional needs of rodents. It should not be surprising that the growth needs of rats are not quite the same as those of humans. For example, birds and rats have high requirements for methionine and cystine, the sulfur-containing amino acids. The sulfur-containing amino acids are important when growing feathers and fur. More recently, the essential amino acid profiles have been updated to reflect more closely the needs of humans. Human breast milk, for example, is lacking if we are considering the nutritional requirements of baby rats, but otherwise ideal when looking at human requirements.

Today, protein scores are computed differently than in the past. They are based on human needs, not rats', and soy protein earns a higher score than beef protein.[39]

Using a computer dietary-analysis program, I tried to compose a natural-foods diet deficient in any required amino acid. It was impossible. Almost any assortment of plant foods contained about 30–40 grams of protein per 1,000 calories. When your caloric needs are met, your protein needs are met automatically. Focus on eating healthy natural foods; forget about trying to get enough protein.

What about the athlete, weight lifter, or pregnant woman? Don't they need more protein? Of course an athlete in heavy training needs more protein. I was on the U.S. World Figure Skating Team in the early 1970s. I often exercised more than five hours daily. Besides all the grueling work on the ice, I did plenty of weight lifting and running. With all that exercise, sure I needed more protein, but I needed lots more of everything, especially calories. When you take in more food, you get the extra protein, extra fat, extra carbohydrates, and the extra nutrients that you need. I loaded up the backseat of the car with huge amounts of fruits, vegetables, raw nuts, and whole grains. I ate lots of food and took in more protein (and everything else) in the process. Your protein needs increase in direct proportion to the increased caloric demands and your increased appetite. Guess what? You automatically get enough. The same is true during pregnancy.

When you meet your caloric needs with an assortment of natural plant foods, you will receive the right amount of protein — not too much, not too little.

Putting the RDAs into Perspective

The RDAs are levels set by our government for various nutrients considered to be desirable for good health. But are they correct? Are these levels appropriate, and will even higher levels of certain nutrients benefit us? Difficult questions to answer, but first we must consider how the RDAs were derived.

The RDAs were first developed when the government began questioning the nutritional value of military rations distributed to our soldiers during World War II. Later, our government's Food and Nutrition Board looked at what foods they *expected* most people to eat. By analyzing the average diet, they came up with a suggested minimum and then added an upward adjustment to theoretically ensure optimal health.

The RDAs are biased in favor of the conventional level of intake. They are not based on how people *should* eat to maintain optimal health; rather, they have been formulated to represent how we *do* eat. They characterize the conventional diet: high in animal products; lots of dairy products and fat; and low in fiber, antioxidants, and other nutrients, such as vitamin C, that are rich in plant foods. The RDAs reflect a diet that caused all the problems in the first place.

So we see a tendency to keep RDAs for plant-based nutrients low while keeping animal-based nutrients high. Take for example the most ridiculous recommendation from the RDA — vitamin C. Any diet utilizing an abundance of unrefined natural plant foods offers a significant quantity of C. The diets I recommend, and consume myself, contain between 500 and 1,500 mg of vitamin C each day, just from food. If you consumed a diet only half as good as I recommend, you would still consume between 250 and 750 mg of vitamin C each day. The RDA of 60 is merely reflective of the inadequacy of the American diet and how impossible it would be to get enough vitamin C if you ate a diet so low in natural plant foods.

You can take 1,000 mg of vitamin C in the form of a pill to make up for how deadly deficient your diet is, but then you would be missing all the other plant-derived antioxidants and phytochemicals that come in the same package as the vitamin C. The government must hold the RDA ridiculously low because it would be inconsistent with the other absurd dietary suggestions and make it impossible to achieve such levels without supplementation.

Most of the dietary recommendations from our government have been discarded and updated over time. Such recommendations, such as the Basic Four Food Group Guide, have always been at least ten years behind current science and strongly influenced by the food manufacturers. The current RDAs should meet the same fate; they are based on outmoded nutritional opinions that do not stand up to scientific scrutiny. Last, and most important, is that thousands of phytonutrients lack RDAs. There are subtle nuances and nutritive interactions that create disease resistance from the synergy of diverse substances in natural food. Like a symphony orchestra whose members play in perfect harmony, the performance of our body depends on the harmonious interaction of nutrients, both known and unknown. By supplying a rich assortment of natural foods, we best maximize the function of the human masterpiece.

Remember the two main messages of this chapter. First, when food is refined and the macronutrients are removed from nature's natural packaging, they assume disease-causing properties. And second, green vegetables ran away with the title and legumes and fresh fruit took home a distant silver and bronze in the nutrient-density Olympics.

Eat to Live Takes On Disease

We are all transformed, not just Rob and me, but a large sea of friends and family who have left the lethal American diet. It was good riddance to my asthma and hypertension. Thanks to you, Dr. Fuhrman, we are all slim and healed!

— Linda and Rob Castagna

Whoever would have guessed that my mother, who lives with me, would lose fifty-eight pounds and no longer need insulin injections after fifteen years of a roller-coaster ride of highs and lows.

— Peggy Fennell

We are living among an addicted population of compulsive eaters, creating allergic and sickly individuals. Eat and live like most Americans and you will eventually suffer from an assortment of ailments, like most Americans.

Good health is not merely the absence of disease. Good health assumes protection from disease in the future and can be predicted only by a healthy lifestyle and diet.

You cannot buy your health; you must earn it through healthy living. Visiting physicians, acupuncturists, chiropractors, homeopaths, naturopaths, osteopaths, and other health providers cannot make you healthy. You can receive *symptomatic* relief for your condition, but treatments do not make you healthy.

For most people, illness means putting their fate in the hands of doctors and complying with their recommendations — recommendations that typically involve taking drugs for the rest of their lives while they watch their health gradually deteriorate. People are completely unaware that most illnesses are self-induced and can be reversed with aggressive nutritional methods.

Both patients and physicians act as though everyone's medical problems are genetic, or assumed to be the normal consequence of aging. They believe that chronic illness is just what we all must expect. Unfortunately, the medical-pharmaceutical business has encouraged people to believe that health problems are hereditary and that we need to swallow poisons to defeat our genes. This is almost always untrue. We all have genetic weaknesses, but those weaknesses never get a chance to express themselves until we abuse our body with many, many years of mistreatment. Never forget, 99 percent of your genes are programmed to keep you healthy. The problem is that we never let them do their job.

My clinical experience over the past ten years has shown me that almost all the major illnesses that plague Americans are reversible with aggressive nutritional changes designed to undo the damage caused by years of eating a disease-causing diet. The so-called balanced diet that most Americans eat causes the diseases Americans get.

These conditions, and many others, can be effectively prevented or treated through superior nutrition. As their medical problems gradually melt away, patients can be slowly weaned off the medications they have been prescribed.

Food Is the Cure

Patients are told that food has nothing to do with the diseases they develop. Dermatologists insist that food has nothing to do with acne, rheumatologists insist that food has nothing to do with rheumatoid arthritis, and gastroenterologists insist that food has nothing to do with irritable and inflammatory bowel disease. Even cardiologists have been resistant to accept the accumulating evidence that atherosclerosis is entirely avoidable. Most of them still believe that coronary artery disease and angina require the invasive treatment of surgery and are not reversible with nutritional intervention. Most physicians have no experience in treating disease naturally with nu-

Dietary-Caused Illnesses with High Prevalence

acne	allergies	angina
appendicitis	asthma	arthritis
atherosclerosis	constipation	colonic polyps
diabetes (adult)	diverticulosis	esophagitis
fibromyalgia	gallstones	gastritis
gout	headaches	hemorrhoids
high blood pressure	hypoglycemic symptoms	indigestion
irritable bowel syndrome	kidney stones	lumbar spine syndromes
macular degeneration	musculoskeletal pain	osteoporosis
sexual dysfunction	stroke	uterine fibroids

tritional excellence, and some physicians who don't know about it are convinced it is not possible.

Not only are common disorders such as asthma associated with increased body weight and our disease-causing diet, but in my experience these diseases are also curable with superior nutrition in the majority of cases.[1] Asthma is an example of a disease considered irreversible that I watch resolve regularly.

My patients routinely make complete and *predictable* recovery from these illnesses, predominantly through aggressive dietary changes. I am always delighted to meet new patients who are ready to take responsibility for their own health and well-being.

You can watch a new you being made by the wisdom of your body, and this new you will result in all your systems and organs, including your brain, functioning better. Depression, fatigue, anxiety, and allergies are also related to our improper diet. The brain and immune system are able to withstand stress better when our body is properly nourished.

I am neither a research scientist nor a writer by profession. I am a practicing physician who sees at least five thousand patients a year. I work with these patients, educating them and motivating them to do more than others have asked them to do. The results I see with my patients are *thrilling*. Diseases that are considered irreversible I see reversed on a daily basis.

Predictable Disease Reversal Is the Rule, Not the Exception

The overwhelming majority of my patients with high blood pressure are able to normalize their readings and eventually go off their medication. The majority of my patients with angina can end their symptoms of coronary artery disease in the first few months on the diet I prescribe. Most of the rest make a recovery, but it takes longer. The point is, they do recover.

More than 90 percent of my Type II diabetics are able to eventually discontinue their insulin within the first month. More than 80 percent of my chronic headache and migraine sufferers recover without medication, after years of looking for relief with various physicians, including headache specialists.

Some people, especially other physicians, may be skeptical. There are so many exaggerated and false claims made in the health field, especially by those selling so-called natural remedies. Nevertheless, it is wrong to underestimate the results obtainable through appropriate but rigorous nutritional intervention. Even many of my patients with autoimmune illnesses (such as lupus, rheumatoid arthritis, asthma, and hyperthyroidism) are able to recover and throw away their medications. The results are so spectacular that I am subjected to skepticism and even periodic expressions of anger from other physicians.

When one of my patients who had a severe case of rheumatoid arthritis went back to her previous physician, a rheumatologist, and told him she was now well and did not require any medication, he replied, "It must just be that you are resting more." She said, "I'm not resting more. In fact, I am more active than ever because my pain is gone, and I stopped the drugs." He replied, "It's just a temporary remission; you'll be back soon with another crisis." She never went back.

On the positive side, more and more physicians are becoming interested in nutritional intervention. Such care is clearly more cost-effective, reduces health-care expenditures, and saves lives. Nothing is more emotionally rewarding for a physician than to watch patients actually get better. How can this not catch on?

An American Has an *Avoidable* Heart Attack Every 30 Seconds

Heart disease is the number one killer in the United States, accounting for more than 40 percent of all deaths. Each year approximately 1.5 million Americans suffer a heat attack or myocardial infarction (MI); nearly 500,000 of them die as a result.[2] Most of these deaths occur soon after the onset of symptoms and well before victims are admitted to a hospital.

Every single one of those heart attacks is a terrible tragedy, as it could have been avoided. So many people die needlessly because of wrong, weak, and practically worthless information from the government, physicians, dietitians, and even health authorities like the American Heart Association. Conventional guidelines are simply insufficient to offer real protection for those wanting to protect themselves from heart disease.

If you are an American over the age of forty, your chance of having atherosclerosis (hardening) of your blood vessels is over 95 per-

Quick Quiz: Heart Disease

1. Percentage of children between the ages of four and eleven who already have signs of heart disease? [3]
   A. None
   B. 10 percent
   C. 40 percent
   D. More than 75 percent

2. Percentage of female heart attack victims who never knew they had heart disease and then die as a result of their first heart attack?[4]
   A. None
   B. 10 percent
   C. 25 percent
   D. More than 75 percent

3. Percentage of heart disease patients who undergo angioplasty and then have their treated arteries clog right back up again within six months? [5]
   A. 5 percent
   B. 10 percent
   C. 30 percent
   D. None of the above

Answers: 1. D   2. C   3.C.

cent. You may think, "Heart disease won't happen to me!" But I have news for you: it has already happened, and your chance of dying from a heart attack because of your atherosclerosis is about 50 percent. Your exercise program and your Americanized low-fat diet won't help you much, either. You need to do more.

American Heart Association Recommendations Are Dangerous

The typical dietary advice, represented by the American Heart Association's guidelines, is still a dangerous diet. It is not likely to protect you from having a heart attack and does not allow heart disease to reverse itself. Moderation kills. The fact is that such dietary advice still allows heart disease to advance in the overwhelming majority of patients.

> **WARNING: Do not merely comply with these overly permissive recommendations of the American Heart Association, or you will most likely die of a heart attack.**
>
> • Total fat intake should be restricted to no more than 30 percent of total calories.
> • Cholesterol intake should be less than 300 mg daily.
> • Salt intake should not exceed six grams of sodium chloride daily.

Just to highlight a small difference between the American Heart Association guidelines and my recommendations: My diets have less than 300 mg of cholesterol and six grams of sodium chloride *per week!* More than a dozen studies have demonstrated that the majority of patients with coronary artery disease who follow an American Heart Association step one or step two diet have their condition worsen.[6] No study has ever shown that the patients who follow an American Heart Association diet can reverse or stop the worsening of coronary artery disease.

In contrast, numerous studies have documented that heart disease is reversible for the majority of patients following a vegetarian diet.[7] Most often these diets, such as the Ornish program, are not even optimal diets, as they do not sufficiently limit processed grains, salt, and other low-nutrient-density processed foods. Nevertheless, they are still effective for most patients.

The medical literature continues to refer to the diet recommended by the National Cholesterol Education Program as "low-fat." By worldwide standards it should be called a high-fat diet, but more important, it should be called a low-nutrient-density diet — one with a dangerously low level of plant-derived nutrients. As a result of following this almost worthless advice, heart disease patients usually eat a diet that derives over 80 percent of its calories from processed foods and animal products.

No matter how poor patients' diet, most claim that they are already on a low-fat diet. They believe that eating a chicken-and-pasta-based diet is in some way healthy merely because they eat less red meat. Yet chicken is almost as dangerous for the heart as red meat; switching from red meat to white meat does not lower cholesterol.[8] Such conventional diets simply do not lower cholesterol sufficiently and do not contain adequate heart-protective factors such as fiber, antioxidants, folate, bioflavonoids, and other phytochemicals.

Another real problem with these so-called low-fat diets is that they are often low in fiber and phytochemical-rich vegetation and may not be carefully designed to include enough of the cardioprotective fats. For example, multiple studies have shown the protective effects of consuming walnuts, which are rich in omega-3 fatty acids. A study of 34,192 Californian Seventh-Day Adventists showed a 31 percent reduction in the lifetime risk of ischemic heart disease in those who consumed raw nuts frequently.[9] The ideal diet for heart disease reversal, then, is free of saturated fat, trans fat, and cholesterol; rich in nutrients and fiber; and low in calories, to achieve thinness. However, it should contain sufficient essential fatty acids, so it is important to add a small amount of nuts and seeds, such as walnuts and flaxseed.

Dramatically Lower Your "Bad" Cholesterol Without Drugs

Some studies published in the past few years have concluded that dietary changes alone are insufficient to alter plasma lipid levels.[10] The message reported in both the lay and medical media is that low-fat diets don't work. This reinforces the concept that there is not much we can do to alter our genetics, except maybe take drugs. Sadly, the diets offered by nutritional authorities are not aggressive enough to offer true protection or to expect predictable recovery in patients with heart disease. These so-called heart-healthy diets are not anything like my diets.

The concern that some medical authorities have regarding "low-fat" diets is that these diets may lower your HDL and raise triglycerides.[11] This is true. Lowering fat intake is not the principal step necessary to achieve a cardioprotective diet. It is not sufficient merely to lower fat intake. If all you do is cut back on fat, you may see little benefit and possibly raise your triglycerides.

However, triglyceride levels increase on low-fat diets only when the diets are *high in refined foods, low in fiber, and unsuccessful in weight reduction.*[12] My observations have been corroborated by other studies.[13] Researchers have compared a high-vegetable-and-fruit diet (like the one recommended in this book) with a grain-based, low-fat diet. Study participants who ate the high-vegetable-and-fruit diet experienced a 33 percent drop in their bad cholesterol (LDL) — a reduction that is greater than most cholesterol-lowering drugs.[14] This reduction is dramatically greater than for subjects eating a grain-rich Mediterranean diet or the modern low-fat diet recommended by the American Heart Association.

I rarely ever see triglycerides rise when patients are placed on my nutrient-dense, high-fiber, low-fat diet. For 95 percent of the patients, triglycerides drop dramatically. This is also because my patients do not overeat; they lose weight because they feel satisfied from all the fiber in the natural foods and because the diet has such a high nutrient-per-calorie density. We watch the triglyceride problem melt away as they lose the unwanted pounds; triglycerides drop precipitously with weight loss.

The conclusion of the nutrition committee of the American Heart Association is something we all agree on:

> There is overwhelming evidence that reduction in saturated fat, dietary cholesterol, and weight offer the most effective dietary strategies for reducing total cholesterol, LDL-C levels, and cardiovascular risk. Decreases in saturated fat should come at the expense of total fat because there is no biological requirement for saturated fat.[15]

So the main difference between my recommendations and those of the American Heart Association is that I adhere more rigorously to these conclusions than they do. You must do what is necessary to achieve the results desired. If you water down the recommendations to make them more politically or socially acceptable, you sell out the people who want real help and are willing to do what is necessary to protect themselves. An example of the results possible with such aggressive dietary intervention is the patient below.

The results I see with my patients are consistently more spectacular than other dietary interventions because my advice is generally

Case Study: Cliff Johnston

Cliff is a chiropractic physician. His father died of heart disease at age forty-seven. Cliff is now forty-five years old. Guess what *he* was headed for? Luckily, he became my patient and was able to get appropriate advice in time.

	8/6/96	9/11/96	% CHANGE
Cholesterol	401	170	−58
Triglycerides	1,985	97	−95
GGT	303	55	−82
Glucose	136	89	−35

The GGT is a parameter of liver function, and the elevated level reflected a degree of fatty infiltration in the liver, negatively affecting its function. The elevated glucose showed the beginning of diabetes. Both were resolved when I placed him on an appropriate diet.

I had originally asked him to wait two months to have his blood redrawn, but he was so enthusiastic and feeling so great because his weight went from 206 to 178 in the one-month period that he came back four weeks early. Can you imagine losing twenty-eight pounds in one month while eating as much food as you like? This is a lot of weight to lose in one month, and is not typical.

more rigorous and takes into account the nutrient-per-calorie density of foods to devise a plant-based diet that is maximally effective.

Some studies from other parts of the world show fairly impressive results, utilizing what they call "anti-atherogenic" vegetarian diets, as illustrated by a Russian study where all types of lipid abnormalities were found to improve significantly.[16]

Caldwell Esselstyn, M.D., of the Cleveland Clinic, offers his patients dietary programs for reversing coronary artery disease. His diet may not be as aggressive as the one I offer my heart disease patients, but he, too, is not satisfied until the total cholesterol is below 150. He has documented his results with consecutive coronary catherizations.[17] The average patient reversed his coronary narrowing by about 7 percent. All of his patients who remained committed to his recommended diet had no further coronary events in the ten years of follow-up. Most of the patients who chose not to follow his aggressive dietary interventions had heart attacks within the decade.

Heart Attack Counterattack

Two things are necessary to predictably reverse heart disease: one is to become thin and superbly nourished, and the other is to get your LDL below 100. Reversal of heart disease then occurs. If one expects to diminish atherosclerotic plaque over time and stabilize the plaque so the chance of having a heart attack significantly decreases, I insist that he or she must strive to achieve the following parameters of normalcy:

- The patient must achieve a normal weight or become thin (less than one inch of abdominal fat in women, and less than three-quarters of an inch in men), or be in the process of steadily losing weight toward this goal.
- The patient must achieve normal cholesterol. My definition of *normal* is an LDL cholesterol below 100 (most authorities are now using this benchmark). Drugs are rarely needed to attain this level when an aggressive nutritional approach is taken.
- The patient's diet must be nutrient-dense. Animal products and detrimental fats must be avoided to prevent the after-meal fat surge.[18] Refined carbohydrates should also be avoided to prevent the after-meal glucose surges and to control triglycerides. Homocysteine levels should be normalized, by supplementation with appropriate nutrients if necessary.
- Blood pressure must return to within the normal range, below 130/85, or be slowly improving and moving toward this minimal goal. The normalization of blood pressure as medications are gradually discontinued represents reversal of atherosclerosis and is an important criterion to predict cardiac safety. The person who has removed his cardiac risk no longer requires blood pressure medication to maintain normal blood pressure readings. The vessels have become more elastic through nutritional intervention.

Angioplasty and Bypasss Surgery Can Be Avoided

My vigorous, nutritionally centered reversal treatment should be started in every patient diagnosed with coronary artery disease before elective revascularization procedures are considered. My experience has shown that most patients will pursue an aggressive regimen when it is supported by a knowledgeable and involved physician who provides sustained guidance and support. After spending adequate time with a doctor reviewing all the risks of the conventional approach and discussing how reversal is possible with aggressive nutritional management, how many patients do you think would choose to have their chests split open with bypass surgery?

Even if you are lucky enough to have no postoperative complications from bypass, some degree of brain injury occurs in almost every patient from the time spent hooked up to the heart-lung machine. On neuropsychological testing six months later, about 20 percent still show deterioration.[19] Brain injury can range from subtle degrees of intellectual impairment or memory loss to personality changes and permanent brain damage.[20]

Even if you do fine after angioplasty, stent placement, or bypass, atherosclerosis develops at a faster rate in those arteries that were subject to bypass or angioplasty — the plaque grows faster after surgery. Approximately one-third of arteries treated by angioplasty clog up again within four to six months.[21] This is called restenosis.

Restenosis is an iatrogenic (physician-caused) disease. Because restenosis involves scarring, it does not behave like native atherosclerosis and does not respond as favorably or as predictably to lifestyle modifications later on. In other words, because of the changes made to the atherosclerotic plaque by the angioplasty treatment, the blockages are less responsive to nutritional intervention when they return. Many patients are worse off after treatment, not better. If they had followed my CAD (coronary artery disease) reversal plan instead, they would be watching their heart get healthier each week.

Stenting attempts to reduce this high risk of restenosis but has not solved the problem.[22] Stents are tiny wire-mesh tubes that are laced in the narrowed segment of arteries that were stretched by balloon angioplasty. The stent may also cause vascular instability or inflammation where the stent ends and the native plaque begins, thus increasing the risk for coronary thrombosis.[23] It would be good to remind patients that revascularization procedures do not influence the underlying disease, because the rest of the coronary vasculature, with diffuse, nonangiographical noticeable atherosclerosis, is still there posing a risk for future cardiac events, whether the procedure is done or not.

Heart attacks most commonly occur when plaque of a lipid-rich segment ruptures. These vulnerable areas of plaque are not necessarily those that are seen as significantly narrowed on catherization.

Heart attacks still occur in the minimally narrowed segments, areas that may appear normal on catherization and stress testing.

Most of an Iceberg Is Hidden Under Water

Your stress test results or cardiac catherization results being normal does not mean you do not have atherosclerosis. You can have a heart attack the day after you are told your vessels are clear. These tests show only advanced disease.

Massive atheromas (fatty deposits) lurking within the vascular wall — outside the view of angiography (cardiac catherization) — account for two-thirds of myocardial infarctions.[24] Most heart attacks occur at sites invisible to the tests done by cardiologists.[25] This is why invasive cardiac procedures relieve pain but do not have an impressive record of reducing the risk of future heart attacks.

Only strong risk-factor control, with aggressive nutritional intervention, can reverse diffuse disease, avoiding the high probability of that heart attack occurring down the road. Your survival depends on risk-factor management — quitting smoking and lowering your weight, blood pressure, glucose, cholesterol, and insulin levels as a result of careful nutrition — not the procedures done by the interventional cardiologist or cardiac surgeon. Only then will beneficial changes occur in the plaque composition, promoting healing of the blood vessel's lining that will stabilize the vessel wall and substantially reduce the risk of a heart attack.

You are deluding yourself if you think chelation or drugs alone will reverse your condition while you remain overweight and nutritionally malnourished. Chelation will not dissolve your atherosclerosis, as claimed. The studies done on this therapy are not impressive.[26] In spite of chelation, patients generally continued to deteriorate unless they changed their diet, lost weight, and lowered their cholesterol. In other words, changes not related to chelation.

The areas of vulnerable plaque that cause heart attacks have a large fatty core of cholesterol. Removing the lipid from the plaque can make it smaller and more resistant to rupture. Use common sense; chelation could no more suck fatty substance out of a coronary artery than it could suck the fat off your left hip. There is no way chelating agents can selectively remove the lipids in atheromas.

These atheromas that form on the inside of our blood vessels are fatty tumors with a fibrous cap. They shrink and become more resistant to rupture proportionally to, and as a result of, weight reduction, caloric restriction, nutritional excellence, and aggressive lipid lowering. The most impressive results of shrinking and removing atheromas occur *after* the person has lost all his excess body fat. Body fat is designed for energy storage. Atheromas are more difficult to remove; they resolve after other fat storage sites have been depleted. Fortunately, the same body that created the atheromas has the ability to disintegrate them.

Many of my patients were first advised by other physicians to undergo angioplasty or bypass. When they refused they were referred to my office and chose aggressive nutritional management. Without exception, they have all done well; chest pain has resolved in almost every case (only one went to repeat angioplasty because of a recurrence of chest symptoms); and none of these patients has died from cardiac disease.

A typical patient is John Pawlikowski. I see patients like him almost every day. John's story is not unusual — but a miracle to him nevertheless. John came to me with a history of steadily worsening angina. His chest pains were increasing. His stress thallium test suggested multivessel coronary artery disease. He underwent a cardiac catherization, which revealed a 95 percent stenosis of the left anterior descending artery, and the left circumflex had diffuse disease, but all less than 40 percent narrowed. He had normal heart function. His cholesterol was 218, he weighed 180 pounds, and he was on two blood pressure medications.

Within a few weeks of following my diet, John's chest pain ceased and he stopped taking nitroglycerin tablets for chest pain relief. In two months his weight dropped to 152 — a loss of 28 pounds in eight weeks. Today, five years later, he still weighs 150, following the same diet. He is well, with no restrictions on his activity, and his blood pressure runs about 128/78. He takes no medication, and his stress test has normalized.

JOHN'S LABORATORY REPORTS

DATE	6/6/94	5/5/99	% CHANGE
Cholesterol	218	161	−26
Triglycerides	140	80	−43
HDL	48	65	35
LDL	144	80	−44
Cholesterol:HDL ratio	4.7	2.4	−49

Revascularization procedures may be necessary in rare circumstances, such as triple vessel disease with reduced cardiac output or an injured (stunned) heart muscle. However, I am convinced that aggressive nutritional therapy with the addition of nutritional supplements (and if needed, medication) will provide a more favorable outcome for the majority of patients than angioplasty, stent placement, and bypass.

One might argue, where are the adequate studies that prove this? But where are the studies to prove revascularization will give a better outcome with a stable patient, without a reduction in cardiac output? The benefits of revascularization procedures for patients with good cardiac function have not been convincingly demonstrated, and there is considerable evidence to suggest that the adverse outcomes outweigh the potential benefits. Furthermore, these dubious results are measured against patients who refuse revascularization and then follow the normal (worthless) dietary recommendations. When we factor in the results I see with very aggressive nutritional management, it seems likely that many patients would be at lower risk if they avoided invasive cardiac procedures and surgery. Fortunately, I am not the only physician in America with this opinion, but it sure seems like it.[27]

Rarely will you find a cardiologist who advises aggressive nutritional therapy before angioplasty or bypass. And physicians who offer medical interventions are usually satisfied if blood pressures are merely below 140/90 and cholesterol levels are under 200. Those levels are not sufficiently normal to offer true protection.

For true protection, do not be satisfied until your total cholesterol is below 150 or your LDL cholesterol below 100. Studies clearly demonstrate that the higher one's cholesterol level, the higher the risk of heart disease; conversely, the lower the cholesterol level, the lower the risk. There is nothing particularly magical about the number 200 — heart disease risk continues to decrease as one's cholesterol level decreases below this level. The *average* cholesterol level in China is 127. The Framingham Heart Study showed that those with cholesterol levels below 150 did not have heart attacks.[28] In fact, most heart attacks occur in patients whose cholesterol runs between 175 and 225, because that is the average range of Americans, and the average American has heart disease. Do you want to be average, or do you want to be healthy?

A more accurate measure of heart disease risk takes into account the proportion of blood cholesterol carried in low density lipoprotein (LDL) and in high density lipoprotein (HDL) particles — the higher the LDL or lower the HDL, the greater the risk of heart disease. So the ratio of LDL to HDL, or the ratio of total cholesterol to HDL, is a better measure of heart disease risk. For example, the typical man in the Framingham study had a total cholesterol:HDL cholesterol ratio of about 5.0, and the typical woman about 4.4.[29] The typical woman who had a heart attack in the Framingham study had a ratio of total cholesterol:HDL cholesterol of about 4.6–6.4, while the typical man had a ratio of about 5.5–6.1. Physicians who ran in the Boston Marathon had an average ratio of 3.4. My patients frequently achieve what would be considered spectacular ratios following my dietary recommendations. It is not unusual for me to see total cholesterol:HDL ratios below 2.0 in those truly eating healthfully. The majority drop below 3.0 after a few years on the program.

Your Doctor Lied: You Do Have High Blood Pressure and High Cholesterol

I know you were told that if your blood pressure is below 140/90, it is normal. Unfortunately, this is not true, either. It is *average* — not *normal*. This number is used because it is the midpoint of adult Americans older than sixty. The risk for strokes and heart attacks starts climbing at 115/70.

In societies where we do not see high rates of heart disease and strokes, we do not see blood pressure increase with age. In rural China the healthy elderly had the same low blood pressure readings as they did when they were kids. Almost all Americans have blood pressure that is unhealthfully high. At a minimum, we should consider blood pressure higher than 125/80 abnormal.

Numerous scientific investigations have shown that the following interventions have some degree of effectiveness in lowering blood pressure:[30]

- Weight loss
- Sodium restriction
- Increased potassium intake
- Increased calcium and magnesium intake
- Alcohol restriction
- Caffeine restriction
- Increased fiber intake
- Increased consumption of fruits and vegetables
- Increased physical activity or exercise

Studies have shown controlling sodium intake and weight loss to be effective in reducing blood pressure, even in the elderly.[31] How can you implement these interventions into your lifestyle? It's simple. Eat many more fruits, vegetables, and legumes; eat less of everything else; and engage in a moderate amount of exercise. High blood pressure is relatively simple to control.

> Though it took a full two years, Rhonda Wilson dropped her weight from 194 to a slim 119. She was also able to come off blood pressure medication as a result of her newfound commitment to a healthful lifestyle. When she first came to me, she was on two medications to control her high blood pressure. These two medications were not sufficient, as her blood pressure was still excessively high. Rhonda did not see normal blood pressure readings for a long time and was not able to stop her blood pressure medication until she became relatively thin. Her story illustrates a common dilemma. It is not unusual for some people to lose some weight, yet still have high blood pressure. Some individuals develop high blood pressure and diabetes even from a small amount of excess body fat. For these individuals, it is even more important to maintain an ideal weight.

I encourage my patients to do what it takes to normalize their blood pressure so they do not require medication. Prescribing medications for high blood pressure has the effect of a permission slip. Medication has a minimal effect in reducing heart attack occurrence in patients with high blood pressure because it does not remove the underlying problem (atherosclerosis), it just treats the symptom. Patients given medication now falsely believe they are protected, and they continue to follow the same disease-causing lifestyle that caused the problem to begin with, until the inevitable occurs — their first heart attack or stroke. Maybe, if high blood pressure medications were never invented, doctors would have been forced to teach healthful living and nutritional disease causation to their patients. It is possible that many more lives could have been saved.

Only You, Not Your Physician, Must Take Full Responsibility

Do not expect to receive valuable health advice from your typical doctor. Physicians usually do not help; they rush through their patient appointments, especially in the current HMO climate, because they are paid so poorly for each visit and are pressured to see as many patients as possible each day. Your physician is likely doing just as poorly as you are and eating just as unhealthfully or worse. After reading this book, you could improve his health and reduce his risk of premature death more than he could help yours. Even when physicians offer their fullest time and effort, their recommendations are invariably too mild to have a significant benefit.

Drs. Randall S. Stafford and David Blumenthal, of Massachusetts General Hospital in Boston, reviewed the records of more than 30,000 office visits to 1,521 U.S. physicians of various specialties and found that doctors measured patients' blood pressure during 50 percent of the visits. However, doctors tested their patients' cholesterol levels only 4.6 percent of the time. Physicians offered patients advice on how to lose weight in 5.8 percent of the visits, and suggestions on how smokers could quit 3 percent of the time. On average, doctors gave patients advice on dietary and other changes that can help lower cholesterol in 4.3 percent of the visits, and advice on exercise in 11.5 percent of the visits. When records were reviewed in those who had cardiovascular disease, the typical (almost worthless) dietary counseling and exercise was usually never even mentioned.[32] Obviously, we have a long way to go.

Diabetes — The Consequence of Obesity

One in twenty people has diabetes in this country, more than 16 million Americans. As our population grows fatter, this figure is climbing. Diabetes is a nutritionally related disease — one that is both preventable and reversible (in the case of Type II diabetes) through nutritional methods.

Diabetes can take a severe toll — causing heart attacks and strokes, as well as other serious complications. More than 70 percent of adults with Type II diabetes die of heart attacks and strokes. The statistics are even more frustrating when you watch people gain weight, become even more diabetic, and develop attendant complications, all while under the care of their physicians.

As our country's weight has risen, diabetes has increased accordingly. The worldwide explosion in diabetes parallels the increase in body weight.

Patients are told to learn to live with their diabetes and to learn to control it because it can't be cured. "No, no, and no!" I say. "Don't live with it, get thin and get rid of it, as many of my patients have!"

There are basically two kinds of diabetes: Type I, or childhood onset diabetes, and Type II, or adult onset diabetes. In Type I, which generally occurs earlier in life, children incur damage to the pancreas — the organ that produces and secretes insulin — so they have an insulin deficiency. In Type II, the most common type, the individual produces near-normal levels of insulin, but the body is resistant to it, so the level of blood sugar, or glucose, rises. The end result is the same in both types — the individual has a high glucose level in his or her blood.

Both types of diabetes accelerate the aging of our bodies. Diabetes greatly promotes the development of atherosclerosis and cardiovascular disease, and it ages and destroys the kidneys and other body systems. Diabetes is the leading cause of blindness in adults and is the leading cause of kidney failure. We witness today a huge number of Type II diabetes patients with terrible complications such as amputations, peripheral neuropathy (painful nerve damage in the legs), retinopathy (the major cause of blindness in diabetics), and nephropathy (kidney damage); it is just as bad as those with Type I diabetes.[33]

Diabetics, regardless of type, have higher levels of triglycerides and increased levels of LDL cholesterol than the general population. Diabetics have more than a 400 percent higher incidence of heart attacks than nondiabetics. One-third of all patients with insulin-dependent (Type I) diabetes die of heart attacks before age fifty. This acceleration of the atherosclerotic process, and the resulting high mortality rate, is present in both types of diabetes.[34]

By simple logic, you would expect that any dietary recommendations designed for diabetics would at least attempt to reduce the risk of heart attack, stroke, or other cardiovascular event. Unfortunately, the nutritional advice given to diabetics is to follow the same diet that has proved not to work for heart disease patients. Such a diet is risky for all people, but for the diabetic it is exceptionally hazardous — it is deadly. The combination of refined grains, processed foods, and animal products guarantees a steady stream of available customers for hospitals and emergency rooms.

When Type I patients take a more aggressive and progressive nutritional approach, they can prevent many of the complications that befall diabetics. They can expect a normal life span, because it is the interaction between diabetes and the disease-causing modern diet that results in such dismal statistics, not merely being diabetic. Type I diabetics will still require some insulin, but often I find my Type I diabetic patients requiring about half as much insulin as they did prior to adopting my lifesaving program. Their sugars don't swing wildly up and down, and since they are using less insulin, they have less chance of developing potentially dangerous hypoglycemic episodes.

Type II diabetics adopting this approach can become undiabetic and achieve wellness and even excellent health. They can be diabetes-free for life! Almost all my Type II diabetic patients are weaned off insulin in the first month. Thanks to their excellent nutrition, these patients have much better (lower) blood sugars than when they were on insulin. The horrors of diabetes about to befall them are aborted.

I have also observed patients who came to me with diabetic retinopathy and peripheral neuropathy gradually improve and eventually resolve their conditions. Dr. Milton Crane reported similar findings in his patients: seventeen out of twenty-one patients who adopted a plant-rich vegan diet obtained complete relief from their peripheral neuropathy.[35]

Insulin for Type II Diabetes Makes Things Worse

Insulin works less effectively when people eat fatty foods or gain weight. Diets containing less fat improve insulin sensitivity, as does weight loss.[36] An individual who is overweight requires more insulin, whether he or she is diabetic or not. In fact, giving overweight diabetic people even more insulin makes them sicker by promoting weight gain. They become even more diabetic. How does this process work? Our pancreas secretes the amount of insulin demanded by the body. A person of normal weight with about a third of an inch of periumbilical fat will secrete X amount of insulin. Let's say this person gains about twenty pounds of fat. His body will now require more insulin, almost twice as much, because fat on the body blocks the uptake of insulin into the cells.

If the person is obese, with more than fifty pounds of additional fat weight, his body will demand huge loads of insulin from the pancreas, even as much as ten times more than a person of normal weight needs. So what do you think happens after five to ten years of forcing the pancreas to work so hard? You guessed it — pancreatic poop-out.

The pancreas begins to secrete less insulin, in spite of the huge demands of the body. Eventually, with less insulin available to move glucose from the bloodstream into the cells, the glucose level in the blood starts to rise and the person gets diagnosed with diabetes. In most cases, these individuals are still secreting an excessive amount of insulin (compared with a person of normal weight), just not enough for them. When they eat a less taxing diet and lose weight, they don't need the extra insulin to control the sugars.

What this means is that typical Type II diabetes is caused by overweight in individuals who have a smaller reserve of insulin-secreting cells in the pancreas. In the susceptible individual, even ten to twenty pounds of excess weight could make the difference. Losing the extra weight enables these individuals to live within the capabilities of their body. Most Type II diabetics still produce enough insulin to maintain normalcy as long as they maintain a thinner, normal weight.

Following my program is the most important thing a diabetic individual can do to extend his or her life span. It has been known for years that intentional weight loss improves diabetics' blood sugars, lipids, and blood pressure. A recent study documented a significant increase in life expectancy, with an average of 25 percent reduced premature mortality when diabetic individuals dropped their body weight.[37] Imagine the results when a program of nutritional excellence achieves the weight loss.

Insulin is a dangerous drug for Type II diabetics. These are people who are overweight to begin with. Insulin therapy will result in further weight gain, accelerating their diabetes. A vicious cycle begins that usually causes patients to require more and more insulin as they put on the pounds. When they come to see me for the first time, they report their sugars are impossible to control in spite of massive doses of insulin, which they are now combining with oral medication. It is like walking around with a live hand grenade in your pocket ready to explode at any minute.

Don't Merely Control Your Diabetes — Get Rid of it For Good

As my patients begin the program I usually cut their insulin in half. The insulin is then gradually phased out over the next few days or weeks, depending on their response and how advanced their condition was when they started. Most patients can stop all insulin within the first few days. The warning I give to patients and their physicians adopting this program is not to underestimate how effective it can be. If the medications, especially insulin, are not dramatically reduced, a dangerous hypoglycemic reaction can occur from overmedication. It is safer to undermedicate and let the glucose levels run a little high at first, then add back a little medication if necessary. This will minimize the risk of hypoglycemia, or driving the blood sugar level too low. Since this diet is so powerfully effective in reversing diabetes and other diseases of nutritional neglect, it is essential you work closely with a doctor who can help you adjust your medication dose downward in a careful fashion.

> Note: No diabetic patient on medication should make dietary changes without the assistance of a physician, as adjusting the medication will be necessary to prevent hypoglycemia, or excessively lowering the blood sugar level.

I typically continue or begin Glucophage (metformin) or other similar drugs. The newer medications that do not interfere with weight loss are safer than the older oral medications diabetics used in the past. Eventually, as more weight is lost, these patients can have normal glucose levels without any medication. They become nondiabetic, though diabetes can recur should they adopt a more stressful and girth-growing diet.

Gerardo Petito is a patient I began seeing about ten months ago. His case exemplifies the outcome I see with other diabetic patients on a regular basis. Gerardo stated that his main reason for coming to me was that he wanted to control his diabetes better. On his first visit, January 18, 2000, he was taking three medications: Accupril 20 mg, for blood pressure, and two medications for diabetes, Glucophage 500 twice daily and fifteen units of insulin twice daily. He had been on insulin for seven years. His fasting glucose in the morning had been running around 175 with this regimen. His blood pressure was 140/85 and he weighed 256 pounds.

After a lengthy discussion, Gerardo agreed to follow my dietary advice. I instructed him to cut back his insulin dose to ten units the evening of the visit and to five units the following morning; after that, he was to take no more insulin.

When Gerardo came back for his second visit two weeks later, he weighed 237, a loss of nineteen pounds in just two weeks. His glu-

cose in the morning was averaging 115, and his blood pressure was down to 125/80. Other than checking his blood test and doing an EKG for the record, I made no changes in his program. He was enjoying the diet and following my advice to the letter.

At Gerardo's third visit the next month, he weighed 221, a loss of thirty-five pounds in fifty-two days. He had just returned from a cruise, where he continued to follow his healthful diet. His morning glucose was averaging around 80 (completely normal), so I stopped the Glucophage. His blood pressure was 88/70, so I discontinued the Accupril, his blood pressure medication.

Ten months after Gerardo's first visit, he weighed 190, a loss of sixty-six pounds, his cholesterol was 134, his blood pressure 112/76. His hemoglobin A1C, a measure of diabetic control, was 5.3, in the nondiabetic range. He was on no medication.

Rather than controlling his blood pressure and diabetes, he chose to follow my advice and get rid of his medical problems altogether.

Advice for the Diabetic Patient

The general advice given in this book is sufficient for most diabetics. The most important goal is how much weight you lose, not whether your glucose is a little higher or lower in the short run. Follow my guidelines for aggressive weight loss in the next chapter. If you follow my program to the letter, it will not be necessary to make your diet complicated by following diabetic food exchanges and counting calories. Most people do not have to measure portions, either. Your goals are the same as the patient with coronary artery disease: get thin and aggressively treat your risk factors. With time, your body will normalize your numbers. Keep the following guidelines in mind:

1. Refined starches such as white bread and pasta are particularly harmful; avoid them completely.
2. Do not consume any fruit juice or dried fruits. Avoid all sweets, except for fresh fruit in reasonable quantities. Two or three fruits for breakfast is fine, and one fruit after lunch and dinner is ideal. The best fruits are those with less sugar — grapefruit, oranges, kiwis, strawberries and other berries, melons, green apples.
3. Avoid all oil. Raw nuts are permitted, but only one ounce or less.

4. The name of your diet is the "greens and beans diet"; green vegetables and beans should make up most of your diet.
5. Limit animal food intake to no more than two servings of fish weekly.
6. Try to exercise regularly and consistently, like dispensing your medication. Do it on a regimented schedule, preferably twice daily. Walking stairs is one of the greatest exercises for weight loss.

As the information in this book becomes your prescription for health, heart attacks and strokes can be avoided. If this diet were adopted by the general public, these illnesses would become rare and diabetes would practically disappear from our society.

The Eat to Live Formula Lowers Triglycerides

Some physicians and nutritionists believe that individuals suffering from obesity, diabetes, and elevated triglycerides may have more effective results in losing weight and controlling the high triglycerides and elevated glucose with a high-protein, low-carbohydrate diet. They believe this because it has been observed that high-carbohydrate diets can raise triglyceride levels.

I agree that a diet high in *refined* carbohydrates is not advised and will worsen this condition. However, I want to make it absolutely clear that these patients can achieve spectacular results without the added dangers of a diet high in animal protein and saturated fat. They merely need advice on how to modify the plant-based diet for their condition. They do so by eating a relatively high protein plant-based diet that reduces the amount of low-fiber carbohydrates. The diet is heavy in beans, raw vegetables, and cooked greens. The results are invariably impressive.

Headaches, Hypoglycemia, and Hunger

It's almost incredible to believe, but almost all patients with headaches and hypoglycemia get well permanently following the formula for health in this book. I believe it has very much to do with *detoxification*.

The body can heal itself when the obstacles to healing or stressors are removed. The reason people can't ever make complete recoveries is that they are addicted to their bad habits and unhealthful ways of eating and drinking.

Imagine if you were drinking ten cups of coffee daily. If you stopped drinking coffee, you would feel ill; you might get headaches, feel weak, even get the shakes. Fortunately, this would resolve slowly over four to six days, and then you would be well.

So, if you were this heavy coffee drinker, when do you think you would feel the worst? Right after eating, upon waking up in the morning, or when delaying or skipping a meal?

You are correct if you answered either upon first waking up or when delaying or skipping a meal. The body goes through withdrawal, or detoxification, most effectively when it is not busy digesting food. A heavy meal will stop the ill feelings, or you'll feel better if you just take another cup of coffee, but the cycle of feeling ill will start all over again the minute the caffeine level drops or the glucose level in the blood starts to go down.

Delaying a meal brings about symptoms most people call "hunger." These symptoms include abdominal cramping, weakness, and feeling ill — *the same as during drug withdrawal.*

This is not hunger. Our dietary habits, especially eating animal-protein-rich foods three times a day, are so stressful to the detoxification system in our liver and kidneys that we start to get withdrawal, or detoxification, symptoms the minute we aren't busy processing such food.

Real hunger is not that uncomfortable. True hunger is mediated by the hypothalamus in the brain. The hunger-related activity of the hypothalamus correlates best with increased sensation of need in the mouth and throat area.[38]

You could feel better by drinking a cup of coffee every three hours, evenly spaced out, to keep your caffeine blood levels constant. Or you could take medications such as Fioricet, Cafergot, Excedrin, Esgic, Fiorinol, Migrainal, Wigraine, and others whose active ingredients are narcotics, barbiturates, ergotamines, or caffeine; or you can just get some amphetamines or cocaine from the alley behind the liquor store. Either way, I hope you understand that temporarily feeling better does not mean getting well. Putting toxic drugs in your body can only compromise your health and lead to further dependence and suffering. In order to detoxify, you need to feel worse, not better; then after the withdrawal symptoms are completed, you will truly become well.

Feeling better can mean becoming sicker. Feeling worse (temporarily) may mean getting well.

In medical school my classmates and I learned from a researcher that animal protein places a detoxification stress on the liver and that the nitrogenous wastes generated are toxic. These metabolic toxins (about fourteen of them) rise in the bloodstream and accompany the rise in uric acid after a meal rich in animal protein. Withdrawal from these toxins can cause uncomfortable symptoms in susceptible individuals, symptoms that many call hypoglycemia.

The word *hypoglycemia* means "low glucose in the bloodstream." It gives people the impression that the low glucose level itself is the cause of the problem.

Certain uncommon medical conditions (such as insulin-secreting tumors), excessive diabetic medication, and other rare illnesses can cause hypoglycemia and even hypoglycemic coma, but I am referring to those people with reactive hypoglycemia. They feel ill when they delay eating, but they do not have a serious medical condition, nor do their blood sugars drop dangerously low. Most people carrying this diagnosis do not have fasting glucoses below 50; when their blood is drawn when they delay eating and feel extremely ill, the blood sugar is usually not low enough to account for their feeling so ill. There seems to be no correlation between the severity of the symptoms and their low glucose levels, but they feel uncomfortable if they try to stop treating themselves with high-protein diets.

It is a massive oversimplification to think that a lower level of glucose in the blood is the sole cause of this problem. I find that the people with the most troublesome symptoms do not even have low glucose levels.

Many doctors learn during their training that if the liver is compromised, such as in cirrhosis, the patient cannot effectively remove these toxins and may consequently feel mentally affected, confused, and even psychotic unless they are fed a low-protein diet, generating a lower level of nitrogenous wastes. For this reason, it is standard medical care to feed a patient with advanced liver disease a low-protein diet.

Most Americans are protein-toxic. Like the patient with cirrhosis (but less so), they are toxic because their body detoxification system struggles under the excessive nitrogen load in addition to all the salt, caffeine, sweets, trans fats, and other noxious chemicals we consume.

So the stomach empties and we feel ill, not hungry. Most people are too toxic to feel hungry. Detoxification symptoms appear first. Most people are driven to eat because it is time to eat or because they feel detoxification discomfort. *Most Americans have never felt* true hunger *in their entire overfed existence.*

Many people come into my office with a diagnosis of hypoglycemia, meaning they feel ill when they delay eating. They are often told to eat a diet with frequent feedings of high-protein food. I insist that this diet is the precise cause of the condition, not the remedy; it is no more a remedy than putting them on a cup of coffee every hour. Sure, they will feel better temporarily, but if they want to make a complete and lasting recovery, they must unscramble their thinking. They must put up with about one week of not feeling so great, but then they can be set free from their discomfort and their addiction to bad habits and a toxic diet.

So this is yet another reason our modern society is so overweight. Most people have lost touch with the ability to detect true hunger; they are driven to eat way before hunger appears, because they are addicted to their unhealthful diets and feel uncomfortable if they don't overeat or eat too often.

When I first begin treating patients with hypoglycemic symptoms, I continue them on snacks between meals and use some raw nuts and beans at each meal. They are forbidden to consume any refined carbohydrates such as bread, pasta, sweets, or fruit juice, to prevent swings in insulin. In some individuals, insulin levels swing up too high and then too low merely because they are eating refined sugars and refined grains, and not natural, unrefined food. These individuals are just sensitive to the junk food eaten by most Americans. The notoriously unreliable glucose tolerance test, in which patients consume about 100 grams of glucose, duplicates eating a huge quantity of junk food. Even normal people can feel ill from this experience.

Invariably, within two or three weeks their symptoms diminish and they gain the ability to delay eating without feeling ill. They can then follow the same diet I recommend for everyone without feeling any ill effects.

If you have this condition, you must also avoid alcohol, coffee, tea, artificial flavorings, and food additives. Fresh fruit does not need to be restricted.

Headache Sufferers Rejoice

Recurrent headaches are not much different. They are almost always the result of nutritional folly and, like other reasons that keep doctors' offices busy, are completely avoidable.

The relationship between food triggers and migraines has been the subject of much debate, with varying results from medical researchers. Headache specialists such as Seymour Diamond, director of the Diamond Headache Clinic of Columbus Hospital, report that about 30 percent of patients can identify food triggers.[39]

My experience in treating migraine and severe-headache patients with a more comprehensive nutritional approach has shown that 90 to 95 percent of patients are able to remain headache-free after the first three-month period. These patients avoid common migraine triggers, but also in the healing phase they adhere to a strict natural-food vegan diet of primarily fruits and vegetables rich in natural starches like potatoes and brown rice. These patients must avoid all packaged and processed foods, which are notorious for containing hidden food additives, even though they are not disclosed on the labels. They also avoid all added salt.

I believe I obtain such impressive results not merely because of avoiding triggers but because the patient becomes healthier and is able to process toxins more effectively. Additionally, when animal-product consumption is significantly lowered or removed from the diet, the liver is not faced with breaking down this heavy toxic load and can perform its normal detoxification function more effectively.

Very often in the initial phase of my program, when patients are on a diet with a lower level of tissue irritants, a headache will be precipitated. In other words, it is possible that the patient will initially feel worse, not better. I encourage such patients not to take medication during this initial phase, if at all possible. Instead, use a cold washcloth draped over the forehead and lie down in a dark room and rest. The prescribed diet, very low in sodium and animal protein, resolves the headaches in the large majority of patients. If it does not, not all is lost, because some fasting usually clears up the problem in most of the remaining headache sufferers.[40]

My patients begin by following a diet along the lines of the one described on page 170. They are instructed not to take any medication after the first week; after that time they are encouraged to control their pain with ice, hot showers, and pressure bands. They will

15 COMMON MIGRAINE TRIGGERS

sweets	dairy and cheese	salted or pickled foods
fermented foods	chocolate	vinegar
pizza	smoked meats	alcohol
monosodium glutamate	nuts	food additives
yeast	hydrolyzed protein	baked goods

never recover if they don't first detoxify themselves of their addiction to pain medications. These medications may offer pain relief, but they perpetuate the headache at the same time. Drugs that are used for headaches, such as acetominophen (Tylenol), barbiturates, codeine, and ergotomines, all cause headaches to recur on a rebound basis as these toxins begin to wash out of the nervous system. Even a little aspirin can cause a chronic, daily headache syndrome.[41]

The first phase of the anti-headache diet is followed strictly for two weeks. Then if the person is headache-free, I expand the diet to include a wider variety of fruits and begin to add beans in the second phase. I usually have the patient avoid nuts for the first few weeks because these bother some people. All dairy and yeast should be avoided as well.

Autoimmune Diseases and All the Rest

If dangerous drugs were the only way for a person to gain relief from suffering, we would be forced to accept the drawbacks of conventional therapy for autoimmune illnesses. The reality is, however, that dietary and nutritional interventions work for autoimmune diseases such as rheumatoid arthritis.

Caring for such patients has been a major portion of my work as a physician for the past ten years. I have seen scores of rheumatoid arthritis, lupus, and connective tissue disease patients recover completely through these interventions. Many of my patients have also made complete recoveries from allergies and asthma. Not every patient obtains a complete remission, but the majority are able to avoid the use of medication.

The key to treating autoimmune illnesses is to obey the H = N/C formula. Only then can the immune system begin to normalize its haywire circuitry.

**Phase One Anti-Headache Diet
with a Greater than 90 Percent Cure Rate**

Breakfast
Melon, apple, or pear
Oatmeal and water, no sweetener
Yeast-free whole-grain bread

Lunch
Large green salad, with one teaspoon of olive oil and one teaspoon of
   flax oil
One starchy vegetable or grain — corn, sweet potato, steamed carrots,
   brown rice
Grapes, pear, or apple

Dinner
Large green salad with tomatoes, with one teaspoon of olive oil and one
   teaspoon of flax oil
One steamed green vegetable — string beans, asparagus, artichokes,
   broccoli, zucchini
One starchy vegetable or grain — butternut or acorn squash, potato,
   millet, whole-wheat pasta
Tomato sauce (unsalted) permitted

Research studies from around the world confirm that this approach is effective, though I admit the research is scant, especially in this country.[42] There is simply no interest. However, all the studies that have been done are predictably positive and document improvement in blood inflammatory markers, as well as patient symptoms. I see this occur on a daily basis.

Here are the main ways to increase the possibility of obtaining remission or improvement in patients with autoimmune diseases:

1. A strict plant-based (vegan), dairy-free, wheat-free, and gluten-free diet is usually necessary; a lower-protein diet is helpful.
2. A high nutrient-per-calorie density with caloric restriction sufficient to obtain a normal weight is essential.
3. Check the arachidonic acid and DHA levels with an essential fatty acid profile; a blood test that can be ordered through Great Smokies Diagnostic Laboratory is often helpful. If the fatty acid balance is abnormal, supplementation with omega-

3 fatty acids (ground flaxseed, flaxseed oil, fish oil) and/or pure plant-derived DHA supplementation to achieve satisfactory balance may be necessary. I try to hold off on using fish oils, usually mixing flax oil and plant-derived DHA together, because too much fish oil is difficult to digest and potentially toxic. Though usually a little more expensive than fish oil, plant-derived DHA is less rancid. High-dose fish oils are still much safer than the medications used for autoimmune illnesses, so if they help, I would not discourage their use.

4. Therapeutic fasting can be an extremely effective adjunct to control the autoimmune response and reset the hyperactive immune system to a more normal (lower) level of activity. Do not fast patients who are dependent on multiple immunosuppressive drugs, such as Methotrexate and Immuran, as it is not safe to fast while on such medication. It is essential that patients contemplating this therapy be properly supervised by a physician. Those more interested in therapeutic fasting for autoimmune illness should read my book *Fasting and Eating for Health: A Medical Doctor's Program for Conquering Disease*. Physicians can request medical journal articles, including cases studies that I wrote about this therapy along with comprehensive medical references, from me via my website (www.drfuhrman. com) or office.

5. Undertake food elimination and challenge to uncover hidden food sensitivities. Most of the offending foods have already been eliminated — animal products, wheat, and dairy — but many patients find other foods that can worsen their condition as well. These foods are not routinely uncovered with allergy testing. It usually requires a short period of fasting and then the gradual introduction of only one new food each day, eliminating any food that causes an increase in pain over the fasted state. I would like to repeat this to make it clear — the elevated levels of IgG and IgE against various foods on allergy tests are indeed common in patients with rheumatoid arthritis and other autoimmune diseases; however, there is not an adequate clinical correlation between those foods and the foods we find to be aggravating the symptoms. Other researchers have noted the same thing.[43] I usually instruct patients to save their money and forgo those tests.

Diet Is the First-Line Defense

Working with patients with autoimmune diseases such as connective tissue disease, myositis, rheumatoid arthritis, and lupus is very rewarding. These patients had been convinced they could never get well and are usually eternally grateful to be healthy again and not require medication. I regularly get notes and letters, such as these unsolicited comments:

"After three months I am off all drugs."

— Richard Arroni

"I would like to shout, Dr. Fuhrman did it."

— Fred Redington

"Six months ago I prayed I would die, now I'm ready to live again."

— Jennifer Fullum

"Thank you for saving my life."

— Harriet Fleming

An aggressive nutritional approach to autoimmune illnesses should always be tried *first* when the disease is in its infancy. Logically, the more advanced the disease is, and the more damage that has been done by the disease, the less likely the patient will respond. My experience with inflammatory diseases such as rheumatoid arthritis is that some patients are more dietary-sensitive than others and that some patients have very high levels of inflammation that are difficult to curtail with natural therapy. Nevertheless, the majority benefit — and since the conventional drugs used to treat these types of illnesses are so toxic and have so many risky side effects, the dietary method should be tried first. Modern drugs often contribute to the disability and misery of patients with an autoimmune illness and increase cancer risk. Studies show that the long-term outcome is poor after twenty years of taking such medication.[44] A recent study in the *British Journal of Rheumatology* showed the major drugs to treat rheumatoid arthritis, such as azathioprine, cyclophosphamide, chlorambucil, and methotrexate, increase the likelihood that the person will die of cancer.[45]

Patients who use drugs that suppress the immune system forgo some protection that the immune system offers against infection and cancer. These individuals need a superior diet, even if they can't stop all medication.

So many of the patients I see, especially the ones who have made recoveries, are angry at their former physicians who did not even suggest nutrition before starting them on medication. These individuals are usually so "sick of being sick," they will do anything to get well. They don't find the diet restrictive and show enthusiasm and determination to recover their health. It is terrifically exciting to see such patients make recoveries and eliminate the need for medication.

Diseases Resolve or Improve with Nutritional Excellence

Other conditions that also respond exceptionally well to dietary modification include menstrual complaints and irritable bowel syndrome.

Researchers testing similar diets to the one I recommend have noted that a low-fat vegetarian diet increases sex-hormone-binding globulin as it reduces estrogen activity.[46] This not only reduces one's risk of breast cancer but also significantly reduces the pain and bloating associated with menstruation.

I also see a large number of patients with irritable bowel syndrome. Some feel better within three days of following this diet, although others take a few weeks or longer to adjust to the comparatively large amount of fiber. Both animal products and flour products are triggers for bowel symptoms in many individuals.[47] British researchers have documented that increased production of methane and other gaseous products representing increased fermentation in the colon from meats, dairy products, and refined grains correlate with bowel complaints. However, there are other mechanisms by which a natural-food diet high in nutrients and fiber reestablishes normal gut motility and tone. It can take time to undo a lifetime of wrong eating; most of my patients need three months to see improvement. Of course, sometimes diets have to be modified for individual uniqueness. In such cases, working with a knowledgeable physician is helpful.

Most chronic illnesses have been earned from a lifetime of inferior nutrition, which eventually results in abnormal function or frequent discomfort. These illnesses are not beyond our control, they are not primarily genetic, and they are not the normal consequence of aging. True, we all have our weakest links governed by genetics; but these weak links need never reveal themselves unless our health deteriorates. Superior health flows naturally as a result of superior nutrition. Our predisposition to certain illnesses can remain hidden.

Certainly, this method of healing is not for everybody. Some would prefer to eat conventionally and take whatever medication is indicated for their condition. That is their inalienable right. However, it is also the right of sick and suffering individuals who seek a natural approach to be aware of how effective aggressive nutritional interventions can be. I would like to take these patients down the streets of Manhattan for a ticker-tape parade to spread the word — you don't have to be sick. Remember, health is your greatest wealth!

8

Your Plan for Substantial Weight Reduction

I attended one of Dr. Fuhrman's two-hour seminars and proceeded to lose 120 pounds that year without ever being seen by him as a patient. Accurate knowledge, not willpower, finally did it for me.

— Linda Migliaccio

What I learned from Dr. Fuhrman is the very best thing that has happened in my life.

— Rhonda Wilson

What have we learned so far? First, eating foods with too few nutrients is bad for your health. Second, a large amount of animal products in your diet correlates with a vast number of diseases. Last, unrefined plant foods offer the best protection against disease. The question is, How can we translate this data into a health program that will help us achieve a healthy weight, maximize our well-being, and let us enjoy meals at the same time? That is, in part, what the rest of this book will answer. The first part of this chapter describes exactly what I want you to do for the next six weeks of your life. Then the rest of the chapter shows how you can incorporate these principles into the rest of your life in a practical and sensible way — the Life Plan — with more flexibility than the Six-Week-Plan. The Life Plan will include both vegetarian and nonvegetarian options.

The Six-Week Plan

Get ready for the most exciting six weeks of your adult life. If you follow my program precisely for the next six weeks, your body will undergo a remarkable transformation and you will be witness to its miraculous self-healing ability. With no compromise for these first six weeks, you will unleash a biochemical and physiological makeover that will change you forever. You will be thrilled with how easily your weight drops and the subtle changes you experience in your physical and emotional well-being. Maybe even more meaningful than the weight loss, you will feel better than you have in years. Your nose won't feel stuffed, your allergies can disappear, and your constipation will go away. Most people quickly find they are no longer aware that their digestive tract even exists, as they no longer experience stomach aches, cramping, and intestinal discomfort. You will no longer require headache remedies, pain pills, digestive aids, and other drugs that attempt to alleviate the suffering caused by unhealthy eating. I always like to compare the health of my patients after this initial six-week intervention with how they felt when they first came in with their typical complaints of diabetes, high blood pressure, and high cholesterol and triglycerides. The results are remarkable when their weight, blood pressure, and blood tests are rechecked. I encourage people to do a scientific test: Do this very strictly for just six weeks and see how much weight you lose. Most get so excited with the results during the six-week "trial" that they are motivated to keep going. Results encourage change, and results motivate. The stricter you are, the more quickly your taste will change.

The Six-Week Plan includes none of those optional, low-nutrient foods described later in this chapter. Whether you have a serious medical condition or not, your body will still undergo an energizing and healing transformation. Your body will overcome food addictions and get the physiological housecleaning it has been yearning for. It will be hard, initially, but the immediate results will help keep you focused.

I know many of you have not succeeded with diets in the past or have been disappointed with your rate of progress. Such will not be the case here. Your life is too important. Your ideal weight is within reach. Give this diet a true test and do as I recommend. See how much weight you lose, how far down you can get your lipids (cholesterol and triglycerides), and how many symptoms such as headache, gastritis, indigestion, and nasal congestion can disappear. Once you see the incredible results, you will be so pleased that you will feel comfortable with only occasional deviation from this ideal diet. *Eat to Live* for the first time in your life and give yourself this life-changing opportunity.

The Six-Week Plan gives your body time to adjust to this new way of eating. At the beginning the weight comes off quickly, but as you approach your target weight, your weight loss will slow down. Your taste buds will change. They will actually become more sensitive to the subtle flavors in natural foods, and six weeks is sufficient time for any symptoms arising from the new diet to subside. Results beget results. After you have lost about twenty-five pounds, you will feel like exercising more and be thrilled to see even more spectacular results when you go to the gym and sculpt the body you have always dreamed of.

It is not unusual for my patients to lose one pound per day over the first ten to fourteen days on this plan. Sometimes more. One patient, George, who came to me with high blood pressure lost eight pounds in the first three days. Much of that was probably water weight from cutting out all the salt in his diet; nevertheless, his blood pressure came down and he continued to lose weight over the next few months at a rate of about ten pounds per month. He had a little turkey on Thanksgiving and a few other minor deviations from the plan, but he found the diet easy, used some of my recommended flavored vinegars and jarred chilies, and continues to lose more and more weight. Soon he will have lost the full 100 pounds he needed to take off.

Raw Vegetables (including Salad)

These foods are to be eaten in unlimited quantities, but think big. Since they have a negative caloric effect, the more you eat, the more you lose. Raw foods also have a faster transit time through the digestive tract and result in a lower glucose response and encourage more weight loss than their cooked counterparts.[1] The object is to eat as many raw vegetables as possible, with a goal of one pound daily. This is an entire head of romaine or the equivalent amount of a green lettuce. Include raw vegetables such as snow peas, sweet red peppers, raw peas, tomatoes, cucumbers, and sprouts. The entire pound is less than 100 calories of food.

Steamed or Cooked Green Vegetables

Eat as much as you can from this group, too. My saying "the more you eat, the more weight you will lose" applies as well to this group. Again, the goal is one pound. The non-green vegetables included in the list below may also be eaten with abandon. One of the keys to your success is to eat a decent portion of food; so when you eat these greens, try to eat a much larger portion than you might have in the past. Completely rethink what your idea of a portion is; make it huge. Go for variety in your cooked vegetables by using string beans, broccoli, artichokes, asparagus, zucchini, kale, collards, cabbage, Brussels sprouts, bok choy, okra, Swiss chard, turnip greens, escarole, beet greens, spinach, dandelion greens, broccoli raab, cauliflower, eggplant, peppers, and water chestnuts.

Beans or Legumes

Legumes are among the world's most perfect foods. They stabilize blood sugar, blunt your desire for sweets, and prevent midafternoon cravings. Even a small portion can help you feel full, but in the Six-Week Plan I encourage you to eat at least one full cup daily. They can be flavored and spiced in interesting ways, and you can eat an unlimited quantity of them. Eat some beans with every lunch. Among your choices are chickpeas, black-eyed peas, black beans, cowpeas, green peas, lima beans, pinto beans, lentils, red kidney beans, soybeans, cannellini beans, pigeon peas, and white beans.

Fresh Fruit

Eat at least four fresh fruits per day, but no fruit juice. Shred or cut up apples and oranges and add them to your salad for flavor; they will help you feel full. Clementines are a nice addition to a green salad. Pineapple is good with vegetables and can be cooked with tomatoes and vegetables for a Hawaiian-flavored vegetable dish. On the Six-Week Plan, no fruit juice is permitted, except for small quantities for salad dressings and cooking. Juicing fruits allows us to quickly consume three times the calories without the fiber to regulate absorption. The nutrient-per-calorie ratio is much higher for the whole food. Frozen fruit is permissible, but avoid canned fruit because it is not as nutritious. If you need to use canned fruit as a condiment (mandarin oranges, pineapple), make sure it is unsweet-

EAT TO LIVE

The Six-Week Plan

UNLIMITED

eat as much as you want

all raw vegetables, including raw carrots (goal: 1 lb. daily)

cooked green vegetables (goal 1 lb. daily)

beans, legumes, bean sprouts, and tofu (1 cup daily)

fresh fruit (at least 4 daily)

eggplant, mushrooms, peppers, onions, tomatoes

LIMITED

not more than one serving (1 cup) per day

cooked starchy vegetables *or* whole grains

(butternut or acorn squash, corn, potatoes, rice, cooked carrots, sweet potatoes, breads, cereals)

raw nuts and seeds (1 oz. max. per day)

avocado (2 oz. max. per day)

ground flaxseed (1 tablespoon per day)

OFF-LIMITS

dairy products

animal products

between-meal snacks

fruit juice, dried fruit

ened. Dried fruits are off-limits on the Six-Week Plan. Exotic fruits are interesting to try and will add variety and interest to your diet. Some of my personal favorites are blood oranges, persimmons, and cherimoyas. Eat a variety of fruit; try to include many of the following: apples, apricots, bananas, blackberries, blueberries, clementines, dates, figs, grapefruits, grapes, kiwis, kumquats, mangoes, melons, nectarines, oranges, papayas, peaches, pears, persimmons, pineapples, plums, raspberries, starfruit, strawberries, and tangerines.

Starchy Vegetables and Whole Grains

These two food categories are grouped together because either can be the culprit for those who have difficulty losing weight. While wholesome high-carbohydrate foods are a valuable addition to a disease-prevention diet, they are more calorically dense than the nonstarchy vegetables. Therefore, cooked, high-starch vegetables should be limited to one serving daily. Diabetics, those who want to lose weight more rapidly, and those who have difficulty losing weight no matter what they do may want to restrict these foods altogether, at least until they have arrived at their target weight. Eating lots of greens makes it difficult to overconsume high-starch vegetables. You just won't have room for that much. Examples of starchy vegetables include cooked carrots, corn, sweet potatoes, white potatoes, butternut squash, acorn squash, winter squash, chestnuts, parsnips, rutabagas, turnips, water chestnuts, yams, and pumpkins. Grains include barley, buckwheat (kasha), millet, oats, quinoa, brown rice, and wild rice. On some days you may choose to have a cup of oatmeal or other whole grain with your breakfast. On other days, save your serving of starch for dinner.

One final note: soaking whole grains, such as brown rice, buckwheat, and quinoa, for a day before cooking them greatly increases their nutritional value.[2] Certain phytonutrients and vitamins are activated as the grain starts to germinate. These include powerful chemopreventive phenols that inhibit the growth of abnormal cells.[3] A twenty-four-hour soak induces the early stage of germination, but you will not see the sprouts. Soaking a day ahead also shortens cooking time.

Nuts and Seeds

Nuts and seeds contain 150–200 calories per ounce. Eating a small amount — one ounce or less — each day, however, adds valuable nutrients and healthy unprocessed fats. Nuts and seeds are ideal in salad dressings, particularly when blended with an orange and spices or vegetable juice (tomato, celery carrot). *Always* eat nuts and seeds raw because the roasting process alters their beneficial fats. Commercially packaged nuts and seeds are often cooked in hydrogenated oils, adding trans fats and sodium to your diet, so these are absolutely off the list. If you find that you tire of eating nuts or seeds raw, try lightly toasting them at home — this process does not deplete their beneficial properties and adds some variety for pleasure. Among the *raw* nuts and seeds you can add to your diet are almonds, cashews, walnuts, black walnuts, pecans, filberts, hickory nuts, macadamias, pignolis, pistachios, sesame seeds, sunflower seeds, pumpkin seeds, and flaxseed.

Spices, Herbs, and Condiments

Use all spices and herbs, except for salt. When using condiments, a little mustard is okay, but pickled foods contain too much salt and should be avoided. If you love to use ketchup or tomato sauce, you may find a lower-calorie, unsweetened ketchup at the health-food store and a tomato sauce made with no oil. Better yet, make your own tomato sauce with onion and garlic but no oil or salt.

Ten Easy Tips for Living with the Six-Week Plan

1. Remember, the salad is the main dish: eat it first at lunch and dinner.

You have the tendency to eat more of whatever you eat first because you are the hungriest. Raw foods have high transit times; they fill you up and encourage weight loss. You can't overeat on them. Successful, long-term weight control and health, as you know by now, is linked to your consumption of raw greens. They are the healthiest food in the world. Many of my patients with obesity or diabetes eat lettuce with every meal, including breakfast. They might have iceberg lettuce with their fruit breakfast, a mixed baby greens salad with lunch, and a romaine-based salad with dinner. You can eat more than a pound if you like, but don't fret if you are too full and can't eat the whole pound. It is merely a goal; just relax and enjoy eating.

2. Eat as much fruit as you want but at least four fresh fruits daily.

Eat as many fruits as you would like with your meals. Four fruits are about 250 calories, but here it is okay to splurge, even during the Six-Week Plan, particularly if you have a sweet tooth. Finish lunch or dinner with watermelon, a whole cantaloupe, grapefruit, or a box of blueberries or strawberries. The best dessert is fruit, or blended frozen fruit. Eating lots of fresh fruit is satisfying and filling and helps win you over to the Eat to Live way.

3. Variety is the spice of life, particularly when it comes to greens.

Variety is not merely the spice of life, it makes a valuable contribution to your health. The nice thing is that you never have to be concerned about overeating raw vegetables, salads, or cooked greens. There are a variety of foods that you can use to make vegetable salads, including the following: lettuce (including romaine, bib, Boston, red leaf, green ice, arugula, radicchio, endive, frisee, iceberg), celery, spinach, cucumbers, tomatoes, mushrooms, broccoli, cauliflower, peppers, onions, radishes, kohlrabi, snow peas, carrots, beets, cabbage, and all kinds of sprouts. Even more vegetables can be eaten cooked. They include broccoli, kale, string beans, artichokes, Brussels sprouts, spinach, Swiss chard, cabbage, asparagus, collards, okra, and zucchini. These vegetables can be flavored in various ways. Greens are always great with mushrooms, onions, garlic, and stewed tomatoes. If you don't have time to cook, just defrost a box of frozen green vegetables. Throw a box of frozen artichoke hearts, asparagus, or peas on your salad. This is less than 150 calories of food. Cooked greens are very low in calories but give you the nutritional power of ten pounds of other foods. Frozen greens such as broccoli and peas are nutritious and convenient — they are flash-cooked and frozen soon after being picked and are just as nutritious as fresh.

4. Beware of the starchy vegetable.

For the Six-Week Plan, limit cooked, high-starch grains and vegetables to one cup a day. Consider any vegetable that is not green to be a high-starch vegetable, (The main exceptions to this rule are eggplant, peppers, onions, and mushrooms.) One cup of a high-starch vegetable would be one corn on the cob, one small- to medium-sized baked potato, or one cup of brown rice or sweet potato. Fill up on the raw vegetables and cooked green vegetables first. However, make most of your starch consumption from starchy vegetables — such as butternut or acorn squash, corn, turnips, parsnips, rutabagas, cooked carrots, sweet and white potatoes — rather than starchy grains. Refined starchy grains (such as bread, pasta, and white rice) should be even more restricted than the vegetable-based starches, which are more nutrient-dense. All whole grains should be considered high-starch foods. If you do use bread, a thin whole-wheat pita is a good choice for sandwiches because it is less bread and can hold healthful fillings such as vegetables, eggplant, and bean spreads. When you eat grains, use whole grains, such as brown and wild rice, and use them in place of a cooked, starchy vegetable at dinner. Restricting the portion size of rice, potato, and other cooked starchy vegetables to one serving is not necessary for everybody to lose weight on the Life Plan, only for those whose metabolism makes it difficult to lose weight. Many can still achieve an ideal body weight by cutting out refined starches only, such as white bread and pasta, without having to limit starchy vegetables to merely one serving. Your diet should be adjusted to your metabolic needs and activity level.

5. Eat beans or legumes every day.

Beans are a dieter's best friend. On the Six-Week Plan the goal is to eat an entire cup of beans daily; you may have more than one cup if you choose. Beans are a powerhouse of superior nutrition. They reduce cholesterol and blood sugar. They have a high nutrient-per-calorie profile and help prevent food cravings. They are digested slowly, which has a stabilizing effect on your blood sugar and a resultant high satiety index. Eggplant and beans, mushrooms and beans, greens and beans are all high-nutrient, high-fiber, low-calorie main dishes. Throw a cup of beans on your salad for lunch. Eat bean soup. Scientific studies show a linear relationship between soup consumption and successful weight loss.[4] As a weight-loss strategy, eating soup helps by slowing your rate of intake and reducing your appetite by filling your stomach.

6. Eliminate animal and dairy products.

For the Six-Week Plan, eliminate animal products completely or, if you must include a little animal products, use only lean fish (flounder, sole, or tilapia) once or twice a week and an egg white (or Egg Beaters) omelette once a week. *No dairy products are permitted in the Six-Week Plan.*

7. Have a tablespoon of ground flaxseed every day.

This will give you those hard-to-find omega-3 fats that protect against diabetes, heart disease, and cancer.[5] The body can manufacture EPA and DHA from these omega-3 fats for those of us who do not consume fish. An additional source of omega-3 fat might be a few walnuts or soybeans. Edamame, those frozen green soybeans in the freezer of most health-food stores, taste great and are a rich source of omega-3 fat. A nutritional supplement containing DHA fat is also a good idea, especially for those who are poor DHA converters (which can be determined via a blood test). Vegetable-derived (from microalgae) DHA fat can be found in most health-food stores.

8. Consume nuts and seeds in limited amounts, not more than one ounce per day.

Pecans, walnuts, macadamia nuts, and others may be rich in calories and fat, but scientific studies consistently report that nuts offer disease protection against heart attacks, stroke, and cancer and also help lower cholesterol.[6] They can be used in larger amounts once you reach your ideal weight. Raw nuts and seeds are ideal foods for kids, athletes, and those who want to *gain* weight. One ounce of nuts is about 200 calories and can fit into a cupped hand, so do not eat more than this one handful of nuts per day. They are great in both fruit salads and green salads.

9. Eat lots of mushrooms all the time.

Mushrooms make a great chewy replacement for meat. Exploring their varieties is a great way to add interesting flavors and textures to dishes. Store them in paper bags, not plastic, as too much moisture speeds spoilage. Try adding them to beans, seasoned with herbs and lemon juice. Even though they are a fungus, and not a real vegetable, mushrooms contain a variety of powerful phytochemicals and have been linked to decreased risk of chronic diseases, especially cancer.

Onions Add Fast Flavor to Foods.

Dried onion powder can be quickly added to any salad dressing, soup, or vegetable dish. Red onions or scallions, sautéed in a little water or raw and sliced extra thin, make great flavor enhancers for salads and vegetable dishes. Leeks are in the onion family, too. Using just the white part and the lower lighter green part, slice and simmer them or roast them with other vegetables.

---

10. Keep it simple.

Use the basic skeleton plan below to devise menu plans so you will know what to eat when there is no time to decide.

Simplify, Simplify, Simplify

Breakfast: fresh fruit
Lunch: salad, beans on top, and more fruit
Dinner: salad and two cooked vegetables (1 lb.), fruit dessert

You do not have to prepare fancy recipes all the time. If you're going to be out for a while, just grab some leftover vegetables, lettuce and tomato on whole-grain bread or stuffed into a whole-wheat pita pocket, and a few pieces of fruit. Wash and dry plenty of heads of romaine lettuce on the weekends or when you have the time.

"The best prescription is knowledge."

— Dr. C. Everett Koop

The Life Plan

This is the Six-Week Plan in a nutshell. However, losing weight will do you no good unless you keep it off. When you adopt the Eat to Live program as a longevity plan, a slim weight will be a by-product of your new commitment to excellent health. Once the first phase is over, you will move on to the Life Plan, which offers more choices. This is a critical juncture. You have lost a great deal of weight; you don't want to revert to your previous unhealthy diet. You need to decide not only how to maintain the benefits you have achieved but how to change your diet forever. Many of my patients have found a good balance by following the 90 percent rule.

The 90 Percent Rule

For longevity and weight loss, the Life Plan diet should aim to be made up of at least 90 percent unrefined plant food. My most successful patients treat processed foods and animal foods as condiments, constituting no more than 10 percent of their total caloric intake.

The obvious corollary to the principle of consuming a large quantity of nutrient-dense foods is that you should consume smaller quantities of low-nutrient foods. Therefore, you must not have significant amounts of animal foods, dairy, or processed foods in your diet. If you desire these foods, use them occasionally or in very small amounts to flavor a vegetable dish. After the Six-Week Plan, if you want to add animal products back into your diet, then add a little white-meat chicken or turkey once a week, and beef even less frequently. This will essentially limit your total animal-product consumption (beef, turkey, fish) to 12 ounces or less per week. In this manner, you can alternate: one night with a small serving of animal product and the next night a vegetarian dinner. Use animal products primarily as *condiments* — to add flavor to soups, vegetables, beans, or tofu — not as the main dish.

Similarly, if after the first six weeks you choose to reintroduce dairy back into your diet, use fat-free dairy only (skim milk, nonfat yogurt) and limit it to 12 ounces per week. You can add an unsweetened fat-free yogurt or soymilk yogurt with your fruit breakfast. Do not eat fruit flavored yogurt, as it contains sugar. Keep a close eye on your weight with both these additions.

How does this work out in terms of calorie consumption? The accepted wisdom is that the "average" woman should consume fewer than 1,500 calories daily, and a man fewer than 2,300 calories. To hold to the 90 percent rule, women should not consume more than 150 calories per day of low-nutrient food, or about 1,000 calories weekly. Men should not consume more than 200 calories of low-nutrient food daily, or about 1,500 calories weekly.

In real life, this means that if you choose to have a bagel for lunch, you use up your 150-calorie allotment of low-nutrient food for the day. If you put one tablespoon of olive oil or a few ounces of animal food on your salad for lunch, then you should have only plant food for dinner, with no added oils, pasta, or bread. Using the 90 percent rule, you are allowed to eat almost any kind of food, even a small cookie or candy bar, as long as all your other calories that day are from nutrient-dense vegetation.

100 Calories of Low-Nutrient Foods Equals

- 2.5 teaspoons of olive oil
- Half a bagel
- Half a cup of pasta
- One small cookie
- 2 ounces of broiled chicken or turkey breast
- 3 ounces of fish
- 1.5 ounces of red meat
- One thin slice of cheese
- One cup of 1 percent or skim milk

In general, the Life Plan dictates that you eat not more than one or two items of low-nutrient foods daily. Everything else must be unrefined plant food. The number of calories consumed will vary from person to person. Those who exercise or who are naturally thin eat more than those who exercise less and have weight problems. Therefore, the number of calories permitted from these low-nutrient foods should decrease as your total caloric intake goes down. For those who have a lot of weight to lose, eat less than 100 calories per day of low-nutrient foods.

Most people are addicted to the foods they grew up with. They feel deprived if their diet denies them the foods they love. With the Life Plan these food loves will become condiments or rewards for special occasions. You will be surprised how much more you will enjoy a healthier diet once you become accustomed to a different way of preparing foods and eating. It will take time; there will be a period of adjustment.

The USDA Food Guide Pyramid that most people are familiar with is designed around the foods Americans choose to eat already. Its goal is to improve the poor eating habits of Americans, but it fails. The USDA pyramid does not encourage the consumption of nutrient-dense plant foods. Anyone following the USDA guidelines, eating six to eleven daily servings of refined grains (breads, cereals, pastas),

THE LIFE PLAN FOOD PYRAMID

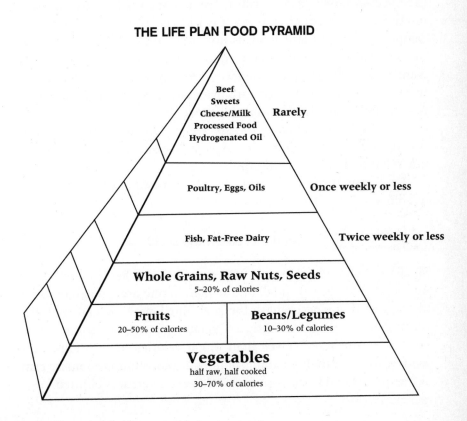

and three to five servings of animal products and dairy, is certain to obtain insufficient antioxidants and phytochemicals, depriving himself or herself of the opportunity to maximize prevention against common diseases. However, I do not recommend a grain-based diet. Potatoes, rice, and even whole grains do not contain the phytochemical power of fruits and vegetables. As I showed earlier, a high intake of refined grains in the diet is linked to common cancers. A high intake of fruit has the opposite effect. Fruits protect powerfully against cancer.[7]

Going for Broke: Serious Health Conditions Require Serious Intervention

Before coming to my office, most of my patients had failed to achieve the results they sought. They had experienced either a worsening of their heart condition or weight gain no matter what program they chose, even those who followed a vegetarian diet. In my care, these same patients were able to achieve impressive results, for the first time because they "did it" 100 percent. For some, "trying" is definitely not good enough; it doesn't work. The 10 percent of optional calories of low-nutrient foods is just that, optional; you might find that you feel better and don't need to include even that much. If you want to lose weight more rapidly; if you have a particularly slow metabolic rate, diabetes, or cardiovascular disease; or if you are a health and longevity enthusiast, kiss even these 150 (low-nutrient) calories good-bye and make the Six-Week Plan your Life Plan. Considering what a struggle it is to make a 90 percent change, it is not much harder to do it all the way.

I will now turn to the most commonly asked questions I hear in my office.

What if I Fall Off the Diet?

Since the goal is to eat at least 90 percent of your diet from nutrient-dense plant foods, if you fall off the plan in one area, make up for it in another. If you accomplish the goal stated above — eating all the recommended amounts of green vegetables, beans, and fruits — you will have consumed fewer than 1,000 calories of nutrient-dense food, with more than 40 grams of fiber. By consuming so many crucial nutrients and fiber, your body's drive to overeat is blunted.

Do you see the difference between these recommendations and those of more traditional authorities who recommend eating less food to lose weight? With my program you are encouraged to eat more food. Only by eating more of the right food can you successfully be healthy and well nourished and feel satisfied. On this plan you consume more than ten times the phytochemicals and ten times the fiber that most Americans consume. Keep in mind that it is the undiscovered nutrients in whole natural foods that offer the greatest protection against cancer.

Is This a Low-Calorie Diet?

Yes. Excess calories don't just make you overweight — they shorten your life. This diet style enables people to feel satiated with 1,000–2,000 calories per day, whereas before it took 1,600–3,000. The simple trick is to receive lots of nutrient bang for each caloric buck.

Of course, those who are considerably active or involved with exercise or sports need more calories, but that's okay — they will have a bigger appetite and need more food to satisfy their hunger. They will get more protein and other nutrients needed for exercise by consuming more food, not a different diet.

Some people can lose weight merely by switching their calories to a healthier plant-based cuisine while maintaining approximately the same caloric consumption. The Chinese consume more calories than do Americans, yet are about 25 percent thinner than Americans. This is because the modern American diet receives about 37 percent of its calories from fat, with lots of sugar and refined carbohydrates. The combination of high fat and high sugar is a metabolic disaster that causes weight gain, *independent* of the number of calories.

Other people are not able to lose weight as easily. They need the entire package: the metabolic benefit of the natural plant foods, along with the satiety that results from both the greater bulk of my "unlimited" foods and the consequent nutrient fulfillment. These patients need even fewer calories. The good news is that they can be satisfied with fewer calories permanently. The Eat to Live diet has both these benefits, making it a powerful weight-normalization plan as well as the healthiest possible diet.

The menus, recipes, and strategies for eating explained in this book also make it possible to achieve the current dietary guidelines of the National Heart, Lung, and Blood Institute (NHLBI) of the National Institutes of Health (NIH) for those desiring to lose weight. According to these guidelines, women should choose a diet with fewer than 1,200 calories a day and men, one with fewer than 1,600.[8]

A computer analysis of many different diets has shown that the Eat to Live diet is the only way to meet the National Institutes of Health guidelines for calories while at the same time supplying adequate nutrients and fiber content. Even the dietary menus for 1,200-calorie and 1,600-calorie diets published in the National Institutes of Health's recent guide for physicians do not meet the RDAs, because the traditional American food choices are too low in nutrients. The NIH diets are too low in important nutrients such as chromium, vitamin K, folate, and magnesium, whereas the Eat to Live diet plans and suggested menus more than meet all RDAs within the NIH's caloric limits.

How Do I Know How Many Calories I Should Eat?

Don't worry about it. Try to follow my rules for a longevity diet and just watch the weight fall off. If you were never able to lose weight in the past, be happy with about one to two pounds per week. If you are not losing weight as fast as you'd like, write down what you eat and how much, to see if you are really consuming a whole pound of raw vegetables a day and an entire pound of steamed green vegetables a day. If you are an overweight female following my guidelines and losing about one to two pounds per week, you are probably consuming about 1,100–1,400 calories a day. You can count calories if you want, but it is not necessary; you will feel sated and content on fewer calories than you were eating before.

My observations over the years have convinced me that eating healthfully makes you drop unwanted pounds efficiently, independent of caloric intake. It's as if the body wants to get rid of unhealthy tissue quickly. I have seen this happen time and time again. Eating the exact same diet, many patients drop weight quickly and easily and then automatically stop losing when they reach an ideal weight. Time and time again, I have seen individuals who were not overweight nonetheless lose weight after the switch. In a few months, however, they gravitated back to their former weight as their health improved. It is as if the body wanted to exchange unhealthy tissue for healthy tissue.

What if My Family Does Not Want to Eat This Way?

Nobody should be made to eat healthfully. Encourage your family to learn about what you are doing and to read this book so that they can help support you. The key is for them to learn what you are doing out of love and respect for you, not because you are trying to force this way of eating down their throats. That will be their decision later. The best way to help other people is by setting an example. Lose the weight, get in great health, and wait for your friends and family to ask how you did it. Very few people object to the presence of healthy foods as long as you do not take away their comfort foods. You can always make healthful meals for yourself and some extra food for the rest of the family. Over time it will get easier. Keep in mind that some people require more time to make changes.

My patient Debra Caruso faced this dilemma. Her teenage son and daughter told her they were definitely not going to eat this way. Debra knew they could all afford to lose weight. There was so much junk food in the house that it was even tempting her. Yet Debra lost more than fifty pounds that first year. Luckily, she had a loving and supportive husband who tried his best to help any way he could. The first thing he did was buy an extra refrigerator that they kept in the garage. Debra and her husband had a family meeting to enforce the rule that any unhealthy food would be kept in one cupboard and in the refrigerator in the garage. If the teenagers wanted something other than the food prepared by their mom, they could make it themselves and clean up after themselves. She agreed to cook their favorite main dishes, whatever they wanted, twice a week. Some off-limits foods such as ice cream, cheese, and other rich desserts would not be allowed in the house. They had to be consumed in another location. Debra and her husband also took the teenagers to the health-food store to purchase healthier snacks. It was important to give the children some say in what they ate. Finally, the entire family came to two of my lectures. After that, Debra's children chose a healthy diet for themselves as well.

It may not work out the same way for you. But the main point to bring home is compromise and patience.

What if I Don't Go All the Way?

The nutrient formula (H = N/C) allows you to approximate the relative disease-fighting power of your diet. If you are like most Americans, whose diets are only 5–6 percent nutrient-dense food, any step you take in the right direction will lessen the risks to your health.

If you improve your diet now, and begin consuming even 60 percent of your calories from nutrient- dense plant food (that's ten times as much vegetation as the average American consumes now), it is reasonable to expect a 60 percent decrease in your risk of cancer or heart attack.

Falling off the plan for one meal should give you more incentive to continue the rest of the week without a setback. Jump right back so that you eat so healthy for the rest of the week to make the one meal off the diet almost meaningless. In other words, follow the 90 percent rule. The 90 percent rule allows you some leeway for imperfection and special occasions or to have a treat once in a while. You can still retain the benefits and your healthy slim body if you follow that less-than-perfect "special occasion meal" with twenty healthy meals.

Focus on Your Actions, the Results Will Follow

You have now received a considerable education in human nutrition by reading this book. In my experience, knowledge about this subject provides the most effective and powerful impetus for change. Superior health and optimal weight are no longer a matter of chance, but a matter of choice. Try not to focus too much on the weight; focus on what you are doing. The weight will drop naturally as a result of eating intelligently, exercising, and adopting a healthy lifestyle. Neither you nor I is totally in control of the amount of weight that you lose or the speed at which you lose it. Your body will set the pace and gravitate toward the ideal weight for you when you eat healthfully. Don't worry if a few days go by without your losing weight; your body will lose at the rate it chooses is best. Weigh yourself as much or as little as you like, but most people find once weekly is sufficient to keep track of their results.

Most people lose weight and then stop losing when they have reached their ideal weight. You are not the judge of your ideal weight; your body is. As almost everyone is overweight, many people think they are too thin when they have reached their best weight. I have many patients who, after following my plan to reverse diabetes or heart disease, report, "Everyone tells me I look too thin now." I then measure their periumbilical fat and check their percentage of body fat, and usually show them that they are still not thin enough.

Stay in Control by Setting a Goal

Be realistic and flexible; give your taste buds time to adjust to the new food choices. Changing your behavior is the key to success. Moderation, however, does not mean it's okay to poison ourselves, abuse our body, and then feel guilty. Moderation means recovering quickly when you have slipped up. Some of us need to plan cheats, once a week or twice a month. Keep to those planned times. A cheat every once in a while is okay if it is moderate, and as long as you go right back to the program immediately and then don't do it again for at least one week.

Many health authorities and diet advisers recommend only small changes; they are afraid that if the change is too radical, dieters will give the whole thing up and gain nothing. I strongly disagree. My work over the past ten years has shown that those who have jumped in with full effort the first six weeks have been the individuals most likely to stick with the plan and achieve results, month after month. Those who try to get into it gradually are the ones most likely to revert back to their former way of eating. Under the gradual approach, they "yo-yo" back and forth between their old bad behaviors and good ones. Change is hard. Why not do more and glean the results you have always been after quickly and permanently?

The Drug of Choice for Most Americans — Food!

Most overweight individuals are addicted to food. This means almost all Americans are food addicts. *Addicted* means that you feel ill or uncomfortable should you not continue your usual habits. Unlike tobacco and drug addiction, however, food addiction is socially acceptable.

Most people thrust into an environment with an unlimited supply of calorie-rich, nutrient-poor food will become compulsive overeaters. That is, the craving for food and the preoccupation with eating, and the resultant loss of control over food intake, are the natural consequences of nutrient paucity. The resulting stress on our system can be toxic.

Obviously, there are complicated emotional and psychological factors that make it more difficult for some to achieve success at overcoming food addiction. Additionally, some physical changes may initially discourage you. Stopping caffeine, reducing sodium, and dropping saturated fat from your diet while increasing fiber and nutrients may result in increased gas, headaches, fatigue, and other withdrawal symptoms. These withdrawal symptoms are temporary and rarely last longer than one week. Eventually the high volume of food and high nutrient content will help prevent long-term food cravings.

The large quantity of food permitted and encouraged on this program makes you less stressed about overeating. Food cravings and addictive symptoms end for almost everyone because this diet satisfies a person's desire to eat more food.

Halting stimulating behavior such as overeating unmasks the fatigue that was always there. The power reserve in a battery is proportional to its use. The less we use it, the more life it has and the stronger it remains. Likewise, when there is continual stress on your body from stimulating foods and caffeine, it gives the false sensation that we have energy, when actually we are using up our nerve energy faster. This ages us. The fatigue is hidden by the stimulating (aging-inducing) effects of sugar, caffeine, and toxic protein load. Now that you are eating in a health-supporting manner, you may be in better touch with the sleep your body needs, and sleep better as a result.

Some cravings and food behaviors have emotional overtones from childhood or compensate for stress and emotional dysfunction. Some food-addicted people eat compulsively in spite of their awareness of the consequences. These people need a more intensive program than a book can provide. Similar to a twelve-week drug-rehabilitation program, an intensive food recovery program should include counseling. Food re-education can work even for the most difficult cases. Please contact me if you require such a program to guarantee your success. You no longer have an excuse to fail; all you need is the commitment.

This program is not for everybody, because added to the desire to lose weight must be the willingness to make a commitment to achieve wellness. Once that commitment is made, however, there need not be any failures; with proper support and this program, everyone can succeed.

Go for it.

9

Sculpting Our Future in the Kitchen
MENU PLANS AND RECIPES

The following menus and recipes are examples of diets and dishes rich in nutrients and fiber, consistent with the basic principles of healthful eating. They include most of my favorite recipes. I eat a quick and easy-to-prepare diet and I eat simply. Most days I eat fruit and nuts for breakfast, and something fast and quick for lunch, such as a salad with a box of frozen broccoli, frozen peas or beans on top, with a light dressing, and a few fruits. Conveniently, it is easy to find a can of vegetable or bean soup and prewashed salad at the health-food store in my area. I can eat healthfully with little work or effort. Likewise, I have tried to make these menus simple. However, you can modify these menus significantly and use your own recipes as long as you obey the guidelines outlined in the previous chapter. The foods or recipes can be switched around and eaten in different combinations or at different meals.

Fourteen days of menu plans and exciting recipes follow. Keep in mind that in the real world you would not make all these different dishes and recipes each week. Most of us make a soup or a main dish and use the leftovers for lunch or even dinner the next day. Remember: you must rethink what you consider a normal portion. Your former side dishes (such as salads, soups, and vegetables) now become the main dishes, and your portion sizes of these lower-calorie foods are now much larger. It is almost impossible to eat too much food, only too much of the wrong food. Make your life simple. Enjoy food, but don't have your life revolve around a menu plan. This diet is delicious; it involves no sacrifice, only different choices.

The vegetarian menus that follow are intentionally strict — for those requiring aggressive or quicker weight loss and for those who have had difficulty losing weight in the past. This kind of vegetarian diet is also appropriate for those looking to reverse heart disease or diabetes. You cannot expect to significantly reverse atherosclerosis (blockages in your arteries), diabetes, or high blood pressure unless you restore yourself to a normal weight. It is the combination of the healthy, nutrient-dense diet and the fat leaving your body that brings about predictable improvement in many health conditions.

For those not wanting to give up the flavor of animal foods, you can cook any vegetable dish in chicken broth or other (unsalted) soup stock. The nonvegetarian menus include a small amount of animal products (less than two ounces per day, or less than twelve ounces per week) and a small amount of oil. A small amount of animal food can be added to any vegetable or bean dish for flavor, if desired.

When the menu or recipes do permit oil, remember not to use more than one teaspoon per day. If your wedding is coming up or you just want to look great in a bathing suit before the summer, follow the seven-day vegetarian plan or, if you're on the less strict nonvegetarian plan, do not use any oil on salads or with any recipes. You can make these nonvegetarian menus stricter and more effective by excluding all oil and further limiting the portion size of the cooked starch.

If stir-frying any vegetable dish, alternatives to oil include vegetable broth, wine, or a little fruit juice, especially pineapple juice. Another option is to create a "wokking sauce" to cook vegetables in. We like to use a handful of dates or dried apricots blended with water and Bragg's Liquid Aminos. Another good mix is tomato sauce and pineapple juice. Just take a can of diced unsweetened pineapple and add some tomato sauce to make a Hawaiian mixed-vegetable dish.

The nonvegetarian menu plans are mostly vegetarian. Even the recipes that include a little animal product can be made totally vegan — if you want to stay on a vegetarian diet, still look through the recipes in the nonvegetarian section so you don't miss out on some great options. I intentionally included recipes that focused on the lower-calorie, more nutrient dense food.

It is advisable to soak beans or legumes overnight and then re-place the soaking water with two to three cups of fresh water for each cup of beans when cooking them. Most beans require about one and a half to two hours of cooking to become soft. Lentils and split peas require only one hour and should not be soaked prior to cooking. Make sure beans are thoroughly cooked, as they are more difficult to digest when undercooked. The bean dishes can be sprin-kled lightly with Beano to aid in digesting the bean oligosaccharides. Keep in mind that as you get in the habit of eating beans regularly, you will digest them better.

I always make large portions of food when I cook so that I have leftovers later. Most of the recipes yield two to four portions, but re-member — you can eat as much as you want. Feel free to experi-ment. Substitute and add the foods and seasonings that you enjoy.

Weekly Shopping List

Always keep a good assortment of healthy food in the house. The key to your success is having the right kind of food available to pre-vent being tempted by the wrong kind of food. I suggest the follow-ing items:

Canned beans — chickpeas, red kidney beans
Canned vegetable and bean soup (from the health-food store or
    health-food section)
Canned Chinese vegetables — water chestnuts, bamboo shoots,
    and others
Tofu
Frozen vegetables — peas, artichokes, asparagus, broccoli,
    mixed Chinese vegetables
Lots of low-sugar fruits — strawberries, kiwis, oranges, grape-
    fruits, melons, apples, lemons
Vinegars of your choice
Fresh vegetables to be eaten raw — carrots, celery, peppers,
    tomatoes, mushrooms, lettuce, snow pea pods
Lots of fresh vegetables for cooking — eggplant, mushrooms,
    tomatoes, cabbage, broccoli, string beans, Swiss chard, kale,
    spinach, onions, garlic cloves
Ingredients for homemade soup — celery, dill, parsley, carrots,

leeks, zucchini, TVP (textured vegetable protein, found in most health-food stores), turnips, parsnips, dried beans, and split peas

Whole-wheat pita bread

Vege Base Instant Soup Mix by Vogue — this is a blend of dehydrated vegetables and mild seasonings that tastes great sprinkled on salad or added to soups or vegetable dishes. I use it frequently in the recipes that follow.

Butter Buds

Fakin Bacon Bits

Nonfat tomato sauce

Low-calorie salad dressings

Spices — Oriental spice mix, Mrs. Dash, mild chili salsa powder, garlic and onion powder, oregano, cayenne

Unhulled sesame seeds, walnuts, and ground flaxseed

Another great option, for those on the go, is to order Ginny's Organic Gourmet, such as Savory Soy Chili, Mexican Fiesta Stew, Roasted Pepper Chili, and Ratatouille. Just open the jars, heat, and eat. Pop open a bag of washed salad, add some chili on top or on the side, and grab a few fruits for dessert. How could designing a filling and satisfying lunch or dinner be simpler?

You can also purchase salsa dips in a jar — those made without oil — at the health-food store. Salsa is just a combination of tomatoes, onions, and peppers (jalapeño peppers, chili peppers, or cilantro). You can make it more spicy, or milder merely by leaving out chili peppers and adding some finely chopped scallions, red onions, parsley, or mint and some lemon or lime juice.

Put your salsa on lettuce, green vegetables, or raw vegetables. It is simple to make your own — just mix 1 cup of diced tomatoes with ¼ cup finely chopped red onion and add the extra ingredients, such as lime juice and finely chopped scallions, parsley, and mint. I like it creamy, made with a quarter mashed avocado added per cup of tomato, almost like a salsa-guacamole dip. Keep this on hand in the refrigerator at all times so you have something quick and easy to snack on. Just take some washed lettuce or frozen vegetables, dip, and eat.

Since this way of eating encourages lots of green salads, I have offered quite a number of healthy, great-tasting salad dressings. Get all the ingredients and try them all in the beginning, then pick out the ones you like the best. Cuisine Perel makes fruit-flavored vinegars, such as, D'Anjou Pear Vinegar, Blood Orange Vinegar, Fig Vinegar, and Spicy Pecan Vinegar that have only five calories per tablespoon and are delicious used alone on a salad. Ordering information on such helpful products can be obtained from my website. Other low-calorie commercial dressings are listed at the end of the "Salads, Dressings, and Dips" section.

Since you are giving up lots of unhealthy foods, treat yourself to those delicious and exotic fruits. This diet permits lots of fresh fruit, since eating fruit is a necessity for optimal health and long life. Persimmons, for example, are a wonderful treat. You must let them ripen until every part, including the bottom rim, is mushy soft before it will be a great-tasting treat. Cherimoyas are another delicious fruit, though quite expensive. Try different varieties of mangoes, as they have different flavors, and don't forget fresh figs.

7 Days of Vegetarian Meal Plans
(For Aggressive Weight Loss)

* = Recipes follow

Day One

BREAKFAST
Strawberries (fresh or frozen)
Orange
Grapefruit

LUNCH
Apple Pie Salad*
Whole-wheat pita pocket stuffed with Tasty Hummus Spread*
   or Grandma Tillie's Eggplant Dip*
Lettuce and tomatoes
1 or 2 fresh fruits

DINNER
Salad with lemon and shredded pear
Steamed Swiss chard and zucchini cooked with onions, mushrooms, and stewed tomatoes
Acorn Squash Supreme*
Blueberries

Day Two

BREAKFAST
>   Oranges
>   1 cup oatmeal
>   1 ounce walnuts
>   1 ounce raisins

LUNCH
>   Raisin Coleslaw*
>   Vegetable or bean soup
>   1 or 2 pieces of fresh fruit

DINNER
>   Salad with Orange/Sesame Dressing*
>   Dr. Fuhrman's Famous Anti-Cancer Soup*
>   Baked potato with nonfat tomato sauce

Day Three

BREAKFAST
>   Baked apple with raisins and cinnamon

LUNCH
>   Salad-stuffed pita with Tasty Hummus Spread*
>   Fresh fruit

DINNER
>   Mixed baby greens, with cracked peppercorn dressing
>   Broccoli and Red Pepper Soup,* slice of seven-grain bread
>   Corn on the cob with Vege Base seasoning

Day Four

BREAKFAST
>   Frozen Banana Fluff* with one tablespoon of ground flaxseed
>   added per person

LUNCH
   Salad with lemon
   Raw vegetables (string beans, carrots, broccoli, peppers), with
      Spicy Bean Dip*
   Fresh or frozen strawberries

DINNER:
   Iceberg lettuce, tomatoes, red onions, with Zesty Tomato-Garlic
      Dressing*
   Lisa's Lovely Lentil Stew*
   Steamed string beans with garlic powder

Day Five

BREAKFAST
   Dried apricots, soaked overnight in soymilk

LUNCH
   Celery stalks stuffed with Spicy Bean Spread*
   Frozen artichoke hearts, dipped in low-calorie dressing
   Frozen blueberries

DINNER
   Romaine lettuce soaked in orange juice
   Tofu Chow Mein*
   Green apple slices in lime juice

Day Six

BREAKFAST
   Whole grapefruit, fresh pineapple
   1 oz. sunflower seeds

LUNCH
   Bean Burgers*
   Green salad with Bloody Delicious Dressing*
   Apple or pear

DINNER

Quick Corn Stew*

Salad with Brainy Blueberry Dressing*

Eggplant Patties*

Day Seven

BREAKFAST

Oranges, green apples

Baby spinach and baby romaine with
    Mango-Pineapple Shazaam Dressing*

LUNCH

Raw veggies, dipped in Grandma Tillie's Eggplant Dip*

Seasonal fresh fruit

DINNER

Tomato Barley Stew*

Broccoli Vinaigrette*

Vegetarian Chili* or one of Ginny's Chilis — Savory Soy Chili or
    Roasted Pepper Chili (Ginny's Organic Gourmet)

Frozen orange juice pops

7 Days of Nonvegetarian Meal Plans
(Less Strict, for Moderate Weight Loss)

Essentially, these are the same basic menus and meal plans as the
preceding ones, except for three things: one, there are a few more
dishes and recipes that include vegetables with a higher starch content; two, a small amount of animal foods may be used to flavor the
vegetable dishes, soups, and casseroles; and three, one teaspoon of
oil daily is an optional inclusion. No cheese is permitted because of
its high saturated fat content, and no more than twelve ounces per
week of animal products is allowed. Most of these recipes and meal
plans can be used for those wishing to stay on a vegetarian diet or
wishing to stay on the more aggressive program — just leave out the
oil and the animal products, and eat smaller portions of the high-
starch vegetables. Almost all the recipes are oil-free.

Day One

BREAKFAST
> 2 cups cooked oatmeal with
>> 1 tbsp. ground flaxseed
>
> 1 banana
> 1 oz. raisins
> ¼–½ cup soymilk or skim milk

LUNCH
> Green salad with low-fat, balsamic vinaigrette and 1 tsp. olive
>> oil, if desired
>
> 1 cup chickpeas or 1 cup frozen peas
> Vegetable or bean soup
> 1 or 2 fresh fruits

DINNER
> Salad with orange juice and lemon
> Oriental Wok* with chicken and tofu
> Steamed string beans with onions and mushrooms

Day Two

BREAKFAST
> Scrambled Tofu*

LUNCH
> Spinach Salad with Orange/Sesame Dressing*
> Rolled Eggplant*
> Fresh pineapple

DINNER
> Salad with 1 tsp. olive oil and Vege Base
> Broiled fish or scallops (4 oz., max.)
> Frozen broccoli
> Strawberry Freeze*

Day Three

BREAKFAST
Fresh pears with soaked prunes or apricots
(dried fruit soaked overnight in regular soymilk or skim milk)

LUNCH
Salad with chickpeas and frozen peas on top, fresh lemon and
   orange squeezed over it
Fresh fruit

DINNER
Salad with sliced oranges and 2 tbsp. sunflower seeds
Steamed and chopped kale with garlic and onion powder
Egg White Omelette*

Day Four

BREAKFAST
Banana-Berry Shake*

LUNCH
Salad soaked with orange and lemon juice
Chicken Optional Veg-Lentil Soup*

DINNER
Mixed green salad with Zesty Tomato-Garlic Dressing*
Broccoli Vinaigrette*
Quick Corn Stew*

Day Five

BREAKFAST
Pita Apple Bake*
Kiwis

LUNCH
Celery, cabbage, and cucumber salad with Tuna Dressing*
Tofu Spinach Pot*

DINNER

Lettuce and tomato (dressing option: ½ tsp. olive oil, ½ tsp. flax oil and balsamic vinegar)
Acorn Squash Supreme*
Portabella Mushrooms and Beans*

Day Six

BREAKFAST

Egg White Omelette* with pan-cooked veggies

LUNCH

Raw veggies; fresh tomatoes, cucumber, and celery with Ginny's Savory Soy Chili (Ginny's Organic Gourmet)
Fruit bowl with pureed mango and 1 oz. crushed walnuts on top

DINNER

Mixed green salad with thin slivers of green apple and thin sliced almonds
Talia's Unmeatballs and Spaghetti*
Spinach and Mushroom Sauce*
Saturday night special dessert — Cara's Apple Cake*

Day Seven

BREAKFAST

Red raspberries, strawberries, or blueberries
1 cup oatmeal with apples, cinnamon, and flaxseed
Light soymilk

LUNCH

Half a toasted whole-wheat pita, with thin slice of turkey breast, lettuce, tomato, and Thousand Lost Island Dressing*
Seasonal fresh fruit

DINNER

Boston lettuce, thinly sliced red onion, white mushrooms, with sliced pear and black fig vinegar
Steamed string beans

Roasted Peppers*
Jenna's Peach Freeze*

The Eat to Live Recipes

Note: All recipes are approximately two servings, unless noted otherwise.

Soups and Stews

CHICKEN OPTIONAL VEG-LENTIL SOUP
BROCCOLI AND RED PEPPER SOUP
DR. FUHRMAN'S FAMOUS ANTI-CANCER SOUP
LISA'S LOVELY LENTIL STEW
TOMATO BARLEY STEW
QUICK CORN STEW

Salads, Dressings, and Dips

GRANDMA TILLIE'S EGGPLANT DIP
SPICY BEAN SPREAD OR DIP
TASTY HUMMUS SPREAD OR DIP
APPLE PIE DRESSING
BRAINY BLUEBERRY DRESSING
BLOODY DELICIOUS DRESSING
MANGO-PINEAPPLE SHAZAAM DRESSING
ORANGE/SESAME DRESSING
RAISIN COLESLAW
THOUSAND LOST ISLAND DRESSING
TUNA DRESSING
ZESTY TOMATO-GARLIC DRESSING
COMMERCIAL DRESSINGS

Main Dishes

ACORN SQUASH SUPREME
BEAN BURGERS

BEAN ENCHILADAS

BLACK AND BLUE BEANS AND GREENS

BROCCOLI VINAIGRETTE

EGGPLANT PATTIES

EGG WHITE OMELETTE

MEDITERRANEAN EGGPLANT AND BEANS

MEXICAN LENTILS

ORIENTAL WOK

PORTOBELLA MUSHROOMS AND BEANS

ROLLED EGGPLANT

ROASTED PEPPERS

SCRAMBLED TOFU

SPINACH AND MUSHROOM SAUCE

TALIA'S UNMEATBALLS AND SPAGHETTI

TOFU CHOW MEIN

TOFU SPINACH POT

VEGETARIAN CHILI

Shakes and Desserts

BANANA-BERRY SHAKE

CARA'S APPLE CAKE

FROZEN BANANA FLUFF OR STRAWBERRY FREEZE

JENNA'S PEACH FREEZE

PITA APPLE BAKE

Soups and Stews

CHICKEN OPTIONAL VEG-LENTIL SOUP

SERVES 4

1½ cups lentils
½ cup barley or couscous, uncooked
1 large onion, chopped
3 celery stalks, diced
3 carrots, chopped
1 tsp. Mrs. Dash seasoning

Mix everything in a large pot with 6 cups of water, bring to boil, and simmer over low flame for 2 hours.

Variation: Use chicken broth instead of water and/or add 2 oz. chicken, diced

BROCCOLI AND RED PEPPER SOUP

2 lbs. of fresh or frozen broccoli, chopped into large pieces
1 large onion, diced
3 garlic cloves, minced
3 tbsp. dried vegetable soup mix (such as Vogue Vege Base)
⅓ cup brown rice (uncooked)
3 red bell peppers
1 lemon, juiced
1 tbsp. vinegar
seasonings, to taste

In a large soup pot, combine the broccoli, onion, garlic, water, Vege Base, and rice in 2 quarts of water. Simmer, covered, over a very low flame. Roast the red peppers in a broiler or on a gas grill until all sides begin to blacken. Quarter and remove the peel and seeds from the peppers, then puree them in a blender with the softened broccoli with some of the soup liquid. Add puree back to the pot. Add the lemon, vinegar, and seasonings to taste (e.g., tarragon, thyme, white or black pepper).

DR. FUHRMAN'S FAMOUS ANTI-CANCER SOUP

SERVES 10

Making this soup involves more time and effort than the other recipes, so you might want to make a huge amount and save it in the refrigerator for the whole week. It tastes so good that a patient of mine who owns a fine restaurant offers it on his menu.

1 cup dried split peas and/or beans
4 medium onions
6–10 zucchini
3 stalks leek
5 lbs. carrots
2 bunches celery
1 cup raw cashews

2 tbsp. Vege Base by Vogue
1 package mushrooms, any type (optional)
6 oz. TVP (textured vegetable protein), optional

Place the beans and 4 cups of water in a very ˡ
cooking them, covered, on the lowest flame possibᵢₑ. ₌₌
skins off the onions and place them in the covered pot. Do not cuₜ
them up, put them in whole. Add the zucchini, uncut. Cut the bottom roots off the leeks and slice them up the side so each leaf can be
thoroughly washed, because leeks have lots of dirt hidden inside.
Throw away the last inch at the green top. Then place the entire leek
(leaves uncut) into the pot. Juice the carrots and celery in a juice ex-
tractor. Add the juice to the pot. While the soup is simmering, chop
up the mushrooms (if desired). By the time you get to this stage, the
zucchini, leeks, and onions should be soft.

This next step only works if you have a Vita-Mix, a powerful
blender, or a food processor. Ladle some of the liquid from the pot
into the machine. Use tongs to remove the soft onions, zucchini, and
leeks. Be careful to leave the beans in the bottom of the pot. In a few
separate batches, completely blend together the onions, zucchini,
and leeks. Add more soup liquid and the cashews to the mixture, and
blend in. Return the blended, creamy mix back to the pot. Add the
TVP and the mushrooms, if desired. Simmer another 20 minutes,
and you have my soup that is famous the world over. I know a doctor who makes and freezes my soup and sells it to his patients to cure
everything from sinusitis to cancer. It's not really a cure, but it sure
does taste great.

The Vita-Mix is also great for making salad dressings, pureeing
vegetables into soup, grinding wheat berries into fresh flour for making homemade bread, and for grinding flaxseed and sesame seeds. It
is a super machine, but expensive. If you want to inquire about pur-
chasing a Vita-Mix at a significant discount, call 1-800-474-9355 and
tell them you were referred by this book.

LISA'S LOVELY LENTIL STEW

1 cup lentils for every 3 cups water
½ medium onion, finely chopped
1 tsp. black pepper (optional)
1 tsp. basil

3 big ripe tomatoes, chopped
1 stalk celery, finely chopped

Cook lentils in water for 30 minutes with onion, pepper, and basil. Add tomatoes and celery and cook for an additional 15 minutes.

TOMATO BARLEY STEW

1 cup celery juice
1 medium onion
2 carrots, diced
1 zucchini
1 baked or boiled potato (no skin)
¼ cup unrefined barley
6 tomatoes, chopped
⅓ cup sun-dried tomatoes, finely chopped
8 oz. white mushrooms, chopped

Heat 1 cup of water and the juice on a low flame. Add the onion, carrots, zucchini and potato. Let simmer about 1 hour and then blend in blender or Vita-Mix. Return pureed mix back to the pot and add the barley, tomatoes, dried tomatoes and mushrooms and simmer for another 45 minutes.

QUICK CORN STEW

2 cups soymilk
1 tbsp. whole-wheat flour
1 medium potato, diced
1 carrot, diced
1 large onion, diced
½ tsp. dulse
2 tbsp. dried vegetable flakes
¼ tsp. Mrs. Dash seasoning
1 tsp. Butter Buds
1 10-oz. bag (or box) frozen corn

Heat 2 cups of water and soymilk together on a low flame. Mix in the flour, dulse, vegetable flakes, and seasoning. Add the diced potato, carrot, and onion and continue to simmer for 5 minutes. Add the frozen corn until it defrosts and the soup comes to a boil again.

Salads, Dressings, and Dips

GRANDMA TILLIE'S EGGPLANT DIP

1 eggplant
1 tomato, diced
1 green or red pepper, diced
1 large onion, diced
dash of Mrs. Dash seasoning

Bake the eggplant in the oven at 350° for 1 hour, or microwave it for 8–11 minutes. In a covered, shallow pan or pot, steam-fry the tomato, pepper, and onion until soft. Scoop out or peel the eggplant and blend it with the steamed vegetables and seasoning.

SPICY BEAN SPREAD OR DIP

1 15-oz. can of beans, any type
1 tsp. mild chili salsa, chili powder, or crushed red chili peppers
1 pinch cumin or turmeric (optional)
¼ tsp. garlic powder, or two garlic cloves, crushed

Mash the beans with a fork, masher, or food processor with about half the liquid from the can. Mix in the spices. Serve with raw or lightly steamed vegetables or toasted pita bread.

TASTY HUMMUS SPREAD OR DIP

1 cup cooked or canned garbanzo beans (chickpeas)
1 tbsp. tahini (sesame seed butter)
2 tbsp. lemon juice
2 garlic cloves, finely chopped
⅓ cup bean liquid (from the can) or water
1 tsp. horseradish (optional)

Blend all ingredients in a blender until creamy smooth. Makes an awesome spread or a dip for raw and lightly steamed vegetables.

APPLE PIE DRESSING

2 peeled apples
¼ cup fresh-squeezed orange juice
cinnamon to taste

Blend together.

I especially like this salad dressing with lettuce, tomatoes, avocados, walnuts, and raisins. Obviously, if you are trying to lose weight, don't add much of the higher-calorie nuts and avocados.

BRAINY BLUEBERRY DRESSING

½ pack frozen blueberries
2 dates
2 tbsp. raspberry vinegar
1 tbsp. lemon juice

Blend together.

BLOODY DELICIOUS DRESSING

¼ cup blood orange vinegar
1 large tomato, or 10 cherry tomatoes

Blend together.

MANGO-PINEAPPLE SHAZAAM DRESSING

1 mango
4 oz. unsweetened canned pineapple
2 tsp. lemon
2 tbsp. red raspberry vinegar or blood orange vinegar
3 oz. silken tofu

Blend together.

ORANGE/SESAME DRESSING

3 tbsp. unhulled sesame seeds
6 raw cashew nuts

½ cup orange juice
2 tbsp. rice vinegar
2 oranges, peeled and diced, or 1 jar unsweetened, mandarin orange slices

Toast the sesame seeds in a dry skillet for 3 minutes, shaking the pan frequently. In a blender or Vita-Mix, combine 2 tbsp. sesame seeds, the cashews, orange juice, and vinegar. Add the diced oranges to the salad and mix in the blended dressing. Sprinkle the remaining sesame seeds on top. This tastes great on a spinach and mushroom salad with thinly sliced red onions, or on a lettuce, tomato, and cucumber salad.

RAISIN COLESLAW

½ cup raisins
½ cup apple juice
½ baked potato, skin removed
1 tsp. mustard
1 tbsp. lemon juice
4 cups cabbage, shredded
2 cups carrots, shredded
1 cup beets, shredded (optional)
2 cups apples, peeled and shredded
¼ cup scallions, finely chopped

Blend or Vita-Mix the raisins, apple juice, potato, mustard, and lemon juice, then mix all the ingredients together. Use this in place of a lettuce salad for lunch or dinner.

THOUSAND LOST ISLAND DRESSING

2 hard-boiled egg whites
⅓ cup chopped celery, cucumber, or chopped steamed string beans
½ tsp. onion powder
3 tbsp. ketchup
1 tbsp. nonfat plain yogurt
⅓ cup chopped red pepper

Blend together.

TUNA DRESSING

1 small cucumber, peeled
½ small can water-packed tuna, with liquid from can
1 tbsp. cider vinegar
2 tsp. fresh dill, finely minced, or 1 teaspoon dried
2 tbsp. nonfat plain yogurt or soy yogurt
1 small tomato

Blend together.

ZESTY TOMATO-GARLIC DRESSING

½ cup tomato or tomato vegetable juice
2 tsp. lemon juice
½ tsp. Italian seasonings
1 garlic clove, chopped, or ¼ tsp. garlic powder
3 oz. low-fat tofu (optional)

Blend together.

Commercial Dressings
with Less than 20 Calories per 2 Tablespoon Serving

Annie's Naturals No-Fat Organic Yogurt Dressing with Dill

Blanchard & Blanchard Balsamic Cracked Peppercorn

Blanchard & Blanchard Balsamic Tomato Herb

Blanchard & Blanchard Balsamic Roasted Garlic

Consorvio Fat-Free Mango Dressing

Consorvio Fat-Free Raspberry and Balsamic

Pritikin Salad Dressings

Rising Sun Farm Oil-Free Roasted Garlic Galore

Rising Sun Farm Oil-Free Pesto Dried Tomato

Rising Sun Farm Oil-Free Raspberry Balsamic

Rising Sun Farm Oil-Free Italian Lovers

Rising Sun Farm Oil-Free Sweet Pepper and Dried Tomato

Southern Sensations Vidalia Onion Tomato — Fat Free

Spectrum Naturals Sweet Onion and Garlic

Spectrum Naturals Toasted Sesame
Spectrum Naturals Creamy Garlic — Fat Free
Spectrum Naturals Creamy Dill — Fat Free (25 cal.)

Main Dishes

ACORN SQUASH SUPREME

1 large acorn squash
4 tbsp. diced dried apricots
2 tbsp. chopped raw cashews
1 (15-oz.) can unsweetened, crushed pineapple, juice reserved
2 tbsp. raisins
cinnamon

Cut squash in half, remove seeds, and bake facedown in ½ inch of water for 45 minutes at 350°.

Cover the apricots in a bowl with some of the pineapple juice. On top, add the pineapple, raisins, and cashews. Let stand and soak while the squash is cooking.

After the squash has cooked, mix up the fruit in the bowl and scoop it into the squash's center. Cover with aluminum foil and bake covered for an additional 30 minutes. Sprinkle with cinnamon, then put it back in the oven for 5 more minutes.

BEAN BURGERS

¼ cup sunflower seeds
2 cups red or pink canned beans (unsalted)
½ cup minced onion
½ tsp. chili powder
2 tbsp. ketchup
1 tbsp. wheat germ or oatmeal

Chop the sunflower seeds in a food processor or hand chopper and mash the beans with a potato masher or food processor and mix. Mix in the remaining ingredients and form the patties. Bake at 350° for 20–25 minutes. Remove from the oven and let cool until you can pick up each patty and compress it firmly in your hands to reform the burger. Then cook for another 15 minutes on each side.

BEAN ENCHILADAS

1 green pepper, sliced
½ cup sliced onion
1 cup nonfat commercial taco sauce or salsa sauce
2 cups canned or cooked pinto or black beans
1 cup frozen corn kernels
1 tsp. cumin
1 tsp. chopped cilantro
6–8 nonfat corn tortillas

Sauté the green pepper and onion in a skillet with 2 tablespoons of the taco sauce, until tender. Stir in the beans, corn, and seasonings. Paint the tortillas with a coating of taco sauce, spoon about ¼ cup of the bean mix on each, and roll up. They can be eaten as is or baked at 375° in the oven for 15 minutes first.

BLACK AND BLUE BEANS AND GREENS

SERVES 4

½ cup black beans
½ cup white beans
1 bay leaf
2 garlic cloves, chopped
½ tsp. Mrs. Dash seasoning
1 tsp. Vege Base by Vogue
one bunch kale, chopped or sliced in strips, stems removed
3 medium white onions
10 oz. spinach, chopped or sliced in strips (or one box frozen spinach)
4 small zucchini
small bunch fresh dill, chopped

Start cooking beans in 3 cups of water with the bay leaf, garlic, and seasonings. Then peel the onions and add them along with the spinach, zucchini, kale, and dill on top of the cooking beans and let simmer over a low flame for at least 2 hours. Then stir up the mixture well, breaking up the zucchini and onion now that they are soft and mushy.

BROCCOLI VINAIGRETTE

1 bunch broccoli
¼ cup seasoned rice vinegar
2 tsp. Dijon mustard
2 large garlic cloves, pressed or minced

Break the broccoli into bite-size florets. Peel stems and slice them into ¼-inch-thick strips. Steam florets and stems for 10 minutes, or until just tender. While the broccoli is steaming, whisk the rest of the ingredients in a bowl. Add broccoli and toss to mix.

EGGPLANT PATTIES

Serves 4

2 eggplants, peeled and sliced
3 tbsp. balsamic vinegar
4 garlic cloves, minced
1 tbsp. finely chopped rosemary
pinch of black pepper
pinch of oregano
1 tbsp. Bragg's Liquid Aminos

Slice eggplant into ⅓-inch-thick patties. Mix together all ingredients in a flat-bottom bowl. Let the eggplant patties marinate in the mixture for 15–20 seconds. Wet napkin with olive oil and wipe down a nonstick baking tray or aluminum foil, creating a thin coat of oil. Then bake the eggplant on the tray or sheet of aluminum foil at 350° for 20–25 minutes. Mushrooms can be used instead of or in addition to the eggplant.

EGG WHITE OMELETTE

½ medium onion, diced
½ medium green or red pepper, diced
½ cup of canned or fresh mushrooms, diced, liquid reserved
½ cup diced tomatoes (optional)
2 egg whites or nonfat egg substitute

Sauté the onions, pepper, and mushrooms in some of the liquid from the canned mushrooms (or instead, with the diced tomato broth), then add egg whites and cook.

MEDITERRANEAN EGGPLANT
AND BEANS

1 eggplant, peeled and diced
1 onion, sliced thinly
1 green pepper, chopped
½ cup raisins
1 tbsp. lemon juice
3 tbsp. ketchup
2 cups garbanzo or other beans, cooked or canned

Steam the eggplant for 10–12 minutes. Cook the onion and pepper over a low flame in a covered skillet with 2 tablespoons of water for 6–8 minutes. Then add the eggplant, raisins, lemon juice, and ketchup and simmer uncovered for another 5 minutes. Mix in the beans.

MEXICAN LENTILS

1 cup lentils, uncooked
1 cup frozen or fresh corn
1 cup nonfat tomato sauce
1 onion, chopped
Mexican seasonings to taste (crushed red chili peppers, garlic, and dill)

Boil the lentils in 2 cups of water for 30 minutes and drain. Combine the remaining ingredients and simmer over low heat for 20 minutes.

ORIENTAL WOK

1 tbsp. sweet mirin seasoning
1 tsp. Mrs. Dash or Oriental seasoning
2 garlic cloves, chopped
¼ cup cooking wine or vegetable broth
10–20 ounces assorted fresh vegetables, or 1–2 (10-oz.) bags frozen
  Oriental vegetables (defrosted)
1 onion, or 3 shallots, chopped
1 can water chestnuts, juice reserved
1 box tofu, diced
2 oz. chopped chicken (optional)

Place the seasoning, garlic, and cooking wine (or broth) in a covered pot or wok and heat. Add the vegetables. If using frozen vegetables, drain off the water and don't use the juice from the water chestnuts because you will not need as much liquid. Fresh vegetables need to cook longer and require more liquid. Any vegetables can be stir-fried in pineapple juice, vegetable broth, flavored vinegar, light soy sauce, or Bragg's Liquid Aminos for a change of flavor.

PORTOBELLA MUSHROOMS AND BEANS

½ tsp. olive oil
1 large onion, chopped
2 garlic cloves, chopped
2 large portobella mushroom caps, sliced thin
⅓ cup red wine (or vegetable broth)
1 large tomato, diced, or 8 halved cherry tomatoes
1 (15-oz.) can garbanzo beans, juice reserved

Heat oil and spread to cover the bottom of a skillet. Add the onion and garlic and sauté for 2 minutes, then add the mushrooms and the red wine or broth. Cook for 5 more minutes. Add the tomatoes and garbanzo beans, plus half the juice from the can. Cook for another 5–10 minutes.

ROLLED EGGPLANT

1 eggplant, peeled and sliced into thin, flat, wide strips
1 pepper, diced (red or green)
1 onion, chopped
2 garlic cloves, chopped
2 cups nonfat tomato sauce

Bake eggplant in a lubricated pan at 350° degrees for 20 minutes, until flexible. Sauté pepper, onion, and garlic in water to make the filling. Take the strips of partially cooked eggplant and roll them up with the filling mix in the middle. Cover with nonfat tomato sauce and bake at 350° for another 30 minutes.

ROASTED PEPPERS

4 red peppers, halved, with seeds scooped out
low-calorie commercial dressing

Rub down the peppers with the salad dressing using your hands and cook in oven on low broil for 10 minutes, or roast in oven at 450° for 30 minutes. Wash hands.

SCRAMBLED TOFU

1 small onion (or several green onions), chopped
½ cup green pepper, finely chopped
2 garlic cloves, chopped
2 cups firm tofu, drained and crumbled
black pepper to taste, or Vege Base or Mrs. Dash seasoning

In a large skillet, sauté onion, green pepper, and garlic in ⅓ cup water for 5 minutes. Add the tofu and pepper (or seasoning) and cook for another 5 minutes. Add a little Vege Base or Mrs. Dash as a flavoring. Note: Vege Base Instant Soup Mix by Vogue is good in salads or in soups to add flavor. It is made from dehydrated vegetables.

SPINACH AND MUSHROOM SAUCE

2 lbs. spinach, washed
1 lb. white mushrooms, divided
¼ cup light soymilk
1 white onion, chopped
½ tsp. garlic powder
2 tbsp. whole-wheat flour

Steam the spinach with half of the mushrooms for 10 minutes, then remove it from the pot and drain. Take the other half of the mushrooms and gently heat in a pot with the soymilk, onion, garlic, and flour for 15 minutes. Blend the heated mixture in a blender, food processor, or Vita-Mix and pour over each separate serving of steamed spinach and mushrooms.

TALIA'S UNMEATBALLS AND SPAGHETTI

SERVES 4

¼ cup light soymilk
1 tbsp. sesame tahini
chopped garlic, dill, oregano, parsley (optional)
1 tbsp. Vege Base by Vogue
¼ cup whole-wheat flour
½ cup oatmeal
1 cup TVP (textured vegetable protein)
¼ cup walnuts, chopped
1 cup firm tofu, chopped or crumbled
2 onions, chopped

Warm the soymilk gently and fold in the tahini to make a sauce. Remove from heat and add the seasonings and Vege Base. Add the flour and oatmeal and mix well. Add the remaining ingredients. Mash it all together and knead the mixture with your hands to form solid ball. Then form the mixture into small balls and lay them on a non-stick baking tray and bake at 375° for 30 minutes.

Serve over baked spaghetti squash, or lentil bean pasta, with plenty of fat-free tomato sauce. You can make your own fat-free, salt-free tomato sauce by gently heating in a pot fresh or canned tomatoes, crushed garlic, chopped onions, chopped scallions, and 2 tablespoons of salt-free Italian seasonings, one teaspoon of lemon juice, and one teaspoon of wine vinegar.

TOFU CHOW MEIN

2 cups cabbage, chopped
2 cups onions, sliced
sesame or almond oil
1 lb. tofu, diced
2 cups peas
2 cups mushrooms, sliced
1 tbsp. arrowroot powder
1 tbsp. low-salt soy sauce, tamari, or Bragg's Liquid Aminos
1 tsp. Oriental seasonings
1 (15-oz.) can water chestnuts
2 cups mung bean sprouts

In a covered pan or wok, sauté the cabbage and onions in 1 teaspoon of sesame or almond oil. Cook for 5 minutes and then add the tofu, peas, and mushrooms. In a separate bowl, mix the arrowroot powder and the soy sauce with 3 tablespoons of the liquid from the cooking mushrooms or from the canned water chestnuts. Add this mixture, the seasonings, the water chestnuts, and the bean sprouts to the sauté mixture and mix well. Cook for 3 more minutes.

TOFU SPINACH POT

1 lb. firm or extra-firm tofu, cubed
1 (10-oz.) box frozen spinach, thawed
3 tomatoes, chopped
2 tbsp. lemon juice
⅛ tsp. cayenne
⅛ tsp. onion powder
½ cup vegetable broth

Sauté all the ingredients in the vegetable broth. Any type of bean may be substituted for the tofu.

VEGETARIAN CHILI

2 cups dry kidney or pinto beans
1 (15-oz.) can crushed tomatoes
2 cups chopped red onion
2 cups chopped green or red peppers
1 cup chopped carrots
1 cup chopped celery
1 cup TVP (textured vegetable protein)
4 garlic cloves, finely chopped
1 tsp. oregano
1 tsp. basil
1 tsp. chili powder
½ tsp. cumin
1 tsp. red wine vinegar
1 tbsp. diced raisins or dates

Wash the beans and soak them in water overnight. Cover with water, simmer for 2 hours, and pour off the water, or use a 15-oz. can of pinto beans instead. Combine all ingredients in a large saucepan and simmer for 1 hour. This can be poured over chopped lettuce or steamed green vegetables such as spinach and kale, or eaten by itself.

Shakes And Desserts

BANANA-BERRY SHAKE

1 banana
1 bag frozen or 1 box fresh strawberries
1 cup regular soymilk or skim milk
1 tbsp. ground flaxseed

Blend all ingredients together in a food processor, blender, or Vita-Mix.

CARA'S APPLE CAKE

SERVES 4

¼ tsp. vanilla
¼ cup apple juice
1 tsp. cinnamon
1 egg white
¼ cup vanilla soymilk
3 apples, peeled and chopped
¼ cup raisins, chopped
½ cup rolled oats or oatmeal flakes

Stir the vanilla into the apple juice. Stir in the cinnamon, egg white, and soymilk. Then add the apples, raisins, and oats. Bake uncovered at 350° for 1 hour. Remove and cover with aluminum foil.

FROZEN BANANA FLUFF
OR STRAWBERRY FREEZE

1 banana
¼ cup vanilla soymilk
dash vanilla extract (optional)

Peel and freeze the ripe banana in a plastic bag or kitchenware. This is a good way to make sure no bananas go to waste — just freeze the ones that start to get too ripe.

Place the soymilk in the food processor, with the S blade in place. Turn the machine on and drop in small slices of frozen banana, one by one. My children like this with ground flaxseed added to the top at the time of serving. The same recipe can be made with other frozen fruit. Try 1 cup of organic frozen strawberries and ½ a banana per person.

JENNA'S PEACH FREEZE

1 frozen banana
2 large dates, or 4 small
3 peaches or nectarines
¼ cup vanilla soymilk
1 tsp. vanilla
⅛ tsp. cinnamon

Cut up the bananas and fruit. Mix all ingredients together in a blender or Vita-Mix.

PITA APPLE BAKE

2 apples, chopped
¼ cup raisins (optional)
2 tbsp. water or apple juice
1 tbsp. ground flaxseed (optional)
¼ tsp. cinnamon
1 whole-wheat pita, split and separated

Heat the apples, raisins (if desired), and water or juice over a low flame for 5 minutes, stirring frequently. Remove from heat and mix in flaxseed and cinnamon. Cut pita in half and fill with apple mixture. Toast in the toaster oven on high for 3 minutes. Try it with other fruits, like pears or peaches, too.

Frequently Asked Questions

Should I take vitamins and other nutritional supplements?

I often recommend that people take a high-quality multivitamin to ensure that they get enough vitamin D, B_{12}, zinc, iodine, and selenium. Very few individuals eat perfectly, and some of us require more of certain nutrients than others. It makes sense to be sure that you ingest adequate amounts of all these important substances. I also recommend a sensibly designed multi because I instruct my patients to avoid salt. Salt is iodinated, making it the primary source of iodine in most people's diets; therefore, a multi can ensure adequate iodine intake for those who avoid salt in their diet.

The main concern with taking a multivitamin is that it may contain a high dose of vitamin A or beta-carotene. Ingesting large amounts of these nutrients may interfere with the absorption of other carotenoids, such as lutein and lycopene, thus potentially increasing the risk of cancer.[1] There is also concern that supplemental vitamin A induces calcium loss in the urine, contributing to osteoporosis. Even though too much vitamin A is known to be toxic to the liver, the most common effect of toxic doses of vitamin A in animals is spontaneous fracture. Apparently, excessive vitamin A is potentially a problem in humans, too — one study comparing vitamin A intake in the .5 mg range to the 1.5 mg range showed a doubling of the hip fracture rate.[2] There are multiple vitamins available today with natural, mixed carotenoids in place of vitamin A and beta-carotene that also contain extra plant-derived phytochemicals. Look for this type of multiple. My office or website can suggest appropriate brands.

Another concern is the current popularity of high-dose vitamin C. Researchers at the University of California found that men who took 500 mg of vitamin C daily had arterial walls 2.5 times thicker than men who did not take the supplement.[3] Arterial thickening increases the risk of hypertension and heart disease. Keep in mind that this is only one study. Hundreds of others have shown benefits of supplemental vitamin C (for those on the vitamin C–deficient diet that the vast majority of Americans eat). So other studies are needed to confirm these findings. However, the diets I recommend are rich in vitamin C, containing 500 mg from food, not supplements. There are only positive effects when vitamin C comes from food in lieu of supplements.

Some nutritional immunologists believe that nutrient supplementation beyond what can be obtained from the diet is necessary to optimize immune function, especially in the elderly.[4] A few others argue that consuming too much of certain nutrients and dietary excess of some substances may have a detrimental effect on the absorption and utilization of other substances, as seems to be the case with vitamin A and beta-carotene. You should also avoid using iron supplements on a regular basis. There is no evidence that other nutrients, in the dosages found in ordinary multivitamin/multimineral preparations, would be harmful.

However, a crucial point that cannot be emphasized enough is that supplements are no substitute for a healthy diet. To the extent they offer some people the confidence to eat less wholesome vegetation, they are hurtful, not helpful.

Could restricting my intake of animal products or eating a strict vegetarian diet cause me to develop vitamin deficiencies?

A strict vegetarian diet is deficient in meeting the vitamin B_{12} needs of some individuals. If you choose to follow a complete vegetarian (vegan) diet, it is imperative that you consume a multivitamin or other source of B_{12}, such as fortified soymilk. My vegetarian menu plans and dietary suggestions are otherwise rich in calcium and contain sufficient iron from green vegetables and beans. They contain adequate protein and are extremely nutrient-dense.

Vitamin D, often called the sunshine vitamin, is another common deficiency I find when I check the blood levels of my patients. Most of us work indoors and avoid the sun or wear sunscreen, which lowers our vitamin D exposure. Some of us don't absorb it as well and just require more. So, given all the data that is available today and my personal experience with patients, I advise most people to consume an appropriate multi.

My observations suggest that vegetarians would be foolish not to play it safe, either by taking a B_{12} supplement or a multi or by consuming foods that have been fortified with vitamin B_{12}. Another option for those who loathe taking vitamins is to have their blood checked periodically. Checking your B_{12} level alone is not sufficient. Methylmalonic acid (MMA) must be checked to accurately gauge if the level of B_{12} in your body is enough for you.

What about supplements or herbs to help me lose weight?

Don't be conned by diet pills, magic in a bottle, or fat absorbers. Anything really effective is not safe, and those that are safe are not effective. To deal with the real problem, you must make real changes. Here is some data on three of the most popular remedies:

Garcinia cambogia (hydroxycitric acid): In spite of an interesting theory and some intriguing animal studies, the human studies are unimpressive. In the best study to date, 135 patients were double-blinded to receive either 1,500 mg per day of hydroxycitric acid or a placebo. They were all placed on a high-fiber, low-calorie diet. After twelve weeks, the placebo group had lost more weight.[5] Conclusion: garcinia cambogia doesn't work.

Chitosan: This form of chitin, derived from the shells of crustaceans, supposedly traps fat in the intestine and is frequently advertised as Fat Absorb. A review of the data available seems to indicate that you would have to consume an entire bottle every day to have much of a reduction in fat absorption. The amount of fat absorbed is minuscule and clinical data shows that Chitosan does not promote weight loss.[6] Conclusion: Chitosan doesn't work.

Ephedra alkaloids (ma huang): Though this natural stimulant has a small effect on reducing appetite, the FDA has issued a warning regarding serious and potentially lethal side effects associated with the use of products containing ephedra, including arrhythmias, heart attacks, strokes, psychosis, abnormal liver function, seizures, rapid heart rate, anxiety, and stomach pain.[7] Ephedra is so dangerous that it has been linked with fatalities — even a low dose has detrimental health effects. Conclusion: it's not worth the risk.

What about drugs for weight loss?

Remember: for anything to be effective, you have to be on it forever. Even if the drugs were remarkably effective, you would have to be prepared to stay on them forever; the minute you stopped, the benefits would slowly be lost. In the long run, it is still your diet that determines your health and your weight. The amphetamine-related appetite suppressants have received much press, and they were quite popular until their dangers became more well known. They were never approved for long-term use, so it wasn't very wise for people to use them.

The two FDA-approved drugs for weight reduction are Meridia (sibutramine) and Xenical (orlistat). Meridia can cause headache, insomnia, constipation, dry mouth, and hypertension and is only slightly helpful.[8] Xenical, the fat inhibitor, can cause abdominal pain and diarrhea, and reduces absorption of the fat-soluble vitamins such as D, E, and K. It may help those who consume an unhealthful, fatty diet, but even then it is hardly worth the side effects. Overall, drugs are drugs — they are a poor substitute for healthy living.

Can't I eat chocolate, ice cream, or other junk food ever again?

You can eat anything you desire, on occasion, but just don't make a habit of it. Try to be very strict the first three months in order to document how much weight you can expect to lose when you eat sensibly. We are all tempted by these treats. It is easier to resist if you get them out of your house completely. All cheats should be done outside of your home. If possible, associate with friends who will support you in recovering your health — or may join you in trying to be healthy.

Once you regain your health and feel great, you are less likely to crave these foods or be so tempted. Then, when you do deviate from a healthful diet, it is likely you will feel poorly, have a persistent dry mouth, and not sleep well. If you go off your diet and eat junk food on occasion, mark it on your calendar and consider it a special occasion that you won't repeat too often.

Nobody is perfect; however, do not let your weight yo-yo. You must adhere to the plan strictly enough so that you never put back on whatever weight you do take off.

Is exercise essential for success in weight loss, and what type of exercise is best?

Exercise is important, but if your ability to be active and exercise is limited, do not despair. My more aggressive menu plans will still enable you to lose weight. Obviously, those unable to exercise require a stricter diet. Some people have health conditions that preclude them from exercising much. However, you should still try to devise an exercise prescription to fit your capabilities. Almost everyone can do something; even those who cannot walk can do arm exercises with light weights and use an arm cycle.

Exercise will facilitate your weight loss and make you healthier. Vigorous exercise has a powerful effect on promoting longevity. If you have the will to adopt this plan and take good care of yourself, you will find the will to exercise. "No time to exercise" is not an excuse. If you have time to brush your teeth, take a shower, or go to the bathroom, you can make some time to exercise. Take frequent five-minute exercise breaks — walk stairs or stand up then sit down slowly in your chair twenty times. Lots of people with no time to exercise or join a health club can usually go up and down stairs in their home or place of work. Try doing as many flights as you can two or three times a day. Walking twenty or more flights a day is an effective way to achieve your goal. Most of my patients have a health club in their house — that is, a stairway leading to the upstairs floor, and most have one going down to the basement as well. I ask them to walk up and down the two flights ten times in the morning before they shower and ten times at night. It takes only five minutes, but it really works.

I also encourage patients to join a real health club and use a variety of equipment to utilize many body parts for maximum results. The more muscle groups that are exercised, the more metabolically active players you have on your team to help you meet your goals. It is definitely helpful to have access to an assortment of exercise equipment, such as ellipse machines, treadmills, steppers, recumbent bicycles, and numerous resistance machines. When you tire of one machine, you can move on to a new one.

Are there other strategies for success in the weight-loss arena?

This is not a book on stress management, social support, or stimulus control. Entire books have been written on these subjects. Clearly, it is difficult to eat healthfully in our crazy world, where it seems that everyone else is on a vendetta to commit suicide with food. That said, some of the following suggestions have proven helpful for people trying to lose weight:

Social support: Include family and friends in your plan. Ask others to read this book — not with the purpose of recruiting them to this way of eating, but so they will support you and understand why you are eating this way. If they are truly your friends, they will support you in your desire to improve your health and will try to have the right food choices available when you are around. Maybe they will even join you on your quest. It is extremely helpful to find at least one friend to join you or support you on your road back to superior health.

Stimulus control: Implement strategies to prevent temptation and exposure to sedentary activities or social eating. The most important stimulus-control technique is structuring your environment. This means removing temptation from your home and stocking your cupboards and refrigerator with the proper foods. Eat only at the kitchen table, not while watching television. When you finish dinner, clean up and leave the kitchen area, then brush and floss your teeth, so you are not tempted to return and snack again. Lay out your exercise clothes for the morning so you are reminded to begin your day with your exercise program.

When going out to social situations, eat first or bring your own food if you cannot arrange in advance to have food that meets your needs. Volunteer to bring food for the other guests, too; then you have something you can eat without distress. Try not to make food the center of your life. Keep active with interests that keep you from thinking about eating.

Positive visualization and other relaxation techniques: Progressive muscle relaxation and meditation are designed to reduce tension and provide a distraction for stressful events.[9] For many, stress is a predictor of relapse and unhealthful eating. We need both exercise and sufficient rest and sleep to best deal with the stress in our lives. If you are not sleeping well, you can become overwhelmed more easily by stressful situations. An audiotape or CD to guide you in relaxation can be very helpful in reducing stress and sleeping better. My friend Ronald Cridland, M.D., a sleep specialist in Canada, and I have both found Eli Bay's tapes extremely useful for our patients. Ordering information can be found on my website.

Self-monitoring: Accept that this diet is a lifetime commitment. The individual most likely to succeed is one who has changed both his habits and mind-set. Food diaries, weekly weigh-ins, physical activity logs, and goal setting are all effective ways to stay on track. The primary purpose of self-monitoring is to become aware of behaviors and factors that either positively or negatively influence your food and activity choices. Research has consistently demonstrated that self-monitoring is a helpful tool that improves outcome.[10]

I suggest you make a list of goals that losing weight will help you accomplish and post it in a visible place where you will see it in your home. Add to it from time to time and check off those accomplishments as you achieve them. Make the goals very specific to you, such as the following:

I will be confident about my ability to resist disease.
I will succeed at losing pounds and regaining excellent health.
I will be able to fit into fashionable clothes, including my favorite blue dress.
My cholesterol will improve at least 50 points.
I will look good in a bathing suit at the pool this summer.
I will have more energy and be able to enjoy bike trips with my children.
My husband/wife/other will find me more attractive.
My job will be less tiring and I will perform better and make more money.
I will save money on health care and will be able to save for my retirement.
I will have a better social life and be in a position to attract John [or Jane].
My knees and back will stop hurting.
I will gain the respect of my peers.
My allergies, constipation, indigestion, headaches, and acne will all resolve.
My fears about a health crisis or death will subside.

Structured coaching: Some individuals do better when another person tracks their results and provides encouragement. Some people maximize success with a variety of aids, including regular visits to a physician, dietitian, or psychologist. When patients see me each month, we review what has been achieved and what will be necessary to achieve the goal for the following month. Improvements in blood pressure, weight, lipid levels, liver function, and diabetic parameters are all helpful to keep people focused on achieving their goals. If you are on medication, it will be necessary to visit your physician regularly to adjust the dose and potentially discontinue those medications that you will no longer need as you lose weight. You can also ask your physician to read this book and work with you, supporting you as you earn your way back to total wellness.

In-patient facilities or health retreats: If you do not succeed, or are not able to do so on your own, you are not a failure. Some individuals require a structured environment to get them started on the road to success. For others it is imperative for their health that they succeed at taking weight off relatively quickly. If you are committed to success, there is no reason why you should be satisfied with anything less than spectacular results in your health, wellness, and physique. Some individuals may require an initial period of supervision that offers a more disciplined and structured program whereby all the food is prepared.

These guests are soon reeducated to proper eating and learn to adjust to the changes that must be made. They can taste many different ways to prepare healthy food and learn healthy food preparation. There are live-in health spa facilities that adhere to these principles and cater to those who need guaranteed weight loss. You can view information about such facilities on my website, www.drfuhrman.com, or contact me (800-474-WELL) if you are in need of such a facility.

Is a vegetarian or vegan diet healthier than a diet that contains a small amount of animal products?

I do not know for sure. A preponderance of the evidence suggests that either a near vegetarian diet or a vegetarian diet is the best. In the massive China-Cornell-Oxford Project, reduction in cancer rates continued to be observed as participants reduced their animal-food consumption all the way down to one serving per week. Below this level there is not enough data available. Some smaller studies suggest that some fish added to a vegetarian diet provides benefit, which is likely a result of the increased DHA fat from fish.[11] This same benefit most likely could be achieved on a strict vegetarian diet by including ground flaxseed and nuts that contain omega-3, such as walnuts. If you want to get the benefit from the additional DHA contained in fish yet remain on a strict vegetarian diet, you can take plant-derived DHA.

Whether or not you are a strict vegetarian, your diet still must be plant-predominant for optimal health and to maximally reduce cancer risk. A vegetarian or vegan diet may be healthy or unhealthy, depending on food choices, but a diet similar to the one most Americans consume — i.e., one containing a significant quantity of animal products — cannot be made healthful. For those not willing to give them up, animal products should be limited to twelve ounces or less per week. Otherwise, the risk of disease increases considerably. Many of my patients choose to eat only vegan foods in their home and eat animal products only as a treat once a week or so when they are out.

Is a high-nutrient, low-calorie diet the best one for everyone?

I do not recommend the same diet for everyone, but the H = N/C formula never changes. On very rare occasions I come across an individual who requires some modification to this diet. There are some illnesses, such as active inflammatory-bowel disease, for which this diet would have to be adjusted because the patient may not tolerate a large amount of raw vegetables and fruit. I do adjust and customize eating plans and nutritional supplements for individuals with unique medical and metabolic needs. If you are one such person, or if you need a healthful way to gain weight, I would hope you would contact me, or another physician with expertise in this area, for more specific advice.

I don't drink six to eight glasses of water daily. Is that bad?

Only those eating an American-style diet, so high in salt and so low in the high-water-content fruits and vegetables, need to drink that much water. On my fiber- and fluid-rich diet, your need for extra water decreases. Three glasses a day is usually sufficient; but if you are exercising or in the heat, then you obviously need to drink more to replenish those liquids lost through perspiration.

How do you modify your recommendations about superior nutrition and disease prevention for children or those not needing to lose weight?

I believe the diet we currently feed our children is the reason we are seeing so many frequent infections and such high levels of allergies, autoimmune disease, and cancer in this country. Unfortunately, what we eat early in life has a more powerful effect on our eventual health (or ill health) than what we eat later in life. I have three daughters and understand the difficulties of trying to raise healthy children in today's insane world. It seems we are in an environment in which parents are enthusiastically and purposely breeding a nation of sickly and diseased adults.

In my community, parents and neighbors unknowingly attempt to poison their children at every opportunity. They don't merely feed their own children a diet chock-full of sugar and trans fats, but at every birthday, athletic event, and social occasion they bring sugar-coated doughnuts, cupcakes, and candy for the entire crowd. The public schoolroom in my community also serves as another avenue for parents and teachers to regularly supply our children with junk food. I would expect, as parents, we all have the same goal of trying to get our children to eat more nutritious foods: more vegetables, fruits, raw nuts and seeds, and legumes and beans. However, no child will eat healthfully if he is allowed to eat unhealthy foods on a regular basis.

The only way to have a child eat healthfully is to clear all unhealthful foods out of the house, so when the children are hungry they are forced to pick from healthy choices. They will at least eat healthfully when they are home if they are presented with only healthy food choices.

Nevertheless, the dietary rules in this book would be too calorie-restricted and too fat-restricted for a child or thin athlete. However, the principles for healthy eating and longevity do not change. All that has to be done to increase the caloric density and fat density of the diet is to add more wholesome sources of fat and calories, such as raw nuts and seeds, nut butters, and avocados. Starchy vegetables and whole grains can be consumed in larger amounts, and vegetable

and grain dishes can be flavored with sauces and dressings made with nuts and seeds.

If you want to gain weight, eating more — or eating differently to bulk up — will add mostly fat to your body. It is exceptionally rare for a person to gain more muscle just from eating more food. Forcing yourself to consume more food than your body wants is not in your best interest. If you want to gain weight, lift weights to add muscle; then the exercise will increase your appetite accordingly. When you eat a healthful diet, nature has you carry only that mass you need; your muscles will enlarge only if additional stress is placed on them. Of course, this book is designed for those who are overweight and desirous of losing weight. Those who are truly excessively thin, and need to gain weight, may have to modify this eating plan somewhat to meet their individual needs.

Is it dangerous to eat more fruits and vegetables because of the increased consumption of pesticides? Do I have to buy organic?

The effects of ingesting pesticides in the very small amounts present in vegetation are unknown. Bruce Ames, Ph.D., director of the National Institute of Environmental Health Sciences Center at the University of California at Berkeley, who has devoted his career to examining this question, believes these minute amounts pose no risk at all.

He and other scientists support this view because humans and other animals are exposed to small amounts of naturally occurring toxins with every mouthful of organically grown, natural food. The body normally breaks down self-produced metabolic wastes and naturally occurring carcinogens in foods, as well as pesticides, and excretes these harmful substances every minute. Since 99.99 percent of the potential carcinogenic chemicals consumed are naturally present in all food, reducing our exposure to the 0.01 percent that are synthetic will not reduce cancer rates.

These scientists argue that humans ingest thousands of natural chemicals that typically have a greater toxicity and are present at higher doses than the very minute amount of pesticide residue that remains on food. Furthermore, animal studies on the carcinogenic potential in synthetic chemicals are done at doses a thousandfold higher than what is ingested in food. Ames argues that a high percentage of all chemicals, natural or not, are potentially toxic in high doses — "the dose makes the poison" — and that there is no evidence of possible cancer hazards from the tiny chemical residue remaining on produce.

Others believe a slight risk may be present, though that risk may be difficult to prove. There certainly is a justifiable concern that some chemicals have increased toxicity and are potentially harmful at lower doses than are used in rodent experiments. No scientist believes that this means we should reduce our consumption of vegetation, but many (including me) believe it prudent to reduce our exposure to the multiple toxic residues present in our food supply. I certainly advocate avoiding the skins of foods that are reported to have the most pesticide residue. And, of course, all fruits and vegetables should be washed before eating.

If you are concerned about pesticides and chemicals, keep in mind that animal products, such as dairy and beef, contain the most toxic pesticide residues. Because cows and steers eat large amounts of tainted feed, certain pesticides and dangerous chemicals are found in higher concentrations in animal foods. For example, dioxin, which is predominantly found in fatty meats and dairy products, is one of the most potent toxins linked to several cancers in humans, including lymphomas.[12] By basing your diet on unrefined plant foods, you automatically reduce your exposure to the most dangerous chemicals.

According to the U.S. Food and Drug Administration (www.fda. gov), the most contaminated produce, ranked from highest to lowest, are:

RANK	SCORE (200 = MOST TOXIC)	
1	strawberries	189
2	green and red bell peppers	155
3	spinach	155
4	cherries (USA)	154
5	peaches	150
6	cantaloupe (Mexico)	142
7	celery	129
8	apples	124
9	apricots	123
10	green beans	122
11	grapes (Chile)	118
12	cucumbers	117

Source: Environmental Working Group, compiled from FDA and EPA data

These twelve foods account for more than half of the total pesticide exposure. They are the key foods to avoid (unless you purchase organically grown ones).

It makes common sense to peel fruits, if possible, and not to eat potato skins unless you are able to purchase them pesticide-free. Remove and discard the outermost leaves of lettuce and cabbage, if not organically grown; other surfaces that cannot be peeled can be washed with soap and water or a commercial vegetable wash. Washing with plain water removes 25–50 percent of the pesticide residue. I personally avoid strawberries completely unless we purchase organic — my children often eat frozen organic strawberries from the health-food store.

Every study done to date on the consumption of food and its relation to cancer, though, has shown that the more fruits and vegetables people eat, the less cancer and heart disease they have. All these studies were done on people eating conventionally grown, not organic, produce. So, clearly, the benefit of conventional produce outweighs any hypothetical risk.

My doctor noted that my complexion had turned yellowish and told me to cut back on foods containing carotene, such as mangoes, carrots, and sweet potatoes.

The slight yellow-orange tinge to your skin is not a problem; it is a marker that you are on a healthy diet. On the contrary, any person who does not have some degree of carotenemia in his or her skin is not eating properly, and such an eating pattern places him or her at risk of cancer — including skin cancer. I drink no carrot juice; however, my skin has a slight yellow hue, especially when contrasted with the skin of people eating conventionally. When my patients eat a nutritionally packed diet, their skin changes color slightly as well. Tell your doctor it is *he* who has the dangerous skin tone. However, I still do not recommend taking vitamin A or high doses of beta-carotene from supplements.

What about the argument about our ancestors being hunter-gatherers who ate lots of meat?

Of course there were primitive populations who ate high-meat diets and there were primitive people who ate plant-predominant diets. Humans were desperate for calories, so they ate whatever they could get their hands on. The two questions we have to look at are: How long did they live on that diet? What diet for humans gives them the best protection against disease and the greatest chance for longevity in modern times?

Personally, I want to do a lot better than our prehistoric ancestors did. A comprehensive overview and a sensible interpretation of the scientific evidence support the conclusion that we can increase human longevity and prevent disease if we make specific food choices. We still retain our primate physiology, a physiology that has a dependence on high vegetation consumption, that is relevant to explain our ability to thrive on a plant-predominant diet.

Dr. Katerine Milton, from the University of California at Berkeley, is among the few nutritional anthropologists in the world who has worked with and studied cultures and primitive peoples not influenced by modern technology. She has concluded that the diet of both primitive people and wild primates is largely plant-based.[13] The main difference between primitive diets and our own is their consumption of nutrient-dense wild plants and the lack of access to low-nutrient, high-fat foods such as cheese and oil, as well as refined grains.

We have a unique opportunity in human history: We have fresh produce being flown into our food stores from all over the planet. We can take advantage of this abundant variety of fresh vegetation to eat a diet with more phytochemical density and diversity than ever before. We have the opportunity to make decisions about what we eat that were not available to our prehistoric ancestors. Fortunately, we have knowledge that they lacked, and we can use this knowledge to live longer than ever before.

I know you do not recommend butter or margarine, so what do we put on bread, vegetables, or corn?

Butter is loaded with a dangerous amount of saturated fat, but stick margarines have hydrogenated oils that contain trans fats that raise LDL, the bad cholesterol. Adjusting the type of fat consumed, researchers found that butter caused the highest cholesterol level and that varying amounts of margarines and oils had various harmful effects.[14] The best answer is to use nothing, or buy whole-grain bread that tastes good without adding a greasy topping. If you love the flavor of butter, try Butter Buds or sparingly use a spread that contains no hydrogenated oil, such as Spectrum Essential Omega Spread, instead. Lots of my patients like no-salt tomato sauce on bread, or a tomato-salsa blend, avocado, or stewed mushrooms. Of course, the best way to get out of the habit of eating those greasy toppings is not to eat bread at all.

Are soy products and soybeans a healthy food to eat?

Soy products such as soy burgers, soymilk, and soy cheeses are much more popular and available today. Recently, the FDA approved soy-containing products as heart-healthy and allowed health claims for soy protein.

Studies have shown soy's beneficial effects on cholesterol and other cardiovascular risk factors. However, there is no reason not to expect the same results from beans of any type — it's merely that more studies have been done on soy than on other beans. There are numerous studies indicating that soybeans are rich in various anti-cancer compounds such as isoflavones. However, soy is not the only bean to contain isoflavones. Most beans are rich in these beneficial anti-cancer compounds, and many different flavonoids with anti-cancer effects are found in beans of various color. I always recommend the consumption of a broad variety of phytochemical-rich foods to maximize one's health. Beans are no exception — try to eat different types of beans, not just soy.

You should be aware that soy nuts, soymilk, and other processed soy products do not retain much of the beneficial compounds and omega-3 fats that are in the natural bean. The more the food is processed, the more the beneficial compounds are destroyed. Remember, though, tofu and frozen or canned soybeans are a good source of omega-3 fat and calcium.

Recently, a few studies appeared showing potentially negative effects of consuming too much soy. One particularly troublesome study done in Hawaii suggested that men with higher tofu intake had more cognitive decline and brain atrophy with aging than men who ate little tofu.[15] This data contradicts evidence that Japanese men, who consume tofu regularly, have better cognitive function and lower rates of Alzheimer's disease than American men.[16] Obviously, more studies are needed to clarify these suggestive findings and to determine if there is something in tofu or related to tofu consumption that may be harmful. After reviewing these findings, Dr. Harris had soy products from Hawaii tested for aluminum levels and found a significantly higher level of aluminum in tofu from Hawaii than in tofu from the mainland. The aluminum factor may be a plausible explanation for the alleged "brain aging" properties of soy.

In any case, the evidence is not sufficient to warrant being fearful of consuming soybeans as part of a healthful diet. However, this brings to mind my basic theme of nutritional biodiversity — eat a variety of plant foods, and do not eat a soy-based diet.

Most of the processed soy products can be tasty additions to a plant-based diet, but they are generally high in salt and are not nutrient-dense foods, so use them sparingly. In conclusion, the soybean is a superior food, containing the difficult-to-find omega-3 fats. Beans in general are superior foods that fight against cancer and heart disease, which is why you will benefit from using a variety of beans in your diet.

How much salt is permissible on this nutritional program?

This book is designed for those who want to lose weight and for those who want to maintain in excellent health and prevent disease. Any excess salt added to food, outside of what is contained in natural foods, is likely to increase your risk of developing disease. Salt consumption is linked to both stomach cancer and hypertension.[17] For optimal health, I recommend that no salt at all be added to any food. The famous DASH study clearly indicates that Americans consume five to ten times as much sodium as they need and that high sodium levels over the years has a predictable effect on raising blood pressure.[18] Just because you don't have high blood pressure now doesn't mean that you won't. In fact, you probably *will* have high blood pressure if you keep eating lots of salt over the years.

Salt also pulls out calcium and other trace minerals in the urine when the excess is excreted, which is a contributory cause of osteoporosis.[19] If that is not enough, high sodium intake is predictive of increased death from heart attacks. In a large prospective trial, recently published in the respected medical journal *The Lancet*, there was a frighteningly high correlation between sodium intake and all-cause mortality in overweight men.[20] The researchers concluded, "High sodium intake predicted mortality and risk of coronary heart disease, independent of other cardiovascular risk factors, including high blood pressure. These results provide direct evidence of the harmful effects of high salt intake in the adult population."

This means that salt has significant harmful effects, independent of its effects on blood pressure. It very likely increases the tendency of platelets to clot. I recommend that people resist adding salt to foods and look for salt-free canned goods and soups. Since most salt comes from processed foods, bread, and canned goods, it shouldn't be that hard to avoid added sodium.

That said, if you desire to salt your food, do so only after it is on the table and you are ready to eat it. It will taste saltier if the salt is right on the surface of the food. You can add lots of salt yet hardly taste it if the salt is added to the vegetables or soup while they are cooking. Vege Base instant soup mix by Vogue has a nice salty flavor and can be added to salads or sprinkled on food. Use herbs, spices, lemon, vinegar, or other non-salt seasonings to flavor food. Condiments such as ketchup, mustard, soy sauce, teriyaki sauce, and relish are very high in sodium, so if you can't resist them, use the low-sodium varieties sparingly.

Ideally, all your foods should have less than one milligram of salt per calorie. Natural foods contain about half a milligram of sodium per calorie. If a food label has a serving size of 100 calories yet contains 400 mg of salt, it is a very high salt food. If it has 100 calories and less than 100 mg of salt, it is a food with hardly any added salt and is an appropriate food for your diet. Try to rarely use products with more than 200 mg per 100 calories. Within these guidelines, you should be able to keep your average daily sodium intake around or below 1,000 mg.

If you don't use salt, your taste buds adjust with time and your sensitivity to taste salt improves. When you are using lots of salt in your diet, it weakens your taste for salt and makes you feel that food tastes bland unless it is heavily seasoned or spiced. The DASH study observed the same phenomenon that I have noted for years — it took some time for one's salt-saturated taste buds to get used to a low sodium level. If you follow my nutritional recommendations strictly, without compromise, avoiding all processed foods or highly salted foods, your ability to detect and enjoy the subtle flavors in fruits and vegetables will improve as well.

What about coffee?

Clearly, excessive consumption of caffeinated beverages is dangerous. Caffeine addicts are at higher risk of cardiac arrhythmias that could precipitate sudden death.[21] Coffee raises blood pressure and raises both cholesterol and homocysteine, two risk factors for heart disease.[22]

One cup of coffee per day is not likely to cause a significant risk, but drinking more than this one-cup maximum can interfere with your health and even your weight-loss goals.

Besides the increased risk of heart disease, there are two other problems. First, caffeine is a stimulant that allows you to get by with less sleep and reduces the depth of sleep. Such sleep deprivation results in higher levels of the stress hormone cortisol and interferes with glucose metabolism, leading to insulin resistance.[23] This insulin resistance, and subsequent higher baseline glucose level, further promotes heart disease and other problems. In other words, caffeine consumption promotes inadequate sleep, and less sleep promotes disease and premature aging. Adequate sleep is also necessary to prevent overeating. There is no substitute for adequate sleep.

The second issue is that eating more frequently and eating more food suppresses caffeine-withdrawal headaches and other withdrawal symptoms. When you are finally finished digesting the meal, the body more effectively cleans house; at this time people experience a drive to eat more to suppress caffeine-withdrawal symptoms. You are prodded to eat again, eating more food than you would if you were not a caffeine addict.

You will never be in touch with your body's true hunger signals while you are addicted to stimulants. For some the problem is that giving up coffee is more difficult than the dietary restrictions. I still would suggest that my recommendation be carefully adhered to without caffeinated beverages for the first six weeks. After that time, when the addiction to caffeine is no longer present, you can decide if you really can't give up that one cup. Keep in mind that it takes four to five days for the caffeine-withdrawal headaches to resolve once you stop drinking coffee. If the symptoms are too severe, try reducing the coffee slowly, by about half a cup every three days.

If a little coffee would make it possible for you to remain true to my dietary recommendations, I would not have a strong objection. Losing weight is a more important goal for your overall health. It is just that higher amounts of caffeine do not make it easier to control your appetite and food cravings, they make it harder. It would be much better if you gave this plan a true test. See how well you feel and how much weight you can lose in six weeks. Maybe by then you will have lost your craving for mind-altering substances.

How much alcohol is permissible?

Moderate drinking has been associated with a lower incidence of coronary heart disease in more than forty prospective studies. This only applies to moderate drinking — defined as one drink or less per day for women, and two drinks or less for men. More than this is associated with increased fat around the waist and other potential problems.[24] Alcohol consumption also leads to mild withdrawal sensations the next day that are commonly mistaken for hunger. One glass of wine per day is likely insignificant, but I advise against higher levels of alcohol consumption.

Alcohol's anti-clotting properties grant some protective effect against heart attacks, but this protective effect is valuable only in a person or population consuming a heart-disease-promoting diet. It is much wiser to avoid the detrimental effects of alcohol completely and protect yourself from heart disease with nutritional excellence. For example, even moderate alcohol consumption is linked to higher rates of breast cancer and to occurrence of atrial fibrillation.[25] Avoid alcohol and eat healthfully if possible, but if that one drink a day will make you stay with this plan much more successfully, then have it.

I feel best when I eat a high-protein diet, with plenty of animal products. Does that mean these recommendations, to eat a plant-based diet, are not for me?

I have thousands of patients eating vegetarian or near vegetarian diets, and over the past fifteen years have noted a very small percentage of the total who initially report that they feel better with significant animal products in their diet and worse on a vegetarian diet. Almost all these complaints resolve with time on the new diet. I believe the main reasons for this are as follows:

A diet heavily burdened with animal products places a toxic stress on the detoxification systems of the body. As with stopping caffeine, cigarettes, and heroin, many observe withdrawal symptoms for a short period, usually including fatigue, weakness, headaches, or loose stools. In 95 percent of these cases, these symptoms resolve within two weeks.

It is more common that the temporary adjustment period lasts less than a week, in which you might feel fatigue, have headaches or gas, or experience other mild symptoms as your body withdraws from your prior toxic habits. Don't buy the fallacy that you "need more protein." The menus in this book offer sufficient protein — and protein deficiency does not cause fatigue. Even my vegan menus supply about 50 grams of protein per 1,000 calories, a whopping amount. Stopping dangerous but stimulating foods causes temporary fatigue.

Increased gas and loose stools are also occasionally observed when switching to a diet containing so much fiber and different fibers that the digestive tract has never encountered before. Over many years, the body has adjusted its secretions and peristaltic waves (digestive-related bowel contractions) to a low-fiber diet. These symptoms also improve with time. Chewing extra well, sometimes even blending salads, helps in this period of transition. Some people must avoid beans initially, and then use them only in small amounts, adding more to the diet gradually over a period of weeks to train the digestive tract to handle and digest these new fibers.

Certain people have increased fat requirements, and the type of vegetarian diet they may have been on in the past was not rich enough in certain essential fats for them. This can occur in those eating a plant-based diet that includes lots of low-fat wheat and grain products. Frequently, adding ground flaxseed or flaxseed oil to the diet to supply additional omega-3 fats is helpful. Some, especially thin individuals, require more calories and more fat to sustain their weight. This is usually "fixed" by including raw nuts, raw nut butters, avocados, and other healthy foods that are nutrient-rich and also high in fat and calories. Even these naturally thin individuals will significantly improve their health and lower their risk of degenerative diseases if they reduce their dependency on animal foods and consume more plant-derived fats, such as nuts, instead.

There is also the rare individual who needs more concentrated sources of protein and fat in his diet because of digestive impairment, Crohn's disease, short gut syndromes, or other uncommon medical conditions. I have also encountered patients on rare occasions who become too thin and malnourished on what I would consider an ideal, nutrient-dense diet. On such occasions, more animal products have been needed to reduce the fiber content, slow transit time in the gut, and aid absorption and concentration of amino acids at each meal. This problem usually is the result of some digestive impairment or difficulty with absorption. I have only seen a handful of such cases in the past ten years of practice. In other words, not even one in 100, in my estimation, requires animal products regularly in his diet. These individuals should still follow my general recommendations for excellent health and can accommodate their individual needs by keeping animal-product consumption down to comparatively low levels.

Do you recommend low-calorie or no calorie sweeteners?

Sweetening agents, such as NutraSweet (aspartame), are added to more than six thousand foods and drugs. Many people use these sweeteners in an effort to control their weight. It doesn't work; it just perpetuates your desire for unhealthy food. When researchers compared the caloric intake of women fed aspartame-sweetened drinks with women given higher-calorie beverages, the women given the aspartame merely consumed more calories later.[26] It is not the solution.

Since these sweeteners cause brain tumors and seizures in animals, a legitimate health concern exists, despite the FDA's declaration that aspartame is safe. In the past twenty years, brain tumor rates have risen in several industrialized countries, including the United States. Aspartame was introduced to the American market several years prior to the sharp increase in brain tumor incidence.[27] This suggests to me that the potential danger of aspartame should be more carefully studied.

Clearly this is a controversial subject because much of the research documenting the so-called safety of aspartame was financed by the aspartame industry, and a huge amount of political and monetary pressure led to eventual FDA approval. My opinion is that the possible dangers of aspartame are still unknown. Utilizing such artificial products is gambling with your health. Aspartame also exposes us to a methyl ester that may have toxic effects. I recommend playing it safe and sticking to natural foods. Getting rid of your addictions to unsafe substances is valuable in achieving long-term success.

Many health gurus recommend substituting Stevia in place of artificial sweeteners. Stevia is natural and its use is permitted in Japan and other countries. Despite its widespread use, there is a surprising lack of human clinical trials evaluating its safety. Unlike with saccharin, no evidence has been reported that stevioside and its metabolites are carcinogenic. However, animal reports of nephrotoxicity do exist, which suggests that Stevia is likely safer than the other sweeteners, but not entirely without risk.[28] The extent of risk is unknown at this time.

Bottom line: try to enjoy your food choices without sweeteners. Fresh fruit and occasionally a little date sugar or ground dates is the safest way to go. I recommend dropping colas, sodas, sweetened teas, and juices. If they don't contain artificial sweeteners, they are loaded with sugar. Eat unrefined food and drink water. Melons blended with ice cubes make delicious, cooling summer drinks.

I certainly believe that if you are significantly overweight, the risk of being overweight probably exceeds any risk associated with these sweeteners. However, I am not convinced that there are many people who have found low-calorie sweeteners to be the solution to their weight problem.

I eat out frequently, which makes sticking with this plan very difficult. How can I make the transition easier?

Choose restaurants that have healthful options, and know the places that will cater to your needs. When possible, speak to the management or chef in advance. When traveling, look for restaurants that have salad bars. This is not an all-or-nothing plan. Every person exposed to these ideas can improve over his or her current diet. People have a tendency to like best the foods to which they have become accustomed. So, keep in mind that eventually you will lose the desire for some of the unhealthful foods you are eating now and you will enjoy the pleasures of healthy, natural foods more. I actually enjoy eating healthy food more than injurious food because it tastes good and I also feel good. Most of my patients report the same sensation. Food preferences are learned; you can learn to enjoy healthy foods, just as you learned to like unhealthy ones.

You can follow this diet on the road if you are committed to your own success — it just takes more diligence to plan where to go and to make sure in advance that there is something available for you. Get in the habit of ordering a double-size green salad, with dressing on the side, and use only a tiny amount of dressing or squeeze a lemon on the salad.

Remember that this is not a temporary diet, it is your life plan. We must consider how our health is affected by what we choose to eat. We all have to make wise choices to get the most out of life. That doesn't mean you must be perfect. It does mean that however you eat, whether you adopt all of my recommendations or just a part of them, your health will certainly be better off as a result of those improvements. After a while, it becomes habit. If you give it a good try, you may find, as others have, that it is not as difficult as you thought, and you will likely grow to enjoy it.

Do you think everyone will eventually embrace this way of eating?

No. The social and economic forces that are pulling our population toward obesity and disease will not be defeated by one book preaching about achieving superior health with nutritional excellence. The "good life" will continue to bring most Americans to a premature grave. This plan is not for everyone. I do not expect the majority of individuals to live this healthfully. However, they should at least make that decision by being aware of the facts rather than having their food choices shaped by inaccurate information or the food manufacturers. Some people will choose to smoke cigarettes, eat unhealthfully, or pursue other reckless habits. They have that inalienable right to live their lives the way they choose. Don't add stress to *your* life by trying to persuade every person you meet to eat the same way you do. Looking good and feeling healthy will still be your best tools of persuasion, without working to convince others.

A common criticism of my eating plan, which all knowledgeable authorities agree is healthy, is that most people won't stick to such restrictive recommendations. This is an irrelevant point. Since when is what the "masses" find socially acceptable the criterion for value? Value or correctness is independent of how many will choose to follow such recommendations; that is a separate issue. The critical question is how effective these recommendations are to guarantee a slim body, long life, and enduring health. All those naysayers have missed the point; the recommendations were not designed to win a popularity contest.

Thousands of enthusiastic individuals who have benefited from this body of knowledge consider this information a special blessing. It is an opportunity that you can put to use to have your life be so much healthier, happier, and enjoyable. We don't feel deprived; rather, we enjoy fantastic-tasting food that is also healthy. We have developed a distaste for "junk food." At this point in our lives, healthy food simply tastes better. Another question is, How enjoyable is life for those plagued with a multitude of serious medical problems?

Choosing to live a healthful or unhealthful lifestyle is a personal decision, but this is not an all-or-nothing plan. As a health professional, it is my job to encourage people to protect their future health.

We can't buy good health; we must earn it. We are given only one body in this lifetime, so I encourage you to take proper care of it. Over time, your health and happiness are inescapably linked. You don't get a new body when you destroy your health with disease-causing foods. I am 100 percent committed to your success and well-being, so please contact me if you are finding roadblocks to recovering your health. I wish you long life and enduring health. It can be yours.

Glossary

Angioplasty expansion of a blood vessel by means of a balloon catheter inserted into the chosen vessel

Arteriosclerosis or atherosclerosis commonly occurring deposits of yellowish plaques containing lipoid material that thicken and stiffen the vessel walls; these deposits may narrow the lumen, causing chest pain (angina), or rupture, causing clots that lead to heart attacks

Angiogram or catheterization passage of a small catheter into the cardiac circulation to release a radiographic dye permitting visualization of the lumen and detection of cardiac abnormalities

Chelation intravenous infusion of a chemical compound that sequesters metallic ions, traditionally used for heavy metal poisoning but controversially promoted as an intervention to reverse arteriosclerosis

Detoxification the body's efforts to reduce its toxic load by changing irritants to a less harmful form or one that can be more readily eliminated, or the body's efforts to force the expulsion of such substances through channels of elimination, such as mucus, urine, or skin

Embolus a clot or plug brought by the blood from its original site to a place where it occludes the lumen of a smaller vessel

Endothelium the layer of cells lining the interior portion of the heart, blood vessels, and other cavities

Epidemiologist one whose field of medicine is the study of factors affecting the frequency and distribution of diseases

First Law of thermodynamics the scientific concept that energy can be changed from one form to another (into work) but cannot be created or destroyed

Gastroplasty surgery to reduce the size of the stomach

Gastric bypass permanent division and separation of the main section (lower segment) of the stomach to create a small stomach pouch with the remaining (upper) segment, which is then reattached to the small intestines

Homocysteine an intermediate protein in the synthesis of cysteine, which elevates as a result of certain nutritional deficiencies (especially B_{12} or folate) or because of biochemical variance; the elevation of homocysteine has been implicated in coronary artery disease and heart attacks

Hypertension high blood pressure

Ischemia deficiency of blood flow and subsequent oxygenation secondary to constriction or obstruction of a blood vessel

Ketosis an abnormally high concentration of ketone bodies in the blood, caused by poorly controlled diabetes (high serum glucose) or prolonged carbohydrate insufficiency, such as in fasting or carbohydrate-restricted diets

Lipids a group of water-insoluble fatty substances that serve biological functions in the body; an expression to represent the group of lipoproteins affecting heart disease risk, such as cholesterol, triglycerides, and their component subtypes

Liposuction the most common cosmetic procedure in the United States, which involves inserting and manipulating a narrow tube to break up and then suction out fat under the skin

Macronutrients fats, carbohydrates, and protein, which supply calories (energy)

and are necessary for growth and normal function

Micronutrients essential dietary elements required in small quantities for various bodily needs, but not a source of calories

Phytochemicals numerous newly discovered micronutrients present in plant foods with substantial ability to maximize the body's defenses against developing disease, including protection from toxins and carcinogens

Receptors a specifically shaped molecule on or within a cell that recognizes or binds with a particular similarly shaped molecule, inducing a specific response within the cell

Revascularization the restoration of normal blood supply by means of a blood vessel graft, as in coronary bypass surgery

Satiated full satisfaction of appetite or thirst without further desire to ingest more food or drink

Sequelae later illnesses or afflictions caused by an initial illness or affliction

Thrombus an aggregation of blood factors forming a clot, frequently causing vascular obstruction at its point of formation

Vascular pertaining to a blood vessel

Notes

Chapter 1: Digging Our Graves with Forks and Knives

1. Bender, R., C. Trautnet, M. Spraul, and M. Berger. 1998. Assessment of excess mortality in obesity. *Am. J. Epidemiol.* 147 (1): 42–48; Wolf, A. M., and G. A. Colditz. 1998. Current estimates of the economic cost of obesity in the United States. *Obes. Res.* 6 (2): 97–106.

2. Foryet, J. Limitations of behavioral treatment of obesity: review and analysis. 1981. *J. Behav. Med.* 4: 159–73.

3. Perri, M. G., S. F. Sears, Jr., and J. E. Clark. 1993. Strategies for improving maintenance of weight loss: toward a continuous care model of obesity management. *Diabetes Care* 16: 200–09.

4. Bouchard, C. 1996. The causes of obesity: advances in molecular biology but stagnation on the genetic front. *Diabetologia* 39 (12): 1532–33.

5. Must, A., J. Spadano, E. H. Coakley, et al. 1999. The disease burden associated with overweight and obesity. *JAMA* 282 (16): 1523–29.

6. *Clinical guidelines on the identification, evaluation, and treatment of overweight and obesity in adults.* 1998. National Heart, Lung, and Blood Institute reprint. Bethesda, Md.: National Institutes of Health.

7. Must, Spadano, et al. Op. cit.; Allison, D. B., K. R. Fontaine, J. E. Manson, et al. 1999. Annual deaths attributable to obesity in the United States. *JAMA* 282 (16): 1530–38.

8. Melissa, J., M. Christodoulakis, M. Spyridakis, et al. 1998. Disorders associated with clinically severe obesity: significant improvement after surgical weight reduction. *South. Med. J.* 91 (12): 1143–48.

9. Papakonstantinou, A., P. Alfaras, V. Komessidou, and E. Hadjiyannakis. 1998. Gastrointestinal complications after vertical banded gastroplasty. *Obes. Surg.* 8 (2): 215–17; Choi, Y., J. Frizzi, A. Foley, and M. Harkabus. 1999. Patient satisfaction and results of vertical banded gastroplasty and gastric bypass. *Obes. Surg.* 9 (1): 33–35; *Guidelines for treatment of adult obesity.* 1998. Second edition. Bethesda, Md.: Shape Up America and the American Obesity Association.

10. Grazer, F. M., and R. H. De Jong. 2000. Fatal outcomes from liposuc-

tion: census survey of cosmetic surgeons. *Plast. Reconstr. Surg.* 105 (1): 436–48.

11. NIH clinical guidelines, op. cit., p. 81.

12. Samaras, K., P. J. Kelly, M. N. Chiano, T. D. Spector, and L. V. Campbell. 1999. Genetic and environmental influences on total-body and central abdominal fat: the effect of physical activity in female twins. *Ann. Intern. Med.* 130 (11): 873–82.

13. Stoll, B. A. 1998. Western diet, early puberty and breast cancer risk. *Breast Cancer Res. Treat.* 49 (3): 187–93.

14. Horinger, P., and R. Imoberdorf. 2000. Junk food revolution or the cola colonization. *Ther. Umsch.* 57 (3): 134–37.

15. Berenson, G. S., W. A. Wattigney, R. E. Tracey, et al. 1992. Atherosclerosis of the aorta and coronary arteries and cardiovascular risk factors in persons aged 6 to 30 years and studied at necropsy (the Bogalusa heart study). *Am. J. Cardiol.* 70: 851–58.

16. Berenson, G. S., S. R. Srinivasan, W. Bao, et al. 1998. Association between multiple cardiovascular risk factors and atherosclerosis in children and young adults. *N. Eng. J. Med.* 338: 1650–56.

17. Berenson, G. S., S. R. Srinivasan, and T. A. Nicklas. 1998. Atherosclerosis: a nutritional disease of childhood. *Am. J. Cardiol.* 82 (10B): 22–29T.

18. Staszewski, J. 1971. Age at menarche and breast cancer. *J. Nat. Cancer Inst.* 47: 935; Frankel, S., D. J. Gunnell, T. J. Peters, et al. 1998. Childhood energy intake and adult mortality from cancer: the Boyd Orr Cohort Study. *BMJ* 316 (7133): 499–504.

19. Gauthier, B. M., J. M. Hicker, and M. N. Noel. 2000. High prevalence of overweight children in Michigan primary care practices. *J. Fam. Pract.* 49 (1): 73–76.

20. Van Itallie, T. B. 1985. Health implications of overweight and obesity in the United States. *Ann. Int. Med.* 103: 983–88.

21. Manson, J. E., W. C. Willett, M. J. Stampfer, et al. 1995. Body weight and mortality among women. *N. Eng. J. Med.* 333: 677–85.

22. Lee, I., J. E. Manson, C. H. Hennekens, and R. S. Paffenbarger. 1993. Body weight and mortality: a 27-year follow-up of middle-aged men. *JAMA* 270 (23): 2823–28.

23. Manson, J. E., M. J. Stampfer, C. H. Hennekens, et al. 1987. Body weight and longevity — a reassessment. *JAMA* 257: 353–58.

24. Folsom, A. R., S. A. Kaye, T. A. Sellers, et al. 1993. Body fat distribution and 5-year risk of death in older women. *JAMA* 269 (4): 483–87.

25. Verdery, R. B., D. K. Ingram, G. S. Roth, and M. A. Lane. 1997. Caloric restriction increases HDL2 levels in rhesus monkeys. *Am. J. Physiol.* 273 (4 pt. 1): E714–19; Ramsey, J. J., E. B. Roecker, R. Weindruch, and J. W. Kemnitz. 1997. Energy expenditure of adult male rhesus monkeys during the first 30 months of dietary restriction. *Am. J. Physiol.* 272 (5 pt. 1): E901–07.

26. Hansen, B. C., N. L. Bodkin, and H. K. Ortmeyer. 1999. Calorie restriction in nonhuman primates: mechanism of reduced morbidity and mortality. *Toxicol. Sci.* 52 (2 supp.): 56–60; Weindruch, R. 1996. The retardation of aging by caloric restriction: studies in rodents and primates. *Toxicol. Pathol.* 24 (6): 742–45; Roth, G. S., D. K. Ingram, and M. A. Lane. 1999. Caloric restriction in primates: will it work and how will we know? *J. Am. Geriatric Soc.* 47 (7): 896–903; McCarter, R. J. 1995. Role of caloric restriction in the prolongation of life. *Clin. Geriatr. Med.* 11 (4): 553–65; Weindruch, R., M. A. Lane, D. K. Ingram, W. B. Ershler, and G. S. Roth. 1997. Dietary restriction in rhesus monkeys: lymphopenia and reduced nitrogen-induced proliferation in peripheral blood mononuclear cells. *Aging* 9 (44): 304–08; Frame, L. T., R. W.

Hart, and J. E. Leakey. 1998. Caloric restriction as a mechanism mediating resistance to environmental disease. *Environ. Health Perspect.* 106 (supp. 1): 313–24; Masoro, E. J. 1998. Influence of caloric intake on aging and on the response to stressors. *J. Toxicol. Environ. Health B. Crit. Rev.* 1 (3): 243–57; Lane, M. A., D. K. Ingram, and G. S. Roth. 1999. Calorie restriction in nonhuman primates: effects on diabetes and cardiovascular disease risk. *Toxicol. Sci.* 52 (2 supp.): 41–48.

27. Carroll, K. K. 1975. Experimental evidence of dietary factors and hormone-dependent cancers. *Cancer Research* 35: 3374–83.

28. Butler, R. N., M. Fossel, C. X. Pan, D. J. Rothman, and S. M. Rothman. 2000. Anti-aging medicine: efficacy and safety of hormones and antioxidants. *Geriatrics* 55: 48–58.

29. Lawton, C. L., V. J. Burley, J. K. Wales, and J. E. Blundell. 1993. Dietary fat and appetite control in obese subjects: weak effects on satiation and satiety. *Int. J. Obes. Metab. Disord.* 17 (7): 409–16; Blundell, J. E., and J. C. Halford. 1994. Regulation of nutrient supply: the brain and appetite control. *Proc. Nutr. Soc.* 53 (2): 407–18; Stamler, J., and T. A. Dolecek. 1997. Relation of food and nutrient intakes to body mass in the special intervention and usual care groups on the Multiple Risk Factor Intervention Trial. *Am. J. Clin. Nutr.* 65 (1 supp.): 366–73S.

30. Mattes, R. 1996. Dietary compensation by humans for supplemental energy provided as ethanol or carbohydrates in fluids. *Physiology and behavior* 59: 179–87.

31. Dennison, B. A., H. L. Rockwell, and S. L. Baker. 1997. Excess fruit juice consumption by preschool-aged children is associated with short stature and obesity. *Pediatrics* 99 (1): 15–22; Dennison, B. A. 1996. Fruit juice consumption by infants and children: a review. *J. Am. Coll. Nutr.* 15 (5 supp.): 4–11S.

32. "Plymouth Colony." 2000. *World Book Millennium.*

33. Weinsier, R. L., T. R. Nagy, G. R. Hunter, et al. 2000. Do adaptive changes in metabolic rate favor weight regain in weight-reduced individuals? An examination of the set-point theory. *Am. J. Clin. Nutr.* 72: 1088–94.

Chapter 2: Overfed, Yet Malnourished

1. Hebert, J. R., J. Landon, and D. R. Miller. 1993. Consumption of meat and fruit in relation to oral and esophageal cancer: a cross-national study. *Nutr. Cancer.* 19 (2): 169–79; Fraser, G. E. 1999. Association between diet and cancer, ischemic heart disease, and all-cause mortality in non-Hispanic white California Seventh-Day Adventists. *Am. J. Clin. Nutr.* 70 (3): 532–38S; Block, G., B. Patterson, and A. Subar. 1992. Fruit, vegetable, and cancer prevention: a review of the epidemiological evidence. *Nutr. Cancer* 18 (1): 1–29.

2. Joseph, J. A., B. Shukitt-Hale, N. A. Denisova, et al. 1999. Reversal of age-related declines in neuronal signal transduction, cognitive, and motor behavioral deficits with blueberry, spinach, or strawberry dietary supplementation. *J. Neurosci.* 19 (18): 8114–21.

3. Cao, G., B. Shukitt-Hale, P. C. Bickford, et al. 1999. Hyperoxia-induced changes in antioxidant capacity and the effect of dietary antioxidants. *J. Appl. Physiol.* 86 (6): 1817–22.

4. Hertog, M. G., H. B. Bueno-de-Mesquita, and A. M. Fehily. 1996. Fruit and vegetable consumption and cancer mortality in Caerphilly Study. *Cancer Epidemiol. Biomarkers Prev.* 5 (9): 673–77.

5. Kantor, L. S. 1999. A dietary assessment of the U.S. food supply. *Nutrition Week* 29 (3): 4–5.

6. Salmeron, J., J. E. Manson, M. J. Stampfer, G. A. Colditz, A. L. Wing, and W. C. Willett. 1997. Dietary

fiber, glycemic load, and risk of non-insulin-dependent diabetes mellitus in women. *JAMA* 277 (6): 472–77.

7. Salmeron, J., A. Ascherio, E. B. Rimm, G. A. Colditz, D. Spiegelman, D. J. Jenkins, M. J. Stampfer, A. L. Wing, and W. C. Willett. 1997. Dietary fiber, glycemic load, and risk of NIDDM in men. *Diabetes Care* 20 (4): 545–50.

8. Trends in the prevalence and incidence of self-reported diabetes mellitus — United States, 1980–1994. 1997. *Morb. Mortal. Wkly. Rep.* 46 (43): 1014–18.

9. Jacobs, D. R., K. A. Meyer, L. H. Kushi, and A. R. Folsum. 1999. Is whole grain intake associated with reduced total and cause-specific death rates in older women? The Iowa Women's Health Study. *Am. J. Public Health* 89 (3): 322–29.

10. Jacobs, D. R., L. Marquart, J. Slavin, and L. H. Kushi. 1998. Whole-grain intake and cancer: an expanded review and meta-analysis. *Nutrition and Cancer* 30 (2): 85–96; Chatenoud, L., A. Tavani, C. La Vecchia, et al. 1998. Whole-grain food intake and cancer risk. *Int. J. Cancer* 77 (1): 24–28.

11. Jacobs, D. R., Jr., K. A. Meyer, L. H. Kushi, et al. 1998. Whole-grain intake may reduce the risk of ischemic heart disease death in postmenopausal women: the Iowa Women's Health Study. *Am. J. Clin. Nutr.* 68: 248–57.

12. Jacobs, D. R., Jr., J. Slavin, and L. Marquart. 1995. Whole-grain intake and cancer: a review of the literature. *Nutr. Cancer* 24 (3): 221–29; Cohen, L. A. 1999. Dietary fiber and breast cancer. *Anticancer Res.* 19 (5A): 3685–88; Williams, G. M., C. L. Williams, and J. H. Weisburger. 1999. Diet and cancer prevention: the fiber first diet. *Toxicol. Sci.* 52 (2 supp.): 72–86; Gerber, M. 1998. Fibre and breast cancer. *Eur. J. Cancer Prev.* 7 (supp. 2): S630S67; La Vecchia, C., M. Ferranoni, S. Franceschi,

et al. 1997. Fibers and breast cancer risk. *Nutr. Cancer* 28 (3): 264–69.

13. Franceschi, S., A. Favero, E. Conti, R. Talamini, R. Volpe, E. Negri, L. Barzan, and C. La Vecchia. 1999. Food groups, oils and butter, and cancer of the oral cavity and pharynx. *Br. J. Cancer* 80 (3–4): 614–20; Jansen, M. C., H. B. Bueno-de-Mesquita, L. Rasanen, et al. 1999. *Nutr. Cancer* 34 (1): 49–55; Levi, F., C. Pasche, C. La Vecchia, et al. 1999. Food groups and colorectal cancer risk. *Br. J. Cancer* 79 (7–8): 1283– 87; Boutron-Ruault, M. C., P. Senesse, J. Faivvre, et al. 1999. Foods as risk factor for colorectal cancer: a case-control study in Burgundy (France). *Eur. J. Cancer Prev.* 8 (3): 229–35; Zhuo, X. G., and S. Watanabe. 1999. Factor analysis of digestive cancer mortality and food consumption in 65 Chinese counties. *J. Epidemiol.* 4: 275–84; Slattery, M. L., J. Benson, and T. D. Berry. 1997. Dietary sugar and colon cancer. *Cancer Epidemiol. Biomarkers Prev.* 6 (9): 677–85; Negri, E., C. Bosetti, C. La Vecchia, F. Fioretti, E. Conti, and S. Franceschi. 1999. Risk factors for adenocarcinoma of the small intestine. *Int. J. Cancer* 82 (2): 171–74; Franceschi, S., C. La Vecchia, A. Russo, et al. 1997. Low-risk diet for breast cancer in Italy. *Cancer Epidemiol. Biomarkers Prev.* 6 (11): 875–79; Favero, A., M. Parpinel, and S. Franceschi. 1998. Diet and risk of breast cancer: major findings from an Italian case-control study. *Biomed. Pharmacother.* 52 (3): 109–15; Josefson, D. 2000. High insulin linked to deaths from breast cancer. *BMJ* 320 (7248): 1496; Stoll, B. A. 1996. Nutrition and breast cancer risk: can an effect via insulin resistance be demonstrated? *Breast Cancer Res. Treat.* 38 (3): 239–46; Chatenoud, L., C. La Vecchia, S. Franceschi, et al. 1999. Refined-cereal intake and risk of selected cancers in Italy. *Am. J. Clin. Nutr.* 70 (6): 1107–10; Levi, F., C. Pasche, F. Lucchini, et al. 2000.

Refined and whole-grain cereals and the risk of oral, oesophageal and laryngeal cancer. *Eur. J. Clin. Nutr.* 54 (6): 487–89; Morris, K. L., and M. B. Zemel. 1999. Glycemic index, cardiovascular disease, and obesity. *Nutr. Rev.* 57 (9 pt. 1): 273–76; Tseng, M., J. E. Everhart, and R. S. Sandler. 1999. Dietary intake and gallbladder disease: a review. *Public Health Nutr.* 2 (2): 161–72; Liu, S., W. C. Willett, M. J. Stampfer, et al. 2000. A prospective study of dietary glycemic load, carbohydrate intake, and risk of coronary heart disease in U.S. women. *Am. J. Clin. Nutr.* 71 (6): 1455–61.

14. Pennington, J. A. 1996. Intakes of minerals from diets and foods: is there a need for concern? *J. Nutr.* 126 (9S): 2304–08S.

15. Dargatz, D. A., and P. F. Ross. 1996. Blood selenium concentration in cows and heifers on 253 cow-calf operations in 18 states. *J. Anim. Sci.* 74 (12): 2891–95.

16. Dennison, B. A., H. L. Rockwell, and S. L. Baker. 1997. Excess fruit juice consumption by preschool-aged children is associated with short stature and obesity. *Pediatrics* 99: 15–22.

17. Dennison, B. A. 1996. Fruit juice consumption by infants and children: a review. *J. Am. Coll. Nutr.* 15 (5): 4–11S.

18. Lonsdale, D., and R. J. Shamberger. 1980. Red cell transketolase as an indicator of nutritional deficiency. *Am. J. Clin. Nutr.* 33: 205–11; Lane, B. C. 1982. Myopia prevention and reversal: new data confirms the interaction of accommodative stress and deficit inducing nutrition. *J. Int. Acad. Prev. Med.* 7 (3): 28.

19. Kantor, op. cit. pp. 4–5.

20. Romanski, S. A., R. M. Nelson, and M. D. Jensen. 2000. Meal fatty acid uptake in adipose tissue: gender effects in nonobese humans. *Am. J. Physiol. Endocrinol. Metab.* 279 (2): E445–62.

21. Popp-Snijders, C., and M. C. Blonk. 1995. Omega-3 fatty acids in adipose tissue of obese patients with non-insulin-dependent diabetes mellitus reflect long-term dietary intake of eicosapentaenoic and docosahexaenoic acid. *Am. J. Clin. Nutr.* 61 (2): 360–65.

22. Kafatos, A., A. Diacatou, G. Voukiklaris, et al. 1997. Heart disease risk-factor status and dietary changes in the Cretan population over the past 30 years: the Seven Countries Study. *Am. J. Clin. Nutr.* 65 (6): 1882–86.

23. Katan, M. B., S. M. Grundy, and W. C. Willett. 1997. Should a low-fat, high-carbohydrate diet be recommended for everyone? Beyond low-fat diets. *N. Eng. J. Med.* 337 (8): 563–67.

24. Pedersen, A., M. W. Baumstark, P. Marckmann, et al. 2000. An olive-oil rich diet results in higher concentration of LDL subfraction particles than rapeseed oil and sunflower oil diets. *J. Lipid Res.* 42 (12): 1901–11.

25. Micheli, A., G. Gatta, M. Sant, et al. 1997. Breast cancer prevalence measured by the Lombardy Cancer Registry. *Tumori* 83 (6): 875–79.

26. Vigilante, K., and M. Flynn. 1999. *Low fat lies, high-fat frauds and the healthiest diet in the world.* Washington, D.C.: Lifeline Press.

27. Kerns, M. A. 1998. Effects of two energy restriction diets on fuel utilization, blood chemistry and body composition. *Medicine and Science in Sports and Exercise* 30: S62.

28. Steinmetz, K. A., and J. D. Potter. 1996. Vegetables, fruit and cancer prevention: a review. *J. Am. Diet. Assoc.* 96 (10): 1027–39; Hertog, M. G., H. B. Bueno-de-Mesquita, A. M. Fehily, et al. 1996. Fruit and vegetable consumption and cancer mortality in the Caerphilly Study. *Cancer Epidemiol. Biomarkers Prev.* 5 (9): 673–77; Block, G., B. Patterson, and A. Subar. 1992. Fruit, vegetables, and cancer: a review of the epidemiological evidence. *Nutr. Cancer* 18 (10): 1–29; Steinmetz, K. A., and J. D. Potter.

1993. Food-group consumption and colon cancer in the Adelaide Case-Control Study. I. Vegetables and fruit. *Int. J. Cancer* 53 (5): 711–19; Steinmetz, K. A., and J. D. Potter. 1991. Vegetables, fruit and cancer. I. Epidemiology. *Cancer Causes Control* 2 (5): 325–57; Franceschi, S., M. Parpinel, C. La Vecchia, et al. 1998. Role of different types of vegetables and fruit in the prevention of cancer of the colon, rectum, and breast. *Epidemiology* 9 (3): 338–41.

29. Linking plants to people: a visit to the laboratory of Dr. Paul Talalay. 1995. *American Institute for Cancer Research Newsletter*. 46: 10–11.

30. Douglass, J. M., I. M. Rasgon, P. M. Fleiss, et al. 1985. Effects of raw food diet on hypertension and obesity. *South. Med. J.* 78 (7): 841–44.

31. Prochaska, L. J., and W. V. Piekutowski. 1994. On the synergistic effects of enzymes in food with enzymes in the human body. A literature survey and analytical report. *Med. Hypothesis* 42 (6): 355–62.

32. Rumm-Kreuter, D., and I. Demmel. 1990. Comparison of vitamin losses in vegetables due to various cooking methods. *J. Nutr. Sci. Vitaminol.* 36: S7–15.

33. Kimura, M., and Y. Itokawa. 1990. Cooking losses of minerals in foods and its nutritional significance. *J. Nutr. Sci. Vitaminol.* 36 (supp. 1): S25–32.

34. Franceschi, S. 1999. Nutrients and food groups and large bowel cancer in Europe. *Eur. J. Cancer Prev.* 9 (supp. 1): S49–52.

35. Favier, M. L., C. Moundras, C. Demigne, and C. Remesy. 1995. Fermentable carbohydrates exert a more potent cholesterol-lowering effect than cholestyramine. *Biochim. Biophys. Acta* 1258 (2): 115–21.

36. Schatzkin, A., E. Lanza, and D. Corle. 2000. Lack of effect of a low-fat, high-fiber diet on the recurrence of colorectal adenomas. *New Eng. J. Med.* 342: 1149–55; Alberts, D. S.,

M. E. Martinez, D. J. Roe, et al. 2000. Lack of effect of a high-fiber cereal supplement on the recurrence of colorectal adenomas. *New Eng. J. Med.* 342: 1156–62.

37. Byers, T. 2000. Diet, colorectal adenomas, and colorectal cancer (editorial). *New Eng. J. Med.* 342 (16): 1206–07.

38. Ludwig, D. S., M. A. Pereira, C. H. Kroenke, et al. 1999. Dietary fiber, weight gain and cardiovascular disease risk factors in young adults. *JAMA* 282 (16): 1539–46.

Chapter 3: Phytochemicals

1. World Health Organization. Food balance sheets, year 1996. http://apps.fao.org.cvs_down.

2. Steinmetz, K. A., and J. D. Potter. 1993. Food-group consumption and colon cancer in the Adelaide Case-Control Study. I. Vegetables and fruit. *Int. J. Cancer* 53 (5): 711–19.

3. USDA Agriculture Fact Book. 1998. Chapter 1–A. www.usda.gov/news/pubs/fbook98/ch1a.htm.

4. *World Health Statistics Annual 1994–1998*. Online version. www.who.int/whosis; Food and Agriculture Organization of the United Nations. Statistical database food balance sheets, 1961–1999. Available online at www.fao.org; National Institutes of Health. Global cancer rates, cancer death rates among 50 countries, 1986–1999. Available online at www.nih.gov.

5. Gillman, M. W., L. A. Cupples, D. Gagnon, et al. 1995. Protective effect of fruits and vegetables on development of stroke in men. *JAMA* 273 (14): 1113–17; Manson, J. E., W. C. Willett, M. J. Stampfer, et al. 1994. Vegetable and fruit consumption and incidence of stroke in women, abstract. *Circulation* 89 (2): 932; Yu, M. W., H. H. Hsieh, W. H. Pan, et al. 1995. Vegetable consumption, serum retinol level, and risk of hepatocellular carcinoma. *Cancer Res.* 55 (6): 1301–05; Giovannucci, E., A. Asherio, E. B. Rimm, et al. 1995. Intake

of carotenoids and retinol in relation to risk of prostate cancer. *J. Nat. Cancer Inst.* 87 (23): 1767–76; Potter, J. D., and K. Steinmetz. 1996. Vegetables, fruit and phytoestrogens as preventive agents. *IARC Sci. Publ.* 139: 61–90.

6. Franceschi, S., M. Parpinel, C. La Vecchia, et al. 1998. Role of different types of vegetables and fruit in the prevention of cancer of the colon, rectum and breast. *Epidemiology* 9 (3): 338–41; Van Den Brandt, P. A. 1999. Nutrition and cancer: causative, protective, and therapeutic aspects. *Ned. Tijdschr. Genneskd.* 143 (27): 1414–20; Fraser, G. E. 1999. Association between diet and cancer, ischemic heart disease, and all-cause mortality in non-Hispanic white California Seventh-Day Adventists. *Am. J. Clin. Nutr.* 70 (3S): 532–38S.

7. Mayne, S. T. 1996. Beta-carotene, carotenoids, and disease prevention in humans. *FASEB* 10 (7): 690–701.

8. Goodman, G. E. 1998. Prevention of lung cancer. *Current Opinion in Oncology* 10 (2): 122–26.

9. Kolata, G. 1996. Studies find beta carotene, taken by millions, can't forestall cancer or heart disease. *New York Times,* January 19.

10. Omenn, G. S., G. E. Goodman, M. D. Thornquist, et al. 1996. Effects of a combination of beta carotene and vitamin A on lung cancer and cardiovascular disease. *N. Eng. J. Med.* 334 (18): 1150–55; Hennekens, C. H., J. E. Buring, J. E. Manson, et al. 1996. Lack of effect of long-term supplementation with beta-carotene on the incidence of malignant neoplasms and cardiovascular disease. *N. Eng. J. Med.* 334 (18): 1145–49.

11. Albanes, D., O. P. Heinonen, P. R. Taylor, et al. 1996. Alpha-tocopherol and beta-carotene supplements and lung cancer incidence in the alpha-tocopherol, beta-carotene cancer prevention study: effects of base-line characteristics and study compliance. *J. Nat. Cancer Inst.* 88 (21): 1560–70; Rapola, J. M., J. Virtamo, S. Ripatti, et al. 1997. Randomized trial of alpha-tocopherol and beta-carotene supplements on incidence of major coronary events in men with previous myocardial infarction. *Lancet* 349 (9067): 1715–20.

12. Nelson, N. J. 1996. Is chemoprevention research overrated or underfunded? *Primary Care and Cancer* 16 (8): 29.

13. Cohen, J. H., A. R. Kristal, and J. L. Stanford. 2000. Fruit and vegetable intakes and prostate cancer risk. *J. Nat. Cancer Inst.* 92 (1): 61–68.

14. Steinmetz, K. A., and J. D. Potter. 1991. Vegetables, fruit and cancer. II Mechanisms. *Cancer Causes Control* 2 (6): 427–42.

15. Roa, I., J. C. Araya, M. Villaseca, et al. 1996. Preneoplastic lesions and gallbladder cancer: an estimate of the period required for progression. *Gastroenterology* 111 (1): 232–36; Kashayap, V., and B. C. Das. 1998. DNA aneuploidy and infection of human papillomavirus type 16 in preneoplastic lesions of the uterine cervix: correlation with progression to malignancy. *Cancer Lett.* 123 (1): 47–52.

16. Woutersen, R. A., M. J. Appel, and A. Van Garderen-Hoetmer. 1999. Modulation of pancreatic carcinogenesis by antioxidants. *Food Chem. Toxicol.* 37 (9–10): 981–84; Yuan, F., D. Z. Chen, K. Liu, et al. 1999. Anti-estrogenic activities of indole-3-carbinol in cervical cells: implication for prevention of cervical cancer. *Anticancer Res.* 19 (3A): 1673–80; Goodman, M. T., N. Kiviat, K. McDuffie, et al. 1998. The association of plasma micronutrients with the risk of cervical dysplasia in Hawaii. *Cancer Epidemiol. Biomarkers Prev.* 7 (6): 537–44; Reddy, B. S. 1998. Prevention of colon cancer by pre- and probiotics: evidence from laboratory studies. *Br. J. Nutr.* 80 (4): S219–23.

17. Kahn, H. A., R. L. Phillips, D. A. Snowdon, and W. Choi. 1984. Asso-

ciation between reported diet and all-cause mortality. *Am. J. Epid.* 119 (5): 775–87.

18. Steinmetz, K. A., and J. D. Potter. 1996. Vegetables, fruit and cancer prevention: a review. *J. Am. Diet. Assoc.* 96: 1027–39.

19. *Consumer Reports* (October): 1991. A pyramid topples at the USDA. 663–66.

20. Harris, W. 1995. *The scientific basis of vegetarianism,* 101–06. Honolulu: Hawaii Health Publishers.

21. Hausman, P. 1981. *Jack Sprat's legacy, the science and politics of fat and cholesterol.* New York: Center for Science in the Public Interest.

22. United States Department of Agriculture, Economic Research Service. 1991. *Provisions of the Food, Agriculture, Conservation and Trade Act of 1990.* Agriculture Information Bulletin no. 624, p. vii. Washington.

23. McCullough, M. L., D. Feskanich, M. J. Stampfer, et al. 2000. Adherence to the dietary guidelines for Americans and risk of major chronic disease in women. *Am. J. Clin. Nutr.* 72 (5): 1214–22; McCullough, M. L., D. Feskanich, E. B. Rimm, et al. 2000. Adherence to the dietary guidelines for Americans and risk of major chronic disease in men. *Am. J. Clin. Nutr.* 72 (5): 1223–31.

24. Steinmetz, K. A., and J. D. Potter. 1996. Vegetables, fruits and cancer prevention: a review. *J. Am. Diet. Assoc.* 96 (10): 1027–39; La Vecchia, C., and A. Tavani. 1998. Fruit and vegetable consumption and human cancer. *Eur. J. Cancer Prev.* 7 (1): 3–8; Tavani, A., and C. La Vecchia. 1995. Fruit and vegetable consumption and cancer risk in a Mediterranean population. *Am. J. Clin. Nutr.* 61 (6 supp.): 1374–77S.

Chapter 4: The Dark Side of Animal Protein

1. Brody, J. 1990. Huge study of diet indicts fat and meat. *New York Times,* May 8, Science Times section, p. 1.

2. Chen, J., T. C. Campbell, J. Li, and R. Peto. 1990. *Diet, life-style and mortality in China: a study of the characteristics of 65 Chinese counties.* Oxford: Oxford University Press; Ithaca, NY: Cornell University Press; Beijing: Peoples Medical Publishing House, p. 894.

3. Campbell, T. C., B. Parpia, and J. Chen. 1998. Diet, lifestyle, and the etiology of coronary artery disease: the Cornell China Study. *Am. J. Cardiol.* 82 (10B): 18–21T.

4. Willett, W. C. 1997. Nutrition and cancer. *Salud Publica Mex.* 39 (4): 298–309; Marks, F., G. Furstenberger, and K. Muller-Decker. 1999. Metabolic targets of cancer chemoprevention: interruption of tumor development by inhibitors of arachidonic acid metabolism. *Recent Results Cancer Res.* 151: 45–67; Staessen L., D. De Bacquer, S. De Henauw, et al. 1997. Relation between fat intake and mortality: an ecological analysis in Belgium. *Eur. J. Cancer Prev.* 6 (4): 374–81; Rose, D. P. 1997. Dietary fatty acids and prevention of hormone-responsive cancer. *Proc. Soc. Exp. Biol. Med.* 216 (2): 224–33.

5. Giovannucci, E., M. N. Pollak, E. A. Platz, et al. 2000. A prospective study of plasma insulin-like growth factor-1 and binding protein-3 and risk of colorectal neoplasia in women. *Cancer Epidemiol. Biomarkers Prev.* 9 (4): 345–49; Bohlke, K., D. W. Cramer, D. Trichopoulos, and C. S. Mantzoros. 1998. Insulin-like growth factor-1 in relation to premenopausal ductal carcinoma in situ of the breast. *Epidemiology* 9 (5): 570–73; Wolk. A., C. S. Mantzoros, S. O. Andersson, et al. 1998. Insulin-like growth factor-1 and prostate cancer risk: a population-based, case-control study. *J. Nat. Cancer Inst.* 90 (12): 911–15.

6. Campbell, T. C., B. Parpia, and J. Chen. 1990. A plant-enriched diet and long-term health, particularly in reference to China. *Hort. Science* 25 (12): 1512–14.

7. Ibid.

8. Descovich, G. C., C. Ceredi, A. Gaddi, et al. 1980. Multicenter study of soybean protein diet for outpatient hyper-cholesterolaemic patients. *Lancet* 2 (8197): 709–12; Carroll, K. K. 1982. Hypercholesterolemia and atherosclerosis: effects of dietary protein. *Fed. Proc.* 41 (11): 2792–96; Sirtori, C. R., G. Noseda, and G. C. Descovich. 1983. Studies on the use of a soybean protein diet for the management of human hyperlipoproteinemias, in Gibney, M. J., and D. Kritchevsky, eds. *Animal and vegetable proteins in lipid metabolism and atherosclerosis.* New York: Liss, 135–48; Sirtori, C.R., C. Zucchi-Dentone, M. Sirtori, et al. 1985. Cholesterol-lowering and HDL-raising properties of lecithinated soy proteins in type II hyperlipidemic patients. *Ann. Nutr. Metab.* 29 (6): 348–57; Gaddi, A., A. Ciarrocchi, A. Matteucci, et al. 1991. Dietary treatment for familial hypercholesterolemia — differential effects of dietary soy protein according to the apoprotein E phenotypes. *Am. J. Clin. Nutr.* 53: 1191–96; Carroll, K. K. 1983. Dietary proteins and amino acids — their effects on cholesterol metabolism, in Gibney, M. J., and D. Kritchevshy, eds. *Animal and vegetable proteins in lipid metabolism and atherosclerosis.* New York: Liss, 9–17; Jenkins, D. J., C. W. Kendall, C. C. Mehling, et al. 1999. Combined effect of vegetable protein (soy) and soluble fiber added to a standard cholesterol-lowering diet. *Metabolism* 48 (6): 809–16; Anderson, J. W., B. M. Johnstone, and M. E. Cook-Newell. 1995. Meta-analysis of the effects of soy protein intake on serum lipids. *N. Eng. J. Med.* 333 (5): 276–82; Satoh, A., M. Hitomi, and K. Igarashi. 1995. Effects of spinach leaf protein concentrate on the serum cholesterol and amino acid concentrations in rats fed a cholesterol-free diet. *J. Nutr. Sci. Vitaminol.* (Tokyo) 41 (5): 563–73.

9. Singh, P. N., and G. E. Fraser. 1998. Dietary risk factors for colon cancer in a low-risk population. *Am. J. Epidem.* 148: 761–74.

10. U.S. Department of Agriculture, Agricultural Research Service. 1999. USDA nutrient database for standard reference, release 13. Nutrient Data Laboratory home page, www.nal.usda.gov/fnic/foodcomp.

11. Sinha, R., N. Rothman, E. D. Brown, et al. 1995. High concentration of the carcinogen 2-amino-1-methyl-6-phenylimidazo-[4,5–b] pyridine (PhIP) occur in chicken but are dependent on the cooking method. *Cancer Res.* 55 (20): 4516–19.

12. Thomson, B. 1999. Heterocyclic amine levels in cooked meat and the implication for New Zealanders. *Eur. J. Cancer Prev.* 8 (3): 201–06.

13. Davidson, M. H., D. Hunninghake, K. C. Maki, et al. 1999. Comparison of the effects of lean red meat vs. lean white meat on serum lipid levels among free-living person with hypercholesterolemia: a long-term, randomized clinical trial. *Arch. Intern. Med.* 159 (12): 1331–38.

14. Campbell, T. C. 1995. Why China holds the key to your health. *Nutrition Advocate* 1 (1): 7–8.

15. World Health Statistics Annual, 1999 Edition. Available online from WHO Statistical Information System (WHOSIS), www.who.int/whosis.

16. Fraser, G. E., K. D. Lindsted, and W. L. Beeson. 1995. Effect of risk factor values on lifetime risk of and age at first coronary event: the Adventist Health Study. *Am. J. Epidemiol.* 142 (7): 746–58; Fraser, G. E. 1999. Associations between diet and cancer, ischemic heart disease, and all-cause mortality in non-Hispanic white California Seventh-Day Adventists. *Am. J. Clin. Nutr.* 70 (3 supp.): 532–38S.

17. Willett, W. C., D. J. Hunter, M. J. Stampfer, et al. 1992. Dietary fat and fiber in relation to risk of breast cancer: An eight-year follow-up. *JAMA* 268: 2037–44.

18. Campbell, T. C., and C. Junshi. 1994. Diet and chronic degenerative diseases: perspective from China. *Am. J. Clin. Nutr.* 59 (5 supp.): 1153–61S.

19. Key, T. J. A., M. Thorogood, P. N. Appleby, and M. L. Burr. 1996. Dietary habits and mortality in 11,000 vegetarians and health conscious people: results of a 17-year follow up. *BMJ* 313: 775–79.

20. Nelson, N. J. 1996. Is chemoprevention research overrated or underfunded? *Primary Care & Cancer* 16 (8): 29–30.

21. Chang-Claude, J., and R. Frentzel-Beyme. 1993. Dietary and lifestyle determinants of mortality among German vegetarians. *Int. J. Epidemiol.* 22 (2): 228–36; Kahn, H. A., R. I. Phillips, D. A. Snowdon, and W. Choi. 1984. Association between reported diet and all cause mortality: twenty-one-year follow up on 27,530 adult Seventh-Day Adventists. *Am. J. Epidemiol.* 119: 775–87; Nestle, M. 1999. Animal v. plant foods in human diets and health: is the historical record unequivocal? *Proc. Nutr. Soc.* 58 (2): 211–28.

22. Barnard, N.D., A. Nicholson, and J. L. Howard. 1995. The medical costs attributed to meat consumption. *Preventive Medicine* 24: 646–55; Segasothy, M., and P. A. Phillips. 1999. Vegetarian diet: panacea for modern lifestyle disease? *QJM* 92 (9): 531–44.

23. Ruckner C., and J. Hoffman. 1991. *The Seventh-Day Adventist diet.* New York: Random House, 1991.

24. Kahn, op. cit., pp. 775–79.

25. Rodriguez, C., E. E. Calle, L. M. Tatheam, P. A. Wingo, et al. 1998. Family history of breast cancer as a predictor for fatal prostate cancer. *Epidemiology* 9 (5): 525–29.

26. Russo, J. and I. H. 1997. Differentiation and breast cancer. *Medicina* 57 (supp. 2): 81–91.

27. Pike, M. C., D. V. Spicer, L. Dahmoush, and M. F. Press. 1993. Estrogens, progestogens, normal breast cell proliferation, and breast cancer risk. *Epidemiol. Rev.* 15 (1): 17–35.

28. Stoll, B. A., L. J. Vatten, and S. Kvinnsland. 1994. Does early physical maturity influence breast cancer risk? *Acta Oncol.* 32 (2): 171–76; Apter, D. 1966. Hormonal events during female puberty in relation to breast cancer risk. *Eur. J. Cancer Prev.* 5 (6): 476–82.

29. Stoll, B. A. 1998. Western diet, early puberty, and breast cancer risk. *Breast Cancer Res. Treat.* 49 (3): 187–93; Trentham-Dietz, A., P. A. Newcomb, B. E. Storer, et al. 1997. Body size and risk of breast cancer. *Am. J. Epidemiol.* 145 (11): 1011–19.

30. Diamandis, E. P., and H. Yu. 1996. Does prostate cancer start at puberty? *J. Clin. Lab. Anal.* 10 (6): 468–69; Weir, H. K., N. Kreiger, and L. D. Marrett. 1998. Age at puberty and risk of testicular germ cell cancer. *Cancer Causes Control* 9 (3): 253–58; United Kingdom Testicular Cancer Study Group. 1994. Aetiology of testicular cancer: association with congenital abnormalities, age at puberty, infertility, and exercise. *BMJ* 308 (6941): 1393–99.

31. Ross, M. H., E. D. Lustbader, and G. Bras. 1982. Dietary practices of early life and spontaneous tumors of the rat. *Nutr. Cancer* 3 (3): 150–67.

32. Tanner, J. M. 1973. Trend toward earlier menarche in London, Oslo, Copenhagen, the Netherlands and Hungary. *Nature* 243: 75–76.

33. Beaton, G. 1976. Practical population indicators of health and nutrition. World Health Organization monograph 62: 500.

34. Register, U. D., and J. A. Sonneberg. 1973. The vegetarian diet. *J. Am. Diet. Assoc.* 45: 537; Hardinge, M. G., A. Sanchez, D. Waters, et al. 1971. Possible factors associated with the prevalence of acne vulgaris. *Fed. Proc.* 30: 300.

35. Cheek, D. B. 1973. Body composi-

tion, hormones, nutrition, and adolescent growth, in Grumbach, M. M., G. D. Brace, F. E. Mayers, eds., *Control of the onset of puberty.* New York: John Wiley and Sons, p. 424.

36. Apter, D., M. Reinila, and R. Vihko. 1989. Some endocrine characteristics of early menarche, a risk factor for breast cancer, are preserved into adulthood. *Int. J. Cancer* 44 (5): 783–87.

37. Chiaffarino, F., F. Parazzini, C. LaVecchia, E. Di Cintio, and S. Marsico. 1999. Diet and uterine myomas. *Obstet. Gynecol.* 94 (3): 395–98.

38. Kralj-Cercek, L. 1956. The influence of food, body build, and social origin on the age of menarche. *Human Biology* 28: 393; Sanchez, A., D. G. Kissinger, and R. I. Phillips. 1981. A hypothesis on the etiological role of diet on age of menarche. *Med. Hypothesis* 7: 1339–45.

39. Burell, R. J. W., M. J. R. Healy, and J. M. Tanner. 1961. Age at menarche in South African Bantu schoolgirls living in the Transkei reserve. *Human Biology* 33: 250.

40. Guo, W. D., W. H. Chow, W. Zheng, J. Y. Li, and W. J. Blot. 1994. Diet, serum markers and breast cancer mortality in China. *Japan J. Cancer Res.* 85: 572–77.

41. Hill, P., L. Garbeczewski, and F. Kasumi. 1985. Plasma testosterone and breast cancer. *Eur. J. Cancer Clin. Oncol.* 21: 1265–66.

42. U.S. Department of Agriculture. Office of Communications. 1998. What do Americans eat? *USDA Agriculture Fact Book.*

43. De Waard, F., and D. Trichopoulos. 1988. A unifying concept of the aetiology of breast cancer. *Int. J. Cancer* 41: 666–69.

44. Decarli, A., A. Favero, C. La Vecchia, et al. 1997. Macronutrients, energy intake, and breast cancer risk: implications from different models. *Epidemiology* 8: 425–28.

45. Nicholson, A. 1996. Diet and the prevention and treatment of breast cancer *Altern. Ther. Health Med.* 2 (6): 32–38.

46. Wynder, E. L., L. A. Cohen, J. E. Muscat, et al. 1997. Breast cancer: weighing the evidence for a promoting role of dietary fat. *J. Nat. Cancer Inst.* 89: 766–75.

47. Ross, M. H., E. Lustbader, and G. Bras. 1976. Dietary practices and growth responses as predictors of longevity. *Nature* 262 (5569): 548–53.

48. Comments in Gunnell, D. J., G. D. Smith, J. M. Holly, and S. Frankel. 1998. Leg length and risk of cancer in the Boyd Orr cohort. *BMJ* 317 (7169): 1950–51.

49. Cheng, Z., J. Hu, J. King, and T. C. Campbell. 1997. Inhibition of hepatocellular carcinoma development in hepatitis B virus transfected mice by low dietary casein. *Hepatology* 26 (5): 1351–54; Torosian, M. H. 1995. Effect of protein intake on tumor growth and cell cycle kinetics. *J. Surg. Res.* 59 (2): 225–28; Youngman, L. D., J. Y. Park, and B. N. Ames. 1992. Protein oxidation associated with aging is reduced by dietary restriction of protein of calories. *Proc. Nat. Acad. Sci.* 89 (19): 9112–16.

50. Hebert, J. R., T. G. Hurley, B. C. Olendzki, J. Teas, Y. Ma, and J. S. Hampl. 1998. Nutritional and socioeconomic factors in relation to prostate cancer mortality: a cross-national study. *J. Nat. Cancer Inst.* 90 (21): 1637–47.

51. Frentzel-Beyme, R., and J. Chang-Claude. 1994. Vegetarian diets and colon cancer: the German experience. *Am. J. Clin. Nutr.* 59 (supp.): 1143–52S.

52. Berkel, J., and F. deWaard. 1983. Mortality pattern and life expectancy of Seventh-Day Adventists in the Netherlands. *Int. J. Epidemiol.* 12: 455–59; Phillips, R. L., and D. A. Snowdon. 1985. Dietary relationships with fatal colorectal cancer

among Seventh-Day Adventists. *J. Nat. Cancer Inst.* 74: 307–17.

53. Corliss, J. 1993. Pesticide metabolites linked to breast cancer. *J. Nat. Cancer Inst.* 85: 602.

54. Fraser, G. E. 1999. Association between diet and cancer, ischemic heart disease, and all-cause mortality in non-Hispanic white California Seventh-Day Adventists. *Am. J. Clin. Nutr.* 70 (3 supp.): 532–38S; Sarasua, S., and D. A. Savitz. 1994. Cured and broiled meat consumption in relation to childhood cancer. *Cancer Causes Control* 5 (2): 141–48; Favero, A., M. Parpinel, and S. Franceschi. 1998. Diet and risk of breast cancer: major findings from an Italian case-control study. *Biomed. Pharmacother.* 52 (3): 109–15; Levi, F., C. Pasche, C. La Vecchia, F. Lucchini, and S. Franceschi. 1999. Food groups and colorectal cancer risk. *Br. J. Cancer* 79 (7–8): 1283–87; Steinmetz, K. A., and J. D. Potter. 1993. Food-group consumption and colon cancer in the Adelaide Case-Control Study: meat, poultry, seafood, dairy foods and eggs. *Int. J. Cancer* 53 (5): 720–27; Levi, F., S. Franceschi, E. Negri, and C. La Vecchia. 1993. Dietary factors and the risk of endometrial cancer. *Cancer* 71 (11): 3575–81; Negri, E., C. Bosetti, C. La Vecchia, F. Fioretti, E. Conti, and S. Franceschi. 1999. Risk factors for adenocarcinoma of the small intestine. *Int. J. Cancer.* 82 (2): 171–74; Chow, W. H., G. Gridley, J. K. McLoughlin, et al. 1994. Protein intake and risk of renal cell cancer. *J. Nat. Cancer Inst.* 86: 1131–39; Kwiatkowski, A. 1993. Dietary and other environmental risk factors in acute leukemias: a case-control study of 119 patients. *Eur. J. Cancer Prev.* 2 (2): 139–46; National Institutes of Health, National Cancer Institute. 1996. *Cancer rates and risks: cancer death rates among 50 countries (age adjusted to the world standard),* 4th ed. U.S. Department of Health and Human Services. Lung cancer, p. 39. Source: World Health Organization data as adapted by the American Cancer Society; Deneo-Pelligrini, H., E. De Stefani, A. Ronco, et al. 1996. Meat consumption and risk of lung cancer; a case-control study from Uruguay. *Lung Cancer* 14 (2–3): 195–205; Zhang, S., D. J. Hunter, B. A. Rosner, et al. 1999. Greater intake of meats and fats associated with higher risk of non-Hodgkins lymphoma. *J. Nat. Cancer Inst.* 91 (20): 1751–58; Cunningham, A. S. 1976. Lymphomas and animal-protein consumption. *Lancet* 27: 1184–86; Franceschi, S., A. Favero, E. Conti, et al. 1999. Food groups, oils and butter, and cancer of the oral cavity and pharynx. *Br. J. Cancer* 80 (3–4): 614–20; Tominaga, S., K. Aoki, I. Fujimoto, et al. 1994. Cancer mortality and morbidity statistics. *Japan and the World.* Boca Raton, Fla.: Japan Scientific Societies Press, CRC Press, 196; Soler, M., L. Chatenoud, C. La Vecchia, S. Franceschi, and E. Negri. 1998. Diet alcohol, coffee and pancreatic cancer: final results from an Italian study. *Eur. J. Cancer Prev.* 7 (6): 455–60; Sung, J. F., R. S. Lin, Y. S. Pu, Y. C. Chen, H. C. Chang, and M. K. Lai. 1999. *Cancer* 86 (3): 484–91; Black, H. S., J. A. Herd, L. H. Goldberg, et al. 1994. Effect of a low-fat diet on the incidence of actinic keratosis. *New Eng. J. Med.* 330: 1272–75.

55. Dietary carcinogens linked to breast cancer. 1993. *Medical World News,* May, p. 13.

56. Peer, P. G., J. A. van Dijck, J. H. Hendriks, et al. 1993. Age dependent growth rate of primary breast cancer. *Cancer* 71 (11): 3547–51.

57. Wright, C. J., and C. B. Mueller. 1995. Screening mammography and public health policy: the need for perspective. *Lancet* 346 (8966): 29–32; Neugut, A. I., and J. S. Jacobson. 1995. The limitations of breast cancer screening for first-degree relatives of breast cancer patients. *Am.*

J. Public Health 85 (6): 832–34; Olsen, O., P. C. Gotzzsche. 2001. Cochrane review on screening for breast cancer with mammography. *Lancet* 358: 1340–42.

58. Le Marchand, L., J. H. Hankin, F. Bach, et al. 1995. An ecological study of diet and lung cancer in the South Pacific. *Int. J. Cancer* 63 (1): 18–23.

59. Gao, C. M., K. Tajima, T. Kuroishi, et al. 1993. Protective effects of raw vegetables and fruit against lung cancer among smokers and ex-smokers: a case-control study in the Tokai area of Japan. *Japan J. Cancer Res.* 84 (6): 594–600.

60. Verreault, R., J. Brisson, L. Deschenes, et al. 1988. Dietary fat in relation to prognostic indicators in breast cancer. *J. Nat. Cancer Inst.* 89: 819–25.

61. Gregorio, D. I., L. J. Emrich, S. Graham, et al. 1985. Dietary fat consumption and survival among women with breast cancer. *J. Nat. Cancer Inst.* 75: 37–41.

62. Holm, L. E., E. Callmer, M. L. Hjalmar, et al. 1989. Dietary habits and prognostic factors in breast cancer. *J. Nat. Cancer Inst.* 81: 1218–23; Newman, S. C., A. B. Miller, G. R. Howe. 1986. A study of the effect of weight and dietary fat on breast cancer survival time. *Am. J. Epidem.* 123: 767–74.

63. Breslow, N., C. W. Chan, G. Dhom, et al. 1977. Latent carcinoma of prostate at autopsy in seven areas. *Int. J. Cancer* 20: 680–88.

64. Giem, P., W. L. Beeson, and G. E. Faser. 1993. The incidence of dementia and intake of animal products: preliminary findings from the Adventist Health Study. *Neuroepidemiology* 12: 28–36.

65. Fellstrom, B., B. G. Daneilson, B. Kerlstrom, et al. 1983. The influence of a high dietary intake of purine-rich animal protein on urinary excretion and supersaturation in renal stone disease. *Clinical Science* 64: 399–405; Robertson, W. G., M. Pea-

cock, and P. J. Heyburn. 1979. Should recurrent calcium oxalate stone formers become vegetarians? *B. J. Urol.* 51: 427–31; Bosch, L. P., A. Saccaggi, A. Lauer, et al. 1983. Renal functional reserve in humans, effect of protein intake on glomerula filtration rate. *Am. J. Med.* 75: 943–50; Effects of acute protein loads of different sources on glomerular filtration rate. 1987. *Kidney International* 32 (22): S25–28; Kerstetter, J. E., and L. H. Allen. 1989. Dietary protein increases urinary calcium. *J. Nutr.* 120: 134–36; Breslau, N. A., L. Brinkley, K. D. Hill, and C. Y. C. Pak. 1988. Relationship of animal protein-rich diet to kidney stone formation and calcium metabolism. *J. Clin. Endocr. and Metab.* 66: 140–46; Chaiffarino, op. cit., p. 395; Wiseman, M. J., R. Hunt, A. Goodwin, et al. 1987. Dietary composition and renal function in healthy subjects. *Nephron.* 46: 37–42; Appleby, P. N., M. Thorogood, J. I. Mann, T. J. Key. 1999. The Oxford Vegetarian Study: an overview. *Am. J. Clin. Nutr.* 70 (3): 525–31S; Nordoy, A., and S. H. Goodnight. 1990. Dietary lipids and thrombosis: relationship to atherosclerosis. *Arteriosclerosis* 10 (2): 149–63.

66. Maggi, S., J. L. Kelsey, J. Litvak, and S. P. Hayes. 1991. Incidence of hip fractures in the elderly: a cross-national analysis. *Osteoporosis Int.* 1: 232–41.

67. Feskanich, D., W. C. Willett, M. J. Stampfer, and G. A. Colditz. 1997. Milk dietary calcium, and bone fractures in women: a 12-year prospective study. *Am. J. Public Health* 87: 992–97.

68. Tucker, K. L., M. T. Hannan, H. Chen, et al. 1999. Potassium, magnesium, and fruit and vegetable intakes are associated with greater bone mineral density in elderly men and women. *Am. J. Clin. Nutr.* 68 (4): 727–36.

69. Feskanich, D., W. C. Willett, M. J. Stampfler, and G. A. Colditz. 1996.

Protein consumption and bone fractures in women. *Am. J. Epidemiol.* 143 (5): 472–79; Itoh, R., and Y. Suyama. 1996. Sodium excretion in relation to calcium and hydroxyproline excretion in a healthy Japanese population. *Am. J. Clin. Nutr.* 63 (5): 735–40; Massey, L. K., and S. J. Whiting. 1993. Caffeine, urinary calcium, calcium metabolism and bone. *J. Nutr.* 123 (9): 1611–14; Harris, S. S., and B. Dawson-Hughes. 1994. Caffeine and bone loss in healthy postmenopausal women. *Am. J. Clin. Nutr.* 60 (4): 573–78; Nguyen, N. U., G. Dumoulin, J. P. Wolf, and S. Berthelay. 1989. Urinary calcium and oxalate excretion during oral fructose or glucose load in man. *Horm. Metab. Res.* 21 (2): 96–99; Bunker, V. W. 1994. The role of nutrition in osteoporosis. *Br. J. Biomed. Sci.* 51 (3): 228–40; Sampson, H. W. 1997. Alcohol, osteoporosis, and bone regulating hormones. *Alcohol Clin. Exp. Res.* 21 (3): 400–03; Villiger, P. M., and R. Krapf. 1996. Osteoporosis of the lumbar spine. *Schweiz. Rundsch. Med. Prax.* 85 (43): 1354–59; Spencer, H., and L. Kramer. 1985. Osteoporosis: calcium, fluoride, and aluminum interactions. *J. Am. Coll. Nutr.* 4 (1): 121–28; Wolinsky-Friedland, M. 1995. Drug-induced metabolic bone disease. *Endocrinol. Metab. Clin. North Am.* 24 (2): 395–420; Melhus, H., K. Michaelson, A. Kindmark, et al. 1998. Excessive dietary intake of vitamin A is associated with reduced bone mineral density and increased risk of hip fracture. *Ann. Intern. Med.* 129 (10): 770–78.

70. Hu, J. F., X. H. Zhao, B. Parpia, and T. C. Campbell. 1993. Dietary intakes and urinary excretion of calcium and acids: a cross-sectional study of women in China. *Am. J. Clin. Nutr.* 58 (3): 398–406.

71. Barzel, U. S., and L. K. Massey. 1998. Excess dietary protein can adversely affect bone. *J. Nutr.* 128 (6): 1051–53; Remer, T., and F. Mantz. 1994. Estimation of the renal net acid excretion by adults consuming diets containing variable amounts of protein. *Am. J. Clin. Nutr.* 59: 1356–61.

72. Feskanich, op. cit.

73. Abelow, B. J., T. R. Holford, and K. L. Insogna. 1992. Cross-cultural association between dietary animal protein and hip fracture: a hypothesis. *Calcif. Tissue Int.* 50 (1): 14–18.

74. Barzel, op. cit.

75. Heaney, R. P. 1998. Excess dietary protein may not adversely affect bone. *J. Nutr.* 128 (6): 1054–57.

76. Whiting, S. J., and B. Lemke. 1999. Excess retinol intake may explain the high incidence of osteoporosis in northern Europe. *Nutr. Rev.* 57 (6): 192–95.

77. Mazess, R. B., and W. Mather. 1977. Bone mineral content of North Alaskan Eskimos. *Am. J. Clin. Nutr.* 27 (9): 916–25; Pawson, I. G. 1974. Radiographic determination of excessive bone loss in Alaskan Eskimos. *Hum. Biol.* 46 (3): 369–80.

78. Weaver, C. M., and K. L. Plawecki. 1994. Dietary calcium: adequacy of a vegetarian diet. *Am. J. Clin. Nutr.* 59 (supp.): 1238–41S.

79. Tucker, K. L., M. T. Hannan, H. Chen, et al. 1999. Potassium, magnesium, and fruit and vegetable intakes are associated with greater mineral density in elderly men and women. *Am. J. Clin. Nutr.* 69 (4): 727–36; New, S. A., S. P. Robins, M. K. Campbell, et al. 2000. Dietary influences on bone mass and bone metabolism: further evidence of a positive link between fruit and vegetable consumption and bone health? *Am. J. Clin. Nutr.* 71 (1): 142–51.

80. Feskanich, D., P. Weber, W. C. Willett, et al. 1999. Vitamin K intake and hip fractures in women: a prospective study. *Am. J. Clin. Nutr.* 69 (1): 74–79.

81. Grant, W. B. 1998. Milk and other dietary influences on coronary heart disease. *Altrn. Med. Rev.* 3: 281–94;

Segall, J. J. 1997. Epidemiological evidence for the link between dietary lactose and atherosclerosis, in Colaco, C., ed. *The glycation hypothesis of atherosclerosis.* Austin, Tex.: Landes Bioscience, pp. 185–209; Artad-Wild, S. M., S. L. Connor, G. Sexton, et al. 1993. Differences in coronary mortality can be explained by differences in cholesterol and saturated fat intakes in 40 countries but not in France and Finland: a paradox. *Circulation* 88: 2771–79.

82. Davies, T. W., C. R. Palmer, E. Ruja, and J. M. Lipscombe. 1996. Adolescent milk, dairy products and fruit consumption and testicular cancer. *Br. J. Cancer* 74 (4): 657–60.

83. Patandin, S., P. C. Dagnelie, P. G. Mulder, et al. 1999. Dietary exposure to polychlorinated biphenyls and dioxins from infancy until adulthood: a comparison between breast-feeding toddler, and long-term exposure. *Environ. Health Perspect.* 107 (1): 45–51.

84. Skrzycki, C., and J. Warrick. 2000. EPA report ratchets up dioxin peril. *Washington Post,* May 17, 2000.

85. Remer, T., and F. Manz. 1995. Potential renal acid load of foods and its influence on urine pH. *J. Am. Diet. Assoc.* 95 (7): 791–97.

86. Grant, W. B. 1999. An ecologic study of dietary links to prostate cancer. *Altern. Med. Rev.* 4: 162–69; Schwartz, G. G., C. C. Hill, T. A. Oeler, M. J. Becich, and R. R. Bahnson. 1995. 1,25-dihydroxy-16-ene-23-yne-vitamin D3 and prostate cancer cell proliferation in vivo. *Urology* 46: 365–69; Cramer, D. W., et al. 1989. Galactose consumption and metabolism in relation to the risk of ovarian cancer. *Lancet* 2: 66–71; Kushi, L. 1999. Lactose and ovarian cancer. *Am. J. Epidemiol.* 149 (1): 21–31; Cramer, D. W., E. R. Greenberg, L. Titus-Ernstoff, et al. 2000. A case-control study of galactose consumption and metabolism in relation to ovarian cancer. *Cancer*

Epidemiol. Biomarkers Prev. 9 (1): 95–101.

87. Chan, J. M., M. J. Stampfer, J. Ma, et al. 2000. Dairy products, calcium, and prostate cancer risk in the Physicians Health Study. Presentation, American Association for Cancer Research, San Francisco, April.

88. Bosetti, C., A. Tzonou, P. Lagiou, et al. 2000. Fraction of prostate cancer attributed to diet in Athens, Greece. *Eur. J. Cancer Prev.* 9 (2): 119–23.

89. Fairfield, K. 2000. Annual Meeting of the Society for General Internal Medicine. Dairy products linked to ovarian cancer risk. *Family Practice News,* June 11, p. 8.

Chapter 5: Are You Dying to Lose Weight?

1. Preboth, M. A., and S. Wright. 1998. Quantum sufficit. *American Family Physician* 58 (3): 639.

2. Mokdad, A. H., M. K. Serdula, W. H. Dietz, et al. 1999. The spread of the obesity epidemic in the United States, 1991–1998. *JAMA* 282 (16): 1519–22.

3. World Health Organization. 1996. Food balance sheets, online at http://apps.fao.org.cvs_down.

4. Tavani, A., C. La Vecchia, S. Gallus, et al. 2000. Red meat and cancer risk: a study in Italy. *Int. J. Cancer* 86 (3): 425–28.

5. De Stefani, E., L. Fierro, M. Mendilaharsu, et al. 1998. Meat intake, "mate" drinking and renal cell cancer in Uruguay: a case-control study. *Br. J. Cancer* 78 (9): 1239–43; Risch, H. A., M. Jain, L. D. Marrett, and G. R. Howe. 1994. Dietary fat intake and risk of epithelial ovarian cancer. *J. Nat. Cancer Inst.* 86 (18): 1409–15; Pillow, P. C., S. D. Hursting, C. M. Duphorne, et al. 1997. Case-control assessment of diet and lung cancer risk in African Americans and Mexican Americans. *Nutr. Cancer* 29 (2): 169–73; Alavanja, M. C., C. C. Brown, C. Swanson, and R. C. Brownson. 1993. Saturated fat in-

266   Joel Fuhrman, M.D.

take and lung cancer risk among nonsmoking women in Missouri. *J. Nat. Cancer Inst.* 85 (23): 1906–16.

6. Kuller, L. H. 1997. Dietary fat and chronic disease: epidemiologic overview. *J. Am. Diet. Assoc.* 97 (7 supp.): S9–15; Willett, W. C. 1997. Nutrition and cancer. *Salud Publica Mex.* 39 (4): 298–309; La Vecchia, C. 1992. Cancer associated with high-fat diets. *J. Natl. Cancer Inst. Monogr.* 12: 79–85; Steinmetz, K. A., and J. D. Potter. 1996. Vegetables, fruit, and cancer prevention: a review. *J. Am. Diet. Assoc.* 96 (10): 1027–39.

7. Brown, L. M., C. A. Swanson, G. Gridley, et al. 1998. Dietary factors and the risk of squamous cell esophageal cancer among black and white men in the United States. *Cancer Causes Control* 9 (5): 467–74; Cheng, K. K., and N. E. Day. 1996. Nutrition and esophageal cancer. *Cancer Causes Control* 7 (1): 33–40; Hirohata, T., and S. Kono. 1997. Diet/nutrition and stomach cancer in Japan. *Int. J. Cancer* supp. 10: 34–36; Kono, S., and T. Hirohata. 1996. Nutrition and stomach cancer. *Cancer Causes Control* 7 (1): 41–45; Terry, P., O. Nyren, and J. Yuen. 1998. Protective effect of fruits and vegetables on stomach cancer in a cohort of Swedish twins. *Int. J. Cancer* 76 (1): 35–37.

8. Willett, W. C., and D. Trichopoulos, eds. 1996. Nutrition and cancer: a summary of the evidence. *Cancer Causes Control* 7: 178–80; La Vecchia, C., and A. Tavani. 1998. Fruit and vegetables, and human cancer. *Eur. J. Cancer Prev.* 7 (1): 3–8; Tavani, A., and C. La Vecchia. 1995. Fruit and vegetable consumption and cancer risk in a Mediterranean population. *Am. J. Clin. Nutr.* 61 (6): 1374–77S.

9. Key, T. J. A., M. Thorogood, P. N. Appleby, and M. L. Burr. 1996. Dietary habits and mortality in 11,000 vegetarians and health conscious people: results of a 17-year follow up. *BMJ* 313: 775–79.

10. Jacobs, D. R., J. Slavin, and L. Marquart. 1995. Whole grain intake and cancer: a review of the literature. *Nutrition and Cancer* 24: 221–29.

11. O'Keefe, S. J., M. Kidd, G. Espitalier-Noel, and P. Owira. 1999. Rarity of colon cancer in Africans is associated with low animal product consumption, not fiber. *Am. J. Gastroenterol.* 94 (5): 1373–80.

12. Sherwood, N. E., R. W. Jeffery, S. A. French, et al. 2000. Predictors of weight gain in the Pound of Prevention study. *Int. J. Obes. Relat. Metab. Disord.* 24 (4): 395–403; Astrup, A. 1999. Macronutrient balances and obesity: the role of diet and physical activity. *Public Health Nutr.* 2 (3A): 341–47.

13. Kahn, H. S., L. M. Tatham, C. Rodriguez, et al. 1997. Stable behaviors associated with adults' 10–year change in body mass index and likelihood of gain at the waist. *Am. J. Public Health* 87 (5): 747–57.

14. Alavanja, op. cit.; Lichtenstein, A. H., E. Kennedy, P. Barrier, et al. 1998. Dietary fat consumption and health. *Nutr. Rev.* 56 (5) pt. 2: S3–28; Kromhout, D., B. Bloemberg, E. Feskens, et al. 2000. Saturated fat, vitamin C and smoking predict long-term population all-cause mortality rates in the Seven Countries Study. *Int. J. Epidemiol.* 29 (2): 260–65; Staessen, L., D. De Bacquer, S. De Henauw, et al. 1997. Relation between fat intake and mortality: an ecological analysis in Belgium. *Eur. J. Cancer Prev.* 6 (4): 374–81.

15. Kasiske, B. L., J. D. Lakatua, J. Z. Ma, and T. A. Louis. 1998. A meta-analysis of the effects of dietary protein restriction on the rate of decline in renal function. *Am. J. Kidney Dis.* 31 (6): 954–61; Holm, E. A., and K. Solling. 1996. Dietary protein restriction and the progression of chronic renal insufficiency: a review of the literature. *J. Intern. Med.* 239 (2): 99–104.

16. Brenner, B. M., T. W. Meyer, and

T. H. Hostetter. 1982. Dietary protein intake and the progressive nature of kidney disease: the role of the hemo-dynamically mediated glomerular injury in the pathogenisis of progressive glomerular sclerosis in aging, renal ablation and intrinsic renal disease. *N. Eng. J. Med.* 307 (11): 652–59.

17. Clark, B. 2000. Biology of renal aging in humans. *Adv. Ren. Replace. Ther.* 7 (1): 11–21.

18. Rosman, J. B. 1995. Protein restriction in diet therapy in chronic kidney insufficiency. *Ther. Umsch.* 52 (8): 515–18; Zeller, K. R. 1991. Low-protein diets in renal disease. *Diabetes Care* 14 (9): 856–66.

19. Fouque, D., P. Wang, M. Laville, and J. P. Boissel. 2000. Low protein diets delay end-stage renal disease in non-diabetic adults with chronic renal failure. *Nephrol. Dial. Transplant* 15 (12): 1986–92.

20. Gin, H., V. Rigalleau, and M. Aparicio. 2000. Lipids, protein intake, and diabetic nephropathy. *Diabetes Metab.* 26 (supp. 4): 45–53.

21. Pedrini, M. T., A. S. Levey, J. Lau, T. C. Chalmers, and P. H. Wang. 1996. The effect of dietary protein on the progression of diabetic and nondiabetic renal disease: a meta-analysis. *Ann. Intern. Med.* 124 (7): 627–32.

22. Bankhead, C. 1998. Ketogenic diet can cause serious adverse effects, data suggests. *Medical Tribune* 39 (17): 23.

23. Licata, A. A., E. Bow, F. C. Bartler, et al. 1979. Effect of dietary protein on urinary calcium in normal subjects and in patients with nephrolithiasis. *Metabolism* 28: 895; Robertson, W. G., P. J. Heyburn, M. Peacock, et al. 1979. The effect of high animal protein intake on the risk of calcium stone formation in the urinary tract. *Clin. Sci.* 57: 285; Brokis, J. G., A. S. Levitt, and S. M. Cruthers. 1982. The effects of vegetable and animal protein diets on calcium, urate and oxalate excretion. *Br. J. Urol.* 54: 590; Robertson, W. G., M. Peacock, P. J. Heyburn, et al. 1981. The risk of calcium stone formation in relation to affluence and dietary animal protein, in Brokis, J. G., and B. Finlayson, eds. *Urinary calculus, International Urinary Stone Conference.* Littleton, Colo.: PSG Publishing, p. 3.

24. Beyers, T. 1993. Dietary trends in the United States. Relevance to cancer prevention. *Cancer* 72 (3 supp.) 1015–18; Lenfant, C., and N. Ernst. 1994. Daily dietary fat and total food-energy intake — Third National Health and Nutrition Examination Survey, phase 1, 1988–91. *MMWR* 43 (7): 116–17, 123–25.

25. Harnack, L. J., R. W. Jeffrey, and K. N. Boutelle. 2000. Temporal trends in energy intake in the United States: an ecological perspective. *Am. J. Clin. Nutr.* 71 (6): 1478–84.

26. Kennedy, E. T., S. A. Bowman, and R. Powell. 1999. Dietary-fat intake in the U.S. population. *J. Am. Coll. Nutr.* 18 (3): 207–12; Kant, A. K. 2000. Consumption of energy-dense, nutrient-poor foods by adult Americans: nutritional and health implications: Third National Health and Nutrition Examination Survey, 1988–94. *Am. J. Clin. Nutr.* 72 (4): 929–36.

27. Astrup, A. 1999. Macronutrient balances and obesity: the role of diet and physical activity. *Public Health Nutr.* 2 (3A): 341–47; Sherwood, op. cit.

28. Van Dam, R. M., A. W. Visscher, E. J. Feskens, et al. 2000. Dietary glycemic index in relation to metabolic risk factors and incidence of coronary heart disease: the Zutphen Elderly Study. *Eur. J. Clin. Nutr.* 54 (9): 726–31.

29. Chandalia, M., A. Garg, D. Lutjoham, et al. 2000. Beneficial effects of high dietary fiber intake in patients with type-2 diabetes mellitus. *N. Eng. J. Med.* 342 (19): 1392–98.

30. Bengmark, S. 2000. Colonic food: pre- and probiotics. *Am. J. Gastroenterol.* 95 (1 supp.): S5–7.

31. Friedman, M. 1998. Fuel partitioning and food intake. *Am. J. Clin. Nutr.* 67: 513–18S.

32. McCarty, M. F. 2000. The origins of western obesity: a role for animal protein? *Med. Hypothees.* 54 (3): 488–94.

33. Torosian, M. H. 1995. Effect of protein intake on tumor growth and cell cycle kinetics. *J. Surg. Res.* 59 (2): 225–28; Youngman, L.D., J. Y. Park, and B. N. Ames. 1992. Protein oxidation associated with aging is reduced by dietary restriction of protein of calories. *Proc. Nat. Acad. Sci.* 89 (19): 9112–16; Carroll, K. K. 1982. Hypercholesterolemia and atherosclerosis: effects of dietary protein. *Fed. Proc.* 41 (11): 2792–96; Carroll, K. K. 1983. Dietary proteins and amino acids — their effects on cholesterol metabolism, in Gibney, M. J., D. Kritchevshy, eds. *Animal and vegetable proteins in lipid metabolism and atherosclerosis.* New York: Liss, pp. 9–17; Willett, W. C. 1997. Nutrition and cancer. *Salud Publica Mex.* 39 (4): 298–309.

34. Ornish, D., L. W. Scherwitz, J. H. Billings, et al. 1998. Intensive lifestyle changes for reversal of coronary heart disease. *JAMA* 280 (23): 2001–07.

35. Scheen, A. J., N. Paquot, M. R. Letiexhe, et al. 1995. Glucose metabolism in obese subjects: lessons from OGTT, IVGTT and clamp studies. *Int. J. Obes. Relat. Metab. Disord.* 19 (supp. 3): S14–20; Tai, E. S., T. N. Lau, S. C. Ho, et al. 2000. Body fat distribution and cardiovascular risk in normal weight women: associations with insulin resistance, lipids and plasma leptin. *Int. J. Obes. Relat. Metab. Disord.* 24 (6): 751–57; Takeshita, Y. 1995. Changes in insulin sensitivity after weight loss in hypertensive patients with obesity. *Nippon Jinzo. Gakkai. Shi.* 37 (7): 384–90; S. Hy, W. H. Sheu, H. M. Chin, et al. 1995. Effect of weight loss on blood pressure and insulin resistance in normotensive and hypertensive obese individuals. *Am. J. Hypertens.* 8 (11): 1067–71.

36. McLaughlin, T., F. Abbasi, M. Carantoni, et al. 1999. Differences in insulin resistance do not predict weight loss in response to hypocaloric diets in healthy obese women. *J. Clin. Endocrinol. Metab.* 84 (2): 578–81.

37. Gould, A. J., D. E. Williams, C. D. Byrne, et al. 1999. Prospective cohort study of the relationship of markers of insulin resistance and secretion with weight gain and changes in regional adiposity. *Int. J. Obes. Relat. Metab. Disord.* 23 (12): 1256–61.

38. McDougall, J. The great debate: high vs. low protein diets. *The McDougall Newsletter* 11:4; 1–4.

39. Pyorala, M., H. Miettinen, M. Laakso, and K. Pyorala. 1998. Hyperinsulinemia predicts coronary heart disease risk in healthy middle-aged men: the 22-year follow-up results of the Helsinki Policemen Study. *Circulation* 98 (5): 398–404.

40. Bernard, R. J., E. J. Ugianskis, and D. A. Martin. 1992. Role of diet and exercise in the management of hyperinsulinemia and associated atherosclerotic risk factors. *Am. J. Cardiol.* 69 (5): 440–44.

41. Tarjan, Z., M. Tonelli, J. Duba, and A. Zorandi. 1995. Correlation between ABO and Rh blood groups, serum cholesterol and ischemic heart disease in patients undergoing coronarography. *Orv. Hetil.* 136 (15): 767–69; Stakishaitis, D. V., L. I. Ivashkiavicheme, and A. M. Narvilene. 1991. Atherosclerosis of the coronary arteries and the blood group in the population of Lithuania. *Vrach. Delo.* 8: 55–57.

42. Meade, T. W., J. A. Cooper, Y. Stirling, et al. 1994. Factor VIII, ABO blood group and the incidence of ischaemic heart disease. *Br. J. Haematol.* 88 (3): 601–07; Whincup, P. H., D. G. Cook, A. N. Phillips, and A. G. Shaper. 1990. ABO blood group and ischaemic heart disease in British men. *BMJ* 300 (6741): 1679–82.

43. Erikssen, J., E. Thaulow, H. Stor-

morken, et al. 1980. ABO blood groups and coronary heart disease (CHD): a study in subjects with severe and latent CHD. *Thromb. Haemost.* 43 (2): 137–40.

44. Barzilai, N., I. Gabriely, M. Gabriely, et al. 2001. Offspring of centenarians have a favorable lipid profile. *J. Am. Geriatr. Soc.* 49 (1): 76–79.

45. Suadicani, P., H. O. Hein, and F. Gyntelberg. 2000. Socioeconomic status, ABO phenotypes and risk of ischaemic heart disease: an 8-year follow-up in the Copenhagen Male Study. *J. Cardiovasc. Risk* 7 (4): 277–83; Contiero, E., G. E. Chinello, and M. Folin. 1994. Serum lipids and lipoproteins association with ABO blood groups. *Anthropol. Anz.* 52 (3): 221–30.

46. Konigsberg, W., J. Goldstein, and R. J. Hill. 1963. The structure of human haemoglobin VII: the digestion of the beta chain of human haemoglobin with pepsin. *J. Biol. Chem.* 238: 2028–33.

47. Bins, M., P. I. Burgers, S. G. Selbach, et al. 1984. Prevalence of achlorhydria in a normal population and its relation to serum gastrin. *Hepatogastroenterology* 31 (1): 41–43.

48. Feldman, M., and C. Barnett. 1991. Fasting gastric pH and its relationship to true hypochlorhydria in humans. *Dig. Dis. Sci.* 36 (7): 866–69.

49. Carmel, R., and C. A. Spencer. 1982. Clinical and subclinical thyroid disorders associated with pernicious anemia: observations on abnormal thyroid-stimulating hormone levels and on a possible association of blood group O with hyperthyroidism. *Arch. Inter. Med.* 142 (8): 1465–69.

50. Abdullaev, F. I., and E. G. de Mejia. 1997. Antitumor effect of plant lectins. *Nat. Toxins* 5 (4): 157–63.

51. Clerc, M., F. Altglas, and J. Martine. 1974. The amount of indican in the urine and its applications. *Bull. Soc. Pathol. Exot. Filiales* 67 (16): 654–62.

52. Kjeldsen-Kragh, J., M. Haugen, C. F. Borchgrevink, and O. Forre. 1994. Vegetarian diet for patients with rheumatoid arthritis — status: two years after introduction of the diet. *Clin. Rheum.* 13 (3): 475–82.

53. Freed, D. L. 1999. Do dietary lectins cause disease? *BMJ* 318 (7190): 1023–24.

54. Kjeldsen-Kragh, J., M. Haugen, C. F. Borchgrevink, et al. 1991. Controlled trial of fasting and one year vegetarian diet in rheumatoid arthritis. *Lancet* 338: 899–902.

Chapter 6: Nutritional Wisdom Makes You Thin

1. Duncan, K. 1983. The effects of high- and low-energy-density diets of satiety, energy intake, and eating time of obese and non-obese subjects. *Am. J. Clin. Nutr.* 37: 763.

2. Campbell, T. C., and J. Chen. 1994. Diet and chronic degenerative diseases, in *Western diseases: their dietary prevention and reversibility.* Edited by M. J. Temple and D. P. Burkitt. Totowa, N. J.: Humana Press, pp. 67–119.

3. Seddon, J. M., U. A. Ajani, R. D. Sperduto, et al. 1994. Dietary carotenoids, vitamins A, C, and E, and advanced age-related macular degeneration. *JAMA* 272: 1413–20.

4. Dwyer, J. H., M. Navab, K. M. Dwyer, et al. 2001. Oxygenated carotenoid lutein and progression of early atherosclerosis: the Los Angeles atherosclerosis study. *Circulation* 103 (24): 2922–27.

5. Mangels, A. R., J. M. Holden, G. R. Beecher, et al. 1993. Carotenoid content of fruits and vegetables: an evaluation of analytic data. *J. Am. Diet. Assoc.* 93 (3): 284–96.

6. Harris, W. 2000. Less grains, more greens. Posted June 11 at www.vegsource.com/harris/ten-categories.htm.

7. Harris, W. 1995. *The scientific basis of vegetarianism.* Honolulu: Hawaii Health Publishers, pp. 98–100.

8. Innis, S. A. 1991. Essential fatty

acids in growth and development. *Prog. Lipid Res.* 30: 39–103.

9. Siguel, E. N., and R. H. Lerman. 1994. Altered fatty acid metabolism in patients with angiographically documented coronary artery disease. *Metabolism* 43: 982–83; Simon, J. A., J. Fong, J. T. Bernoert Jr., and W. S. Browner. 1995. Serum fatty acids and the risk of stroke. *Stroke* 26 (5): 778–82; Fatty acid reportedly lowers stroke risk. 1995. *Medical Tribune*, June 8, p. 20; Harbige, L. S. 1998. Dietary n-6 and n-3 fatty acids in immunity and autoimmune disease. *Proc. Nutr. Soc.* 67 (4): 555–62; Horrobin, D. F. 2000. Essential fatty acid metabolism and its modification in atopic eczema. *Am. J. Clin. Nutr.* 71 (1 supp.) 367s–72s; Adams, P. B., S. Lawson, A. Sanigorski, and A. J. Sinclair. 1996. Arachidonic acid to eicosapentaenoic acid ratio in blood correlates positively with clinical symptoms of depression. *Lipids* 31 Supp.: s157–61; Edwards, R., M. Peet, J. Shay, and D. Horribin. 1998. Omega-3 polyunsaturated fatty acid levels in the diet and in red blood cell membranes of depressed patients. *J. Affect. Disord.* 48 (2–3): 149–55; Rose, D. P. 1997. Effects of dietary fatty acids on breast and prostate cancers: evidence from in vitro experiments and animal studies. *Am. J. Clin. Nutr.* 66 (6 supp.): 1513s–22s.

10. Simopoulos, A. P. 1999. Essential fatty acids in health and chronic disease. *Am. J. Clin. Nutr.* 70 (3): 560–69.

11. Huges, D. A., and A. C. Pinder. 2000. N-3 polyunsaturated fatty acids inhibit the antigen-presenting function of human monocytes. *Am. J. Clin. Nutr.* 71 (1 supp.): 357s–60s; Purasiri, P., A. McKechnie, S. D. Heys, and O. Eremin. 1997. Modulation in vitro of human natural cytotoxicity, lymphocyte proliferation response to mitogens and cytokine production by essential fatty acids. *Immunology* 92 (2): 166–72.

12. Joseph, A. 1993. Manifestations of coronary atherosclerosis in young trauma victims — an autopsy study. *J. Am. Coll. Cardiol.* 22: 459.

13. Ascherio, A., E. B. Rimm, M. J. Stampfer, et al. 1995. Dietary intake of marine n-3 fatty acids, fish intake, and the risk of coronary disease among men. *N. Eng. J. Med.* 332 (15): 977–82; Katan, M. 1995. Fish and heart disease. *N. Eng. J. Med.* 332 (15): 1024–25.

14. Siscovick, D. S., T. E. Raghunathan, I. King, et al. 1995. Dietary intake and cell membrane levels of long-chain n-3 polyunsaturated fatty acids and the risk of primary cardiac arrest. *JAMA* 274:. 1363–67.

15. Siguel, E. N. 1996. Dietary sources of long-chain n-3 polyunsaturated fatty acids. *JAMA* 275: 836.

16. Siguel, E. N., and M. Macture. 1987. Relative enzyme activity of unsaturated fatty acid metabolic pathways in humans. *Metabolism* 36: 664–69.

17. Salonen, J. T., K. Seppanen, K. Nyyssonen, et al. 1995. Intake of mercury from fish, lipid peroxidation, and the risk of myocardial infarction and coronary, cardiovascular, and any death in eastern Finnish men. *Circulation* 91: 645–55.

18. Ihanainen, M., R. Solonen, R. Seppanen, and J. F. Salonen. 1989. Nutrition data collection in the Kuopio Ischaemic Heart Disease Risk Factor Study: nutrient intake of middle-aged eastern Finnish men. *Nutr. Res.* 9: 597–604; WHO Monica Project. 1989. WHO monica project: assessing CHD mortality and morbidity. *Int. J. Epidemiol.* 18: S38–45.

19. Salonen, op. cit.

20. Some fish found to contain high levels of contaminants. 1989. *Family Practice News*, June 15–30: 46.

21. Shamlaye, C. F., D. O. Marsh, G. J. Myers, et al. 1995. The Seychelles Child Development Study on neu-

rodevelopmental outcomes in children following in utero exposure to methylmercury from a maternal fish diet: background and demographics. *Neurotoxicology* 16 (4): 597–612; Rylander, L., U. Stromberg, and L. Hagmar. 1996. Dietary intake of fish contaminated with persistent organochlorine compounds in relation to low birthweight. *Scand. J. Work Environ. Health* 2 (4): 260–66; Does methylmercury have a role in causing developmental disabilities in children? 2000. *Environ. Health Perspect.* 108 (supp. 3): 413–20.

22. Clarkson, T. W. 1997. The toxicology of mercury. *Crit. Rev. Clin. Lab. Sci.* 34 (4): 369–403.

23. Meydani, S. N., A. H. Lichtenstein, S. Cornwall, et al. 1993. Immunologic effects of national cholesterol education panel step-2 diets with and without fish-derived n-3 fatty acid enrichment. *J. Clin. Invest.* 92 (1): 105–13.

24. Chiang, T. A., P. F. Wu, L. F. Wang, et al. 1997. Mutagenicity and polycyclic aromatic hydrocarbon content of fumes from heated cooking oils produced in Taiwan. *Mutat. Res.* 381 (2): 157–61; Sheerin, A. N., C. Silwood, E. Lynch, and M. Grootveld. 1997. Production of lipid peroxidation products in culinary oils and fats during episodes of thermal stressing: a high field 1 H NMR investigation. *Biochem. Soc. Trans.* 25 (3): 495s; Warner, K. 1999. Impact of high-temperature food processing on fats and oils. *Adv. Exp. Med. Biol.* 459: 67–77.

25. Posner, B., J. L. Cobb, A. Belanger, L. A. Cupples, R. B. D'Agostino, and J. Stokes. 1991. Dietary lipid predictors of coronary heart disease in men. *Arch. Intern. Med.* 151: 1181–87; Gillman, M. W., L. A. Cupples, B. E. Millen, R. C. Ellison, and P. A. Wolf. 1997. Inverse association of dietary fat with development of ischemic stroke in men. *JAMA* 278:

2145–50; Iso, H., M. J. Stampfer, J. E. Manson, et al. 2001. Prospective study of fat and protein intake and risk of intraparenchymal hemorrhage in women. *Circulation* 103: 856.

26. Gillman, M. W., L. A. Cupples, B. Posner, R. C. Ellison, W. Castelli, and P. Wolf. 1995. Protective effects of fruits and vegetables on development of stroke in men. *JAMA* 273: 1113–17; Gey, K. F., H. B. Stahelin, and M. Eichholzer. 1993. Poor plasma status of carotene and vitamin C is associated with higher mortality from ischemic heart disease and stroke. *Clin. Invest. Med.* 71: 3–6; Ascherio, A., E. B. Rimm, M. A. Herman, et al. 1998. Intake of potassium, magnesium, calcium, and fiber and risk of stroke among U.S. men. *Circulation* 17: 366–70.

27. Perry, H. M., Jr., B. R. Davis, T. R. Price, et al. 2000. Effects of treating isolated systolic hypertension on the risk of developing various types and subtypes of stroke: the Systolic Hypertension in the Elderly Program (SHEP). *JAMA* 284 (4): 465–71.

28. Simon, J. A., J. Fong, J. T. Bernert Jr., and W. S. Browner. 1995. Serum fatty acids and the risk of stroke. *Stroke* 26: 778–82; Shimokawa, T., A. Moriuchi, T. Hori, et al. 1988. Effect of dietary alpha-linolenate/linoleate balance on mean survival time, incidence of stroke and blood pressure of spontaneously hypertensive rats. *Life Sci.* 43: 2067–75.

29. Sasaki, S., X. H. Zhang, and H. Kesteloot. 1995. Dietary sodium, potassium, saturated fat, alcohol, and stroke mortality. *Stroke* 26 (5): 783–89.

30. Perez-Jimenez, F., P. Castro, J. Lopez-Miranda, et al. 1999. Circulating levels of endothelial function are modulated by dietary monounsaturated fat. *Atherosclerosis* 145 (2): 351–58.

31. Fraser, G. E. 1999. Association between diet and cancer, ischemic heart disease, and all-cause mortal-

ity in non-Hispanic white California Seventh-day Adventists. *Am. J. Clin. Nutr.* 70 (3 supp.): 532S–38S.

32. Ascherio, A., and W. C. Willett. 1997. Health effects of trans fatty acids. *Am. J. Clin. Nutr.* 66 (4 supp.): 1006S–10S.

33. Judd, J. T., B. A. Clevidence, R. A. Muesing, et al. 1994. Dietary trans fatty acids: effects on plasma lipids and lipoproteins of healthy men and women. *Am. J. Clin. Nutr.* 59 (4): 861–68; Mensink, R. P., and M. B. Katan. 1990. Effects of dietary trans fatty acids on high-density and low-density lipoprotein cholesterol levels in healthy subjects. *N. Eng. J. Med.* 323 (7): 439–45.

34. Valenzuela, A., and N. Morgado. 1999. Trans fatty acid isomers in human health and in the food industry. *Biol. Res.* 32 (4): 273–87.

35. Willett, W. C., M. J. Stampfer, J. E. Manson, et al. 1993. Intake of trans fatty acids and risk of coronary heart disease among women. *Lancet* 341: 581–85; Ascherio, A., C. H. Hennekens, J. E. Buring, et al. 1994. Trans-fatty acids intake and risk of myocardial infarction. *Circulation* 89 (1): 94–101; Lichtenstein, A. H. 2000. Trans fatty acids and cardiovascular disease risk. *Curr. Opin. Lipidol.* 11 (1): 37–42.

36. Kohlmeier, L., N. Simonsen, P. Van't Veer, et al. 1997. Adipose tissue trans fatty acids and breast cancer in the European Community Multicenter Study on Antioxidants, Myocardial Infarction, and Breast Cancer. *Cancer Epidmiol. Biomarkers Prev.* 6 (9): 705–10.

37. Hu, F. B., M. J. Stampfer, J. E. Manson, E. Rimm, G. A. Colditz, B. A. Rosner, C. H. Hennekins, and W. C. Willett. 1997. Dietary fat intake and the risk of coronary heart disease in women. *N. Eng. J. Med.* 337 (21): 1491–99.

38. Hegsted, D. 1968. Minimum protein requirements of adults. *Am. J. Clin. Nutr.* 21: 3520.

39. Schaafsma, G. 2000. The protein digestibility — corrected amino acid score. *J. Nutr.* 130 (7): 1865S–67S; Henley, E. C., and J. M. Kuster. 1994. Protein quality evaluation by protein digestibility corrected amino acid scoring. *Food Technology* 48 (4): 74–77.

Chapter 7: Eat to Live Takes On Disease

1. Carnargro, C. A., S. T. Weiss, S. Zhang, W. C. Willett, and F. E. Speizer. 1999. Prospective study of body mass index, weight change, and risk of adult-onset asthma in women. *Arch. Intern. Med.* 159: 2582–88.

2. Mintz, E. 1997. Emergency department management of acute myocardial infarction. *Mt. Sinai Journal of Medicine* 64: 258–74.

3. Berenson G. S., W. A. Wattigney, W. Bao, S. R. Srinivasan, and B. Radhakrishnamurthy. 1995. Rationale to study the early natural history of heart disease: the Bogalusa Heart Study. *Am. J. Med. Sci.* 310 (S1): S22–28.

4. Marrugat, J., J. Sala, R. Masia, et al. 1998. Mortality differences between men and women following first myocardial infarction. *JAMA* 280: 1405–09.

5. Meier, B., S. B. King, A. R. Gruentzig, et al. 1984. Repeat coronary angioplasty. *J. Am. Coll. Cardiol.* 4: 463.

6. Ramsey, L. E., W. W. Yeo, and P. R. Jackson. 1991. Dietary reduction of serum cholesterol concentration: time to think again. *BMJ* 303: 953–57.

7. Ornish, D., S. E. Brown, L. W. Scherwitz, et al. 1990. Can lifestyle changes reverse coronary heart disease? *Lancet* 336 (8708):129–33; Ellis, F. 1997. Angina and vegan diet. *Am. Heart J.* 93 (6): 803–05.

8. Davidson, M. H., D. Hunninghake, K. C. Maki, P. O. Kwiterovich Jr., and S. Kafonek. 1999. Comparison of the effects of lean red meat vs.

lean white meat on serum lipid levels among free-living persons with hypercholesterolemia: a long-term, randomized clinical trial. *Arch. Intern. Med.* 159 (12): 1131–38.

9. Fraser, G. E. 1999. Association between diet and cancer, ischemic heart disease, and all-cause mortality in non-Hispanic white California Seventh-Day Adventists. *Am. J. Clin. Nutr.* 70 (3 supp.): 532S–38S.

10. Stefanick, M. L., S. Mackey, M. Sheehan, et al. 1998. Effects of diet and exercise in men and postmenopausal women with low levels of HDL cholesterol and high levels of LDL cholesterol. *N. Eng. J. Med.* 339: 12–20.

11. Lichtenstein, A. H., and L. Van Horn. 1998. Very low fat diets. *Circulation* 98 (9): 935–39.

12. O'Dea, K., K. Traianedes, P. Ireland, et al. 1989. The effects of diet differing in fat, carbohydrate, and fiber on carbohydrate and lipid metabolism in type II diabetes. *J. Am. Diet. Assoc.* 89: 1076–86; Schaefer, E. J., A. H. Lichtenstein, S. Lamon-Fava, et al. 1995. Body weight and low-density lipoprotein cholesterol change after consumption of a low-fat ad libitum diet. *JAMA* 274: 1450–55.

13. Turley, M. L., C. M. Skeaff, J. I. Mann, and B. Cox. 1998. The effect of low-fat, high-carbohydrate diet on serum high density lipoprotein cholesterol and triglycerides. *Eur. J. Clin. Nutr.* 52 (10): 728–32.

14. Jenkins, D. J., C. W. Kendall, D. G. Popovich, et al. 2001. Effects of a very-high-fiber vegetable, fruit and nut diet on serum lipids and colonic function. *Metabolism* 50 (4): 494–503.

15. Lichtenstein, op. cit.

16. Ivanov, A. N., I. L. Medkova, and L. I. Mosiakina. 1999. The effect of an anti-atherogenic vegetarian diet on the clinico-hemodynamic and biochemical indices in elderly patients with ischemic heart disease. *Ter. Arkh.* 71 (2): 75–78.

17. Esselstyn, C. B., S. G. Ellis, S. V. Medendorp, and T. D. Crowe. 1995. A strategy to arrest and reverse coronary artery disease: a 5-year longitudinal study of a single physician's practice. *J. Fam. Pract.* 41 (6): 560–68.

18. Ishikawa, T. 1999. Postprandial lipemia as an atherosclerotic risk factor and fat tolerance test. *Nippon Rinsho* 57 (12): 2668–72.

19. Koeford, B. G., A. L. Gullov, and P. Peterson. 1995. Cerebral complications of surgery using cardiopulmonary bypass. *Ugeskr Laeger* 157 (6): 728–34.

20. Brain damage and open-heart surgery. 1989. *Lancet,* August 12, pp. 364–66.

21. Meier, op. cit.

22. Schalcher, C., G. Sutsch, and F. W. Amann. 1999. To stent or not to stent. *Schweiz. Med. Wochenschr.* 129 (45): 1679–96; Park, S. J., S. W. Park, C. W. Lee, et al. 1999. Immediate results and late clinical outcomes after new CrossFlex coronary stent implantation. *Am. J. Cardiol.* 83 (4): 502–06; Pieniazek, P., T. Przewlocki, K. Zmudka, et al. 1998. Stents for treatment of transluminal percutaneous coronary angioplasty (PTCA) complications. *Przegl. Lek.* 55 (7–8): 373–77; Savage, M. P., J. S. Douglas Jr., D. L. Fishman, et al. 1997. Stent placement compared with balloon angioplasty for obstructive coronary bypass grafts. *N. Eng. J. Med.* 337: 740–47.

23. Cequier, A., J. Mauri, J. A. Gomez-Hospital, et al. 1997. Intracoronary stents in the treatment of angioplasty complications. *Rev. Esp. Cardiol.* 50 (supp. 2): 21–30; Craver, J. M., A. G. Justicz, W. S. Weitraub, et al. 1995. Coronary artery bypass grafting in patients after failure of intracoronary stenting. *Ann. Thorac. Surg.* 60 (1): 60–65.

24. Bates, B. 2001. Angiograms miss most atheromas. *Family Practice News* 31 (14): 1,4.

25. Schoenhagen, P., K. M. Ziada, D. G.

Vince, S. E. Nissen, and E. M. Tuzcu. 2001. Arterial remodeling and coronary artery disease: the concept of "dilated" versus "obstructive" coronary atherosclerosis. *J. Am. Coll. Cardiol.* 38 (2): 297–306.

26. Elihu, N., S. Anandasbapathy, and W. H. Frishman. 1998. Chelation therapy in cardiovascular disease: ethylenediaminetetraacetic acid, deferoxamine, and dexrazoxane. *J. Clin. Pharmacol.* 38 (2): 101–05; Ernst, E. 1997. Chelation therapy for peripheral arterial occlusive disease: a systematic review. *Circulation* 96 (3): 1031–33; Lewin, M. R. 1997. Chelation therapy for cardiovascular disease. Review and commentary. *Tex. Heart. Inst. J.* 24 (2): 81–89; Can chelation therapy cure heart disease? *Johns Hopkins Med. Lett. Health After 50.* 1999. 10 (4): 8.

27. Gould, K. L. 1998. New concepts and paradigms in cardiovascular medicine: the noninvasive management of coronary artery disease. *Am. J. Med.* 104 (6A): 2S–17S; Franklin, B. A., and J. K. Kahn. 1996. Delayed progression or regression of coronary atherosclerosis with intensive risk factor modification: effects of diet, drugs and exercise. *Sports Med.* 22 (5): 306–20.

28. Kannel, W. B. 1995. Range of serum cholesterol values in the population developing coronary artery disease. *Am. J. Cardiol.* 76 (9): 69c–77c; Castelli, W. P., K. Anderson, P. W. Wilson, and D. Levy. 1992. Lipids and risk of coronary heart disease: the Framingham Study. *Ann. Epidemiol.* 2 (1–2): 23–28.

29. Kinosian, B., H. Glick, and G. Garland. 1994. Cholesterol and coronary heart disease: predicting risks by levels and ratios. *Ann. Int. Med.* 121 (9): 641–47.

30. Miller, E. R., T. P. Erlinger, D. R. Young, G. P. Prokopowicz, and L. J. Appel. 1999. Lifestyle changes that reduce blood pressure: implementation in clinical practice. *J. Clin. Hypertens.* 1: 191–98; Stassen, J., R. Fagard, P. Lijnen, et al. 1989. Body weight, sodium intake and blood pressure. *J. Hypertens.* 7: S19–S23; Appel, L. J., T. J. Moore, E. Obarzanek, et al., for the DASH Collaborative Research Group. 1997. A clinical trial of the effects of dietary patterns on blood pressure. *N. Eng. J. Med.* 336: 1117–24.

31. Whelton, P. K., L. I. Appel, M. A. Espeland, et al. 1998. Sodium reduction and weight loss in the treatment of hypertension in older persons: a randomized controlled trial of nonpharmacologic interventions in the elderly. *JAMA* 279: 839–46.

32. Stafford, R. S., and D. Blumenthal. 1998. Specialty differences in cardiovascular disease prevention practices. *J. Am. Coll. Cardiol.* 32 (5): 1238–43.

33. Gaster, B., and I. B. Hirsh. 1998. The effects of improved glucose control on complications in type 2 diabetes. *Arch. Intern. Med.* 158: 134–40.

34. Stamler, J., O. Vaccaro, J. D. Neaton, et al. 1993. Diabetes, other risk factors, and 12-year cardiovascular mortality for men screened in the multiple risk factor intervention trial. *Diabetes Care* 16: 434–44; Haffner, S. M., S. Lehto, T. Ronnemaa, et al. 1998. Mortality from coronary heart disease in subjects with type 2 diabetes and in nondiabetic subjects with and without prior myocardial infarction. *N. Eng. J. Med.* 339 (4): 229–34; Janka, H. U. 1996. Increased cardiovascular morbidity and mortality in diabetes mellitus: identification of the high risk patient. *Diabetes Res. Clin. Pract.* 30 (supp.): 85–88.

35. Crane, M. 1994. Regression of diabetic neuropathy with total vegetarian (vegan) diet. *J. Nutr. Med.* 4: 431.

36. Lovejoy, J. C., M. M. Windhauser, J. C. Rood, and J. A. De La Bretonne. 1998. Effects of a controlled high-fat versus low-fat diet on insulin sensitivity and leptin levels in African-American and Caucasian women. *Metab.* 47: 1520–24.

37. Williamson, D. F., T. J. Thompson, M. Thun, et al. 2000. Intentional weight loss and mortality among overweight individuals with diabetes. *Diabetes Care* 23 (10): 1499–1504.

38. Tataranni, P. A., J. F. Gautier, K. Chen, et al. 1999. Neuroanatomical correlates of hunger and satiation in humans using positron emission tomography. *Proc. Natl. Acad. Sci. USA* 96 (8): 4569–74; Friedman, M. I., P. Ulrich, and R. D. Mattes. 1999. A figurative measure of subjective hunger sensations. *Appetite* 32 (3): 395–404.

39. Diamond, S. 1995. Migraine headache: recognizing its peculiarities, precipitants and prodromes. *Consultant*, August, 1190–95.

40. Fuhrman, J. 1995. *Fasting and eating for health, a medical doctor's program for conquering disease.* New York: St. Martins Press.

41. Stephenson, J. 1993. Detox is crucial in chronic daily headache. *Family Practice News*, July 1, 2.

42. Fujita. A., Y. Hashimoto, K. Nakahara, T. Tanaka, T. Okuda, and M. Koda. 1999. Effects of a low-calorie vegan diet on disease activity and general condition in patients with rheumatoid arthritis. *Rinsho Byori* 47 (6): 554–60; Haugen, M. A., J. Kjeldsen-Kragh, K. S. Bjerve, A. T. Hostmark, and O. Forre. 1994. Changes in plasma phospholipid fatty acids and their relationship to disease activity in rheumatoid arthritis patients treated with a vegetarian diet. *Br. J. Nutr.* 72 (4): 555–66; Peltonen, R., M. Nenonen, T. Helve, et al. 1997. Faecal microbial flora and disease activity in rheumatoid arthritis during a vegan diet. *Br. J. Rheumatol.* 36 (1): 64–68; Kjeldsen-Kragh, J. 1999. Rheumatoid arthritis treated with vegetarian diets. *Am. J. Clin. Nutr.* 70 (3 supp.): 594S–600S; Haddad, E. H., L. S. Berk, J. D. Kettering, R. W. Hubbard, and W. R. Peters. 1999. Dietary intake and biochemical, hematologic, and immune status of vegans compared with nonvegetarians. *Am. J. Clin. Nutr.* 70 (3 supp.): 586S–93S.

43. Kjeldsen-Kragh, J., M. Hvatum, M. Haugen, O. Forre, and H. Scott. 1995. Antibodies against dietary antigens in rheumatoid arthritis patents treated with fasting and a one-year vegetarian diet. *Clin. Exp. Rheumatol.* 13 (2): 167–72.

44. Scott, D., D. P. Symmons, B. L. Coulton, and A. J. Popert. 1987. Long-term outcome of treating rheumatoid arthritis: results after 20 years. *Lancet* 1 (8542): 1108–11.

45. Jones, M., D. Symmons, J. Finn, and F. Wolfe. 1996. Does exposure to immunosuppressive therapy increase the 10-year malignancy and mortality risk? *B. J. Rheum.* 35 (8): 738–45.

46. Barnard, N. D., A. R. Scialli, D. Hurlock, and P. Berton. 2000. Diet and sex-hormone binding globulin, dysmenorrhea, and premenstrual symptoms. *Obstet. Gynecol.* 92 (2): 245–50.

47. King, T. S., M. Elia, and J. O. Hunter. 1998. Abnormal colonic fermentation in irritable bowel syndrome. *Lancet* 352 (9135): 1187–89.

Chapter 8: Your Plan for Substantial Weight Reduction

1. Gustafsson, K., N. G. Asp, B. Hagander, et al. 1995. Influence of processing and cooking of carrots in mixed meals on satiety, glucose and hormonal reponse. *Int. J. Food Sci. Nutr.* 46 (1): 3–12.

2. Lintschinger, J., N. Fuchs, H. Moser, et al. 1997. Uptake of various trace elements during germination of wheat, buckwheat and quinoa. *Plant Foods Hum. Nutr.* 50 (3): 223–37.

3. Hudson, E.A., P. A. Dinh, T. Kokubun, et al. 2000. Characterization of potentially chemopreventive phenols in extracts of brown rice that inhibit the growth of human breast and colon cancer cells. *Cancer Epidemiol. Biomarkers Prev.* 9 (11): 1163–70.

4. Jordan, H. A., L. S. Levitz, K. L. Utgoff, et al. 1981. Role of food characteristics in behavioral change and weight loss. *J. Am. Diet. Assoc.* 79: 24; Foreyt, J. P., R. S. Reeves, L. S. Darnell, et al. 1986. Soup consumption as a behavioral weight-loss strategy. *J. Am. Diet. Assoc.* 86: 524–26.

5. Simopoulos A. P. 1999. Essential fatty acids in health and chronic disease. *Am. J. Clin. Nutr.* 70 (3): 560–69S.

6. Iwamoto, M., M. Sato, M. Kono, et al. 2000. Walnuts lower serum cholesterol in Japanese men and women. *J. Nutr.* 130: 171–76; Morgan, W. A., and B. J. Clayshulte. 2000. Pecans lower low density lipoprotein cholesterol in people with normal lipid levels. *J. Am. Diet. Assoc.* 100: 312–18; Zambon, D., J. Sabate, S. Munoz, et al. 2000. Substituting walnuts for monounsaturated fat improves the serum lipid profile of hypercholesterolemic men and women: a randomized crossover trial. *Ann. Intern. Med.* 132: 538–46.

7. Jansen, M.C., H. B. Bueno-de-Mesquita, L. Rasanen, et al. 1999. Consumption of plant foods and stomach cancer mortality in the seven country study: is grain consumption a risk factor? *Nutr. Cancer.* 34: 49–55.

8. National Heart, Lung, and Blood Institute, National Institute of Diabetes and Digestive and Kidney Diseases. 1998. Clinical guidelines on the identification, evaluation, and treatment of overweight and obesity in adults: the evidence report. Washington, D.C.: U.S. Government Press. Guidelines available online at www.nhlbi.nih.gov/guidelines/obesity/ob_gdlns.htm.

Chapter 10: Frequently Asked Questions

1. Mayne. S. T. 1996. Beta-carotene, carotenoids, and disease prevention in humans. *FASEB* 10 (7): 690–701; Goodman, G. E. 1998. Prevention of lung cancer. *Current Opinion in Oncology* 10 (2): 122–26; Kolata, G. 1996. Studies find beta carotene, taken by millions, can't forestall cancer or heart disease. *New York Times,* January 19; Omenn, G. S., G. E. Goodman, M. D. Thornquist, et al. 1996. Effects of a combination of beta carotene and vitamin A on lung cancer and cardiovascular disease. *N. Eng. J. Med.* 334 (18): 1150–55; Hennekens, C. H., J. E. Buring, J. E. Manson, et al. 1996. Lack of effect of long-term supplementation with beta carotene on the incidence of malignant neoplasms and cardiovascular disease. *N. Eng. J. Med.* 334 (18): 1145–49; Albanes, D., O. P. Heinonen, P. R. Taylor, et al. 1996. Alpha-tocopherol and beta-carotene supplements and lung cancer incidence in the Alpha-Tocopherol, Beta-Carotene Cancer Prevention Study: effects of base-line characteristics and study compliance. *J. Nat. Cancer Inst.* 88 (21):1560–70; Rapola, J. M., J. Virtamo, S. Ripatti, et al. 1997. Randomized trial of alpha-tocopherol and beta-carotene supplements on incidence of major coronary events in men with previous myocardial infarction. *Lancet* 349 (9067): 1715–20.

2. Whiting, S. J., and B. Lemke. 1999. Excess retinol intake may explain the high incidence of osteoporosis in northern Europe. *Nutr. Rev.* 57 (6): 192–95; Melhus, H., K. Michaelson, A. Kindmark, et al. 1998. Excessive dietary intake of vitamin A is associated with reduced bone mineral density and increased risk of hip fracture. *Ann. Intern. Med.* 129 (10): 770–78.

3. Supplemental vitamin C may hasten atherosclerosis. 2000. *Geriatrics* 55 (5): 15–16.

4. Meydani, S. N., M. P. Barklund, S. Liu, M. Meydani, R. A. Miller, J. G. Cannon, F. D. Morrow, R. Rocklin, and J. B. Blumberg. 1990. Vitamin E supplementation enhances cell-mediated immunity in healthy eld-

erly subjects. *Am. J. Clin. Nutr.* 52: 557–63; Meydani, S. N., D. Wu, M. S. Santos, and M. G. Hayek. 1995. Antioxidants and immune response in aged persons: overview or present evidence. *Am. J. Clin. Nutr.* 62: 1462–76S.

5. Heymsfield, S. B., D. B. Allison, J. R. Vasselli, et al. 1998. Garcinia cambogia (hydroxycitric acid) as a potential antiobesity agent. *JAMA.* 280 (18): 1596–1600.

6. Lengsfeld, H., A. Fleury, M. Nolte, et al. 1999. Effect of orlistat and chitosan on faecal fat excretion in young healthy volunteers. *Obesity Research* 7 (supp. 1): 50S; Heymsfield, S. B. 1999. Safety and efficacy of herbal treatments for obesity. *Obesity Research* 7 (supp. 1): 8S.

7. Walsh, N. 2001. Epheda users may lose health, not just weight. *Family Practice News*, March 1: 23.

8. Lean, M. E. J. 1997. Sibutramine: a review of clinical efficacy. *Int. J. Obes. Relat. Metab. Disord.* 21 (supp. 1): S30–36.

9. Everly, G. S. 1989. *A clinical guide to the treatment of the human stress response.* New York: Plenum Press.

10. Boutelle, K. N., and D. S. Kirschenbaum. 1998. Further support for consistent self-monitoring as a vital component of successful weight control. *Obes. Res.* 6: 219–24.

11. Pauletto, P., M. Puato, M. G. Caroli, et al. 1996. Blood pressure and atherogenic lipoprotein profiles of fish-diet and vegetarian villagers in Tanzania: the Lugaiawa Study. *Lancet* 348: 784–88; Key, T. J., G. E. Fraser, M. Thorogood, et al. 1999. Mortality in vegetarians and nonvegetarians: detailed findings from a collaborative analysis of 5 prospective studies. *Am. J. Clin. Nutr.* 70 (3): 516–24S.

12. EPA report ratchets up dioxin peril. 2000. *Washington Post,* May.

13. Report from Loma Linda University's Carbophobia Conference. 2000. *Vegetarian Nutrition and Health Letter,* 3 (5): 4.

14. Lichtenstein, A. H., L. M. Ausman, S. M. Jalbert, and E. J. Schaefer. 1999. Effects of different forms of dietary hydrogenated fats on serum lipoprotein cholesterol levels. *N. Eng. J. Med.* 340: 1933–40.

15. White, L. R., H. Petrovitch, G. W. Ross, et al. 2000. Brain aging and midlife tofu consumption. *J. Am. Coll. Nutr.* 19 (2): 242–55.

16. Graves, A. B., I. Rajaram, J. D. Bowen, et al. 1999. Cognitive decline and Japanese culture in a cohort of older Japanese Americans in King County, WA: the Kame Project. *J. Gerontol. B. Psychol. Sci. Soc. Sci.* 54 (3): S154–61.

17. Joossens, J. V., M. J. Hill, P. Elliot, et al. 1996. Dietary salt, nitrate and stomach cancer mortality in 24 countries: European Cancer Prevention (ECP) and the INTERSALT Cooperative Research Group. *Int. J. Epidemiol.* 3: 494–504.

18. Obarzanek, E., F. M. Sacks, T. J. Moore, et al. 2000. *Dietary approaches to stop hypertension (DASH) — sodium trial.* Paper presented at Annual Meeting of the American Society of Hypertension, May 17, New York, NY.

19. Itoh, R., and Y. Suyama. 1996. Sodium excretion in relation to calcium and hydroxyproline excretion in a healthy Japanese population. *Am. J. Clin. Nutr.* 63 (5): 735–40.

20. Tuomilehto, J., P. Jousilahti, D. Rastenyte, et al. 2001. Urinary sodium excretion and cardiovascular mortality in Finland: a prospective study. *Lancet* 357 (9259): 848–51.

21. Mehta, A., A. C. Jain, M. C. Mehta, and M. Billie. 1997. Caffeine and cardiac arrhythmias: an experimental study in dogs with review of literature. *Acta Cardiol.* 52 (3): 273–83.

22. Nurminen, M. L., L. Niittymen, R. Korpela, and H. Vapaatalo. 1999. Coffee, caffeine and blood pressure: a critical review. *Eur. J. Clin. Nutr.* 53 (11): 831–39; Christensen, B., A. Mosdol, L. Retterstol, et al. 2001.

Abstention from filtered coffee reduces the concentration of plasma homocysteine and serum cholesterol — a randomized controlled trial. *Am. J. Clin. Nutr.* 74 (3): 302–07.

23. Spiegel, K., R. Leproult, and E. V. Van Cauter. 1999. Impact of sleep debt on metabolic and endocrine function. *Lancet* 354 (9188): 1435–39.

24. Dallongeville, J., N. Marecaux, P. Ducmetiere, et al. 1998. Influence of alcohol consumption and various beverages on waist girth and waist-to-hip ratio in a sample of French men and women. *J. Obes. Relat. Metab. Disord.* 22 (12): 1178–83.

25. Wright, R. M., J. L. McManaman, and J. E. Rapine. 1999. Alcohol-induced breast cancer: a proposed mechanism. *Free Radic. Biol. Med.* 26 (3–4): 348–54; Dorgan, J. F., D. J. Baer, P. S. Albert, et al. 2001. Serum hormones and the alcohol-breast cancer association in postmenopausal women. *J. Natl. Cancer Inst.* 93 (9): 710–16; Jancin, B. 2002. Just a few drinks raise risk of atrial fibrillation. *Family Physician News,* January 11: 4.

26. Lavin, J. H., S. J. French, and N. W. Read. 1997. The effect of sucrose- and aspartame-sweetened drinks on energy intake, hunger and food choice of female, moderately restrained eaters. *Int. J. Obes. Relat. Metab. Disord.* 21 (1): 37–42.

27. Olney, J. W., N. B. Farber, E. Spitznagel, and L. N. Robins. 1996. Increasing brain tumor rates: is there a link to aspartame? *J. Neuropathol. Exp. Neurol.* 55 (11): 1115–23.

28. Toskulkao, C., et al. 1997. Acute toxicity of stevioside, a natural sweetener, and its metabolite, steviol, in several animal species. *Drug Chem. Toxicol.* 20 (31): 31–44.

Acknowledgments

My gratitude and thanks to:

So many wonderful people who have permitted me to use their real names and case histories in this book. They make this book come alive, giving others hope, enthusiasm, and motivation to achieve their own success stories.

Lisa Fuhrman, my loving wife, who always believed in and encouraged my career dreams, my message, and my vision. Her continual assistance and input in all my work resulted in many contributions to this manuscript.

My four children, Talia, Jenna, Cara, and Sean, all wonderful and uniquely talented, they have all been understanding of my need to frequently work alone on this manuscript while at home.

Mark Da Cunha, my very gifted friend and webmaster, who made numerous contributions to this manuscript, including designing all the graphs and illustrations.

Steve Acocella, D.C., my close friend, who is always willing to help me. He spent many tedious hours collecting and compiling disease and food-consumption data from around the world and made phone calls to foreign health officials just to clarify or corroborate statistics for me.

Jeff Novick, R.D., a friend and colleague, who helped me in numerous ways, including supplying research assistance and dietary analysis.

The National Health Association, which has supported my work over the years and contributed a research grant to aid in data collection for this book.

Marian Fanok, who has helped me many times, proofreading my writing.

William Harris, M.D., whose insight and scientific advice has greatly aided my work.

Mary Ann Naples, my agent, who did more than an agent was expected to do. Her professionalism and ability exceed my expectations. Her advice and editorial help were invaluable.

Deborah Baker, my editor at Little, Brown and Company, who from the very beginning understood the value of my message to society. She had the foresight to see what this book could be and the knowledge to help bring it to fruition.

Index

dairy products (*continued*)
nutrient density of, 121
and osteoporosis, 84–90
prohibited in Six-Week Diet, 183
reintroduced, 186
See also animal foods
DASH study, 240, 241
DDT, 81
dementia, 84
depression, x, 126, 127, 144
desserts, recipes for, 223–24
detoxification. *See* withdrawal symptoms
DHA (docosahexainoic acid)
deficiency of, 123–24, 126
from fish, 126, 127, 128, 233
plant-derived, 171, 183, 233
testing for, 170
diabetes
adult-onset (Type II), 159
advice for the patient, 163–64
body weight and, 16, 21, 158–61, 163
childhood (Type I), 159
complications from, 158, 159–60
fatty acid ratio and, 124, 125
high-protein diet and, 98
incidence of, x, 31
mortality rate, 32, 50, 54
medication for, 3, 160
and diet plan, 4, 11, 162
phasing out, 161–62
reduction or elimination of risk, x, 25, 75, 101, 145, 160, 196
refined foods and, 31–32, 33
avoidance of, in diet, 163, 164, 167
starchy vegetables and, 180
See also insulin
Diamond, Seymour, and Diamond Headache Clinic, 168
diet
American, *see* MAD (modern American diet)
low-carbohydrate, 164
medical-pharmaceutical attitude toward, 143
7 days of nonvegetarian, 202–6
7 days of vegetarian, 199–202
See also low-calorie diet; low-fat diet; vegetarian diet
dietary-caused illnesses (table), 144
dietary guidelines, xi, 53–54, 189–90
diet plans
Atkins diet, 5, 42, 92–98
and changing behavior, 193

D'Adamo (blood-type), 107–13
dangerous, 5, 17–18, 41–45, 92–115
deviation from, 228–29
failure of, 5, 15–16, 17, 29, 115
"heart-healthy," 148
Life Plan, 175, 185–94
low-nutrient, 18, 114
NIH, 190
one pound–one pound rule, 120, 177, 178, 190
plant-food-based, American acceptance of, 247–48
Six-Week, 175, 176–85, 188
Sugar Busters, 42
suggested reading list, 113
Zone diet (Sears), 92, 99–105
diet supplements, 55–56, 95, 225–28
for the elderly, 226
iron, avoidance of, 55, 226
See also vitamins
dioxin, 88–89, 236
dips, recipes for, 211
diverticulosis, 84
DNA
prevention of damage to, 54, 58, 59
repair enzymes enhanced, 25
Dr. Atkins' Health Revolution (Atkins), 92, 93
drugs. *See* medication
Dunkin' Donuts, 133

Eades, Michael and Mary, 92
Eat More, Weigh Less (Ornish), 113
Eat Right for Your Type (D'Adamo), 107–13
edamame (soybeans), 183. *See also* vegetables
EFAs (essential fatty acids), 123–24
eggs
fat content of, 135
egg whites or Egg Beaters, 183
eicosanoids, 99, 103
elderly, the
diet supplements for, 226
lowering blood pressure in, 157
embolus, 128, 132
empty-calorie food. *See* junk food; processed (refined) food
EPA (eicospentainoic acid), 123, 124, 128, 183
ephedra alkaloids (ma huang), 227–28
Eskimos, hip-fracture rate of, 87
Esselstyn, Caldwell, 150